D0849716

COMMUNICATIONAL STRUCTURE:

ANALYSIS OF A PSYCHOTHERAPY TRANSACTION

COMMUNICATIONAL STRUCTURE:

ANALYSIS OF A PSYCHOTHERAPY TRANSACTION

ALBERT E. SCHEFLEN, M.D.

INDIANA UNIVERSITY PRESS

Bloomington and London

Published in Canada by Fitzhenry & Whiteside Limited, Don
Mills, Ontario

Library of Congress catalog card number: 75-165050
ISBN: 0-253-35490-0

Manufactured in the United States of America

To Ray L. Birdwhistell

Dr. Birdwhistell is best known for his work in
non-language communication but he has also
been a prime architect in human communication
theory and behavioral science in general. He
taught me the structural approach and much
more. He has been a close colleague and a good
friend for a dozen years.

TABLE OF CONTENTS

DIAGRAMS

Preface

The major effort of ten years of my career has been the analysis of this thirty-minute transaction and the publication of the method and results. In fact, publication has been the knottiest problem of our research. It is surprising and disturbing to notice how few publications in this field are available to the average reader. An outsider would not know that dozens of researchers have been doing analyses like this one for over a decade. (An unbelievably detailed analysis done in 1955 at Stanford, for example, is still awaiting publication.)

There are some familiar reasons for this situation. Nontraditional approaches to research are difficult to fund, and, with no established body of readers interested, publishers hesitate to take the risk. Also, it takes a long time to formulate new approaches in a clear and readable way. Further, the painstaking requirements of film analysis and the cultural taboos against looking closely at other persons have caused many workers to drop out and leave their work uncompleted.

But there is an obstacle to publication that is even more critical. Many events and behaviors in communication are almost entirely outside the realm of language and consciousness. There are no words for them, and these infrasystems of behavior are so complex that few readers will wade through a systematic description of their integration. Thus, intricate nonlinguistic behaviors must be transformed into the system of speech and metabehavior, and the major effort of this research and others like it has been, not the detailed observation, but the search for a way to tell what the slowmotion analysis of a film has revealed. I have needed as much help in describing the observations and promulgating the ideas as I did in learning the viewpoint and studying the film.

A number of lines of thought that have come together in current concepts and behavioral systems can be traced back for generations. For example, we can trace the basic systems concepts from Maxwell to Einstein to Lewin to Redfield and Bertalanffy, while the general notion of holism in the psychological sciences has precedence among Gestalt theorists like Kofka and Koehler, along with the clinical naturalists like Freud, Bleuler, Meyer, and many others. The history of the concept of behavioral patterns stretches from Boaz to Benedict and Mead in anthropology and from Sapir to Pike in structural linguistics.

I consider the primary architects of the current behavioral systems emphasis to be Kenneth Pike, Ray L. Birdwhistell, Gregory Bateson, Erving Goffman, and the ethologists from Lorenz to the younger non-Europeans like Klopfer and McBride. The development of methods for synthesis is indebted to the work of Pike in linguistics, Schneirla in biology, and the 1955 explication of context analysis by Bateson, Birdwhistell, Brosin, Hockett, Fromm-Reichmann, and McQuown.

A number of people have initiated and guided projects in which younger men have been able to learn and carry out research in this tradition. Henry Brosin has sustained the tradition at Western Psychiatric Institute in Pittsburgh for over a decade and O. Spurgeon English sponsored the work at Temple University in Philadelphia. In fact, English organized or sustained each of the early projects in which this particular work was developed. Brosin, Kubie, Mead, Bateson, Bacon, and others have continuously advised, taught, and supported these programs.

The prime contributor to the actual work in this volume has been Ray Birdwhistell. He taught me the method and participated daily for almost a decade in the analysis and formulation of the data. Although Birdwhistell is best known for his microanalysis of kinesic behavior, he actually has played a primary role in conceptualizing and teaching the broad ideas of systems, behavioral integration, and communication. Others also have contributed. Mr. Jacques vanVlack, the project cinematographer, supplied technical advice and equipment to improve the screening of the films, and our artist, Mr. Sherl Winter, made the drawings for this volume. Miss Libby Goldstein and Mr. Robert Armstrong worked with the transcripts and Drs. Warren Hampe, Arthur Auerback, and Paul Watzlawick helped with the analysis.

A staff of associates and assistants has struggled with me to solve the problem of publication of results. Draft after draft of the manuscript was typed by Josephine Dixon, Susie Slutski,

Barbara Catena, and John Vila. A number of colleagues have
read manuscripts and contributed ideas and encouragement, including Glen McBride, Thomas Sebeok, Charles Kaufman, Adam
Kendon, Joseph Schaeffer, and Andrew Ferber. But the major
task of boiling down data into concise, readable, and interesting
form fell to my wife, Alice Scheflen, research assistant and ed-
itor of the original project. She repeatedly reworked the ideas,
inventing key devices to make explicit operations of search and
testing which previously had been largely intuitive.

Still another kind of contribution has been necessary —
that of the subjects who have been willing to be filmed and studied. I appreciate the willingness of Mrs. V., Marge, Whitaker,
and Malone to be filmed. The willingness of Whitaker and
Malone was a sophisticated sacrifice. They knew that their
work would be judged by clinical colleagues and that their every
muscle twitch would be scrutinized and written about. Both were
willing to tell us anything they could about their behavior;
Whitaker, especially, has supported me in this write-up even
though he did not agree with all of my comments. I feel another,
less obvious, kind of gratitude to these men. They have willing-
ly allowed their clinical work to be used for a nonclinical purpose. They served as guinea pigs in a study which does not primarily deal with their contributions to psychotherapy. It is as
though we asked an outstanding musician to play for us, then
used his work to make an analysis of the physics of sound waves.

Finally, other filmed subjects made a necessary contribution to this research, even though the text does not describe the
transactions in which they were involved. For example, we
first filmed Dr. John Rosen, who not only fostered our efforts
to develop film analysis by serving as a subject but also helped
us raise the money for the study. At Dr. Rosen's request, Mr.
Laurence Rockefeller and Mrs. Edwin Webster put up the first
funds from their own pockets. Later, O. Spurgeon English,
Barnard Holland, Jules Masserman, Milton Erickson, Ross
Spark, Nat Ackerman, Murry Bowan, and others permitted
themselves to be filmed and studied to prove us with recorded
psychotherapy sessions to compare with Session I.

The original research for this volume was done in Philadelphia in the Department of Psychiatry, Temple University
Medical School, and at the Eastern Pennsylvania Psychiatric
Institute. The research at Temple was financially supported by
the Rockefeller Brothers Fund and the Benjamin Rosenthal Foundation. The work at Eastern Pennsylvania Psychiatric Institute
was greatly aided by the administration of Drs. William Phillips
and Richard Schultz and financially supported by a grant from
the Commonwealth Research Foundation of the Commonwealth
of Pennsylvania.

xiv

The first printing of this book, entitled <u>Stream</u> <u>and</u> <u>Structure</u> <u>in Psychotherapy</u> (Scheflen 1965) was sold out before the publication was announced. In 1966, Dr. Thomas A. Sebeok, Professor of Linguistics and Chairman of the Research Center for the Language Sciences at Indiana University, recommended that the volume be revised for the use of the behavioral science reader. At his suggestion, I have prepared the present edition for publication by Indiana University Press. The revision was begun at the Center for Advanced Study in the Behavioral Sciences at Stanford, California, during 1967-68 and completed at the Bronx State Hospital and at the Jewish Family Services of New York. Work on the revised edition has been sponsored by the Center for Advanced Studies in the Behavioral Sciences at Stanford and the Bronx State Hospital.

COMMUNICATIONAL STRUCTURE:

ANALYSIS OF A PSYCHOTHERAPY TRANSACTION

Introduction

A. HISTORICAL BACKGROUND AND FOUNDATION OF THIS RESEARCH

This book is about small group (or face-to-face) communication and the analytical operations on which the views in the
following pages are based. The study is not primarily about
psychotherapy, even though a sound motion picture of a psychotherapy session provides the illustrative data. Certainly the
orientation is never psychological or sociological in the classical sense. It is, rather, a study of behavioral integration — a
study of how communicative behaviors are integrated to enact
social process.

A basic tenet of the method is that the meaning of an event
may be abstracted by seeing it in context. This research and
viewpoint have evolved in a context of major change in the sciences of man. Since the contextual changes which give this book
its orientation are not universally known, and because these
operations and the assumptions behind them cannot be taken for
granted as they might be in a more traditional method, I must
begin by describing the background to this study.

When this analysis began, a decade ago, only a few researchers were doing work with this general orientation. Since then, a
general theory of communication has been taking shape through
the shared effort of a number of theorists, and more and more
people have come to use context analysis or similar approaches.
I have been continuously in touch with many of these researchers
during this decade, and this volume is my attempt at making a

synthesis. I would like to emphasize, however, that the ideas at issue reflect the joint contributions of a number of linguists, anthropologists, sociologists, social biologists, and psychological scientists.

I have not wanted to write an abstract account of methods and theory. It seems more useful to illustrate principles with some data, even though it is data from a single transaction. After all, a cardinal principle of behavioral systems approaches is that we show behavioral events and not simply present our beliefs about them. Therefore I will describe specific behaviors from the filmed session at the end of each chapter. Since I am not sure that we can adequately describe our own research operations, I relegate my metaconceptions of the method to Appendix B.

Two major changes in orientation and a series of minor ones have occurred during the history of this research. We started with a psychological approach to psychotherapy. In the mid-fifties, a social-science era, we enlarged our field of observation in order to understand processes at the social level of organization. Then during the late 1950s we shifted step by step to a focus on direct observation, cinematographic recording, and behavioral analysis. Each of these developments was guided and spurred by an increasing reliance on systems concepts.

We did not necessarily know what we were doing in making these changes. At least, we did not always have words for the methods or conscious rationale for making the changes. In the main, we simply were dissatisfied with the research methods we had been using and designed other approaches which might eliminate the difficulties. But our methods merely reflected trends of the social science and behavioral science phases of the systems movements. Soon these approaches appeared also in the research of other behaviorally-oriented workers.

Thus, the account of the research projects reported here represents an evolution of operations and views which have become general during the last generation. In this Introduction I will describe my own research experiences and relate them briefly to broader trends, and thus provide an introduction to the principles of context analysis and the theory of human communication elaborated in this volume.

Classical Research in Psychotherapy

In the early 1950s a group of us began to do research in psychotherapy. We were faced with certain classical problems of psychological research. We relied either on subjects and judges to interpret the events of psychotherapy, or on our own experiences as participant observers. We had reservations about the objectivity of subjectivist reports, a problem which was then being recognized. A series of research strategies were developed to deal with it.

The first method we tried was very popular at the time. We conducted structured interviews with therapists and patients, or else we had them fill out rating scales and questionnaires. Then we tried to determine statistically whether the various raters had achieved consensual validation.

This procedure caused us endless difficulties. We were never certain that various subjects and raters attributed similar meaning to the items. We could obtain a statistically significant consensus only among raters who had been trained in psychoanalysis by the same training analyst. And a broader doubt always hung in the background. Suppose various subjects did agree. Consensus in a belief system may mean only that members of culture share the same myth — a hundred or a hundred million Americans can be as wrong as any one person. Our objective was twofold: we were trying to objectify belief systems about psychotherapy and we were trying to find out what happened during psychotherapy.

In 1955 we had an opportunity to take a step forward. Dr. John Rosen invited us to observe at first hand his method of psychotherapy for schizophrenic patients, and we received a large grant from the Rockefeller Brother Fund to carry out research on the process. As a result, a group of experienced psychoanalysts, psychologists, and social scientists watched sessions of Dr. Rosen's method of direct analysis every day for three years and discussed the observations in great detail.

The problem of reaching consensus, however, remained with us. Each of the observers noted different facets of the complex processes of psychotherapy and used a different frame of reference to express his observations (Scheflen 1958). Consequently, the various researchers disagreed strongly, and each published his own report (Brody 1959; English, Bacon, Hampe, and Settlage, 1961; Scheflen 1961). Not only did we disagree about conclusions, but we disagreed as well about what actually took place.

Again we attempted to supply our observer reporters with objective measures and definitions. We worked out careful operational definitions, frameworks, and terms, and again we applied rating scales and other instruments. We made the chain of subjectivist reporting more direct, but we did not solve the problem of abstraction.

We employed still another strategy. We isolated, counted, measured, and correlated variables of behavior themselves. We studied head nods, foot wiggles, noun-verb ratios, and the like.

But the scientific (or scientistic) gain in objectivity afforded by
these measurements did not bring us closer to a view of the larger
behavioral or communicational processes themselves. We had
achieved the dilemma that characterized many sciences of man in
the 1950s: we were caught between subjectivism and reductionism.
The conceptions of experienced clinicians could capture a view of
the whole but these overviews were not replicable or explicable.
On the other hand, the behavioral tidbits we measured brought us
a degree of objectivity about the tidbits but not a picture of psychotherapeutic processes as a whole.

Finally, we decided that if we took a motion picture of the
psychotherapy session, we could insure at least that all of the observers looked at and noted the same behaviors as a basis for
inference and abstraction. When in 1956 we started to film-
record sessions, we were not the first. Bateson (1954) had filmed interviews of psychiatric patients in their homes and a group
in Chicago had filmed psychoanalytic sessions (Carmichael and
Hazzard 1955). Within a year or so, many investigators had filmed psychotherapy.

The films did not immediately help us. The clinicians did
not want to look at them, and we still did not know how to study
the behaviors recorded on film in a systematic and integrated way.
The films began to collect in storage vaults as tape recordings had
in the early 1950s. We didn't realize that we had the makings of
an operational breakthrough.[1] But an era of direct behavioral research had begun.

Focus On The Social Level

Interest in social-level phenomena virtually exploded in the
late 1950s. Science, industry, government, and the people of
common culture suddenly became interested in togetherness, interaction, communication, and social relations. Words like talk
and answer were replaced in everyday middle-class lingo by communicate and feedback. Social psychology, social psychiatry,
social medicine, and social biology developed, and the existing
social sciences were greatly expanded.

Those of us trained in the organismic sciences — medicine,
psychology, psychoanalysis, etc. — slowly came to a critical
realization. Through study of only the individual participants in
psychotherapy we could not grasp all of the phenomena of the
process. We had to look at the relations between patient and therapist, as well as the organismic processes within these participants.

When we first talked about interpersonal relationships in psychotherapy, it seemed some kind of heterodoxy. Social theory

appeared to be somehow opposed to psychological theory as an alternative hypothesis. We used to speak, for instance, of individual versus social behavior. We did not yet have a clear idea about
levels of organization, as the general systems concepts were still
relatively unknown (Bertalanffy 1950, 1960; Redfield 1942; Miller
1965).

Consequently, psychological theorists were trying to deal or-
ganismically with social-level concepts like communication. As
psychoanalysts, for example, we thought of communication as the
individual expression of instinct or motivation or defense. The
experimental psychologist tried to squeeze communicational processes into an S-R paradigm (Percy 1961). Steven (1950), for
example, defined communication 'as the discriminatory response
to a stimulus.' In each of the classical disciplines, the first consequence of the social science era was the reformulation of phenomena like communication in the traditional framework of that
discipline. Consequently, as many theories of communication
developed as there were classical disciplines in the sciences of
man.[2] We did not realize that a new frame of reference was
emerging which would permit an extensive synthesis and blur old
disciplinary boundaries.

By 1957 a great many social-psychological projects were
underway. Communication was being examined by looking 'between group members' rather than 'into' individuals. But the
long involvement with organismic-centered concepts constrained our efforts. We developed models of communication that focused upon interaction between individuals and we concentrated
on groups as collections of individuals. Two popular ideas about
communication came into prominence that were still limited by
reductionistic viewpoints.

1. The action-reaction approach. People in a group sometimes take turns talking and listening. If the observer looks first
to one speaker and then to the next one, he will see dialogue as an
alternative, sequential activity. Thus, A speaks and B responds,
then A speaks again, and so on. Often B reacts to what A has
said. A's action was seen as a stimulus to B, and B's action was
seen as a response to A. Thus S-R paradigms were wired in series to develop a model of human communication. Such a model
can be called an action-reaction model.

This model lends itself to the lingo of information theory and
cybernetics (Shannon and Weaver 1949; Wiener 1961). Mr. A
can be said to encode a message which he transmits to Mr. B who
decodes and transmits this message to Mrs. B who decodes this
message and encodes a response to A, and so forth. In this approach the participants in communication are likened to telegraph-
ic or other electronic devices which transmit and receive signals

(Cherry 1961). In the 1950s certain social-psychological theorists had such machinomorphic concepts of psychotherapy that they spoke of exchanges of signals between therapists and patients (Colby 1960; Menninger 1958).

2. Social network concepts. Similarly, we could observe a group of people and decide which members talked to or contacted each other, or we could examine research questions such as who talked first or whose commands dominated the others. Such approaches were popular in the sociological sciences in the 1950s and can loosely be called network concepts (Cherry 1961; Chappel 1949; Haley 1959).

There are serious limitations to these individual-centered frames of reference. First of all, the interactional model at best depicts certain linguistic events in a formal conversation. In general, people do not take turns talking and listening to each other. They do not respond only to what someone has just said. Rather, they act within broader systems of events — to what has been said hours or even months before, to something unsaid, to what might be said, and to matters unrelated to the immediate transaction. And their nonspeech behavior is continuous. All participants hold postures and facial expressions at all times and they move together.

There is yet a broader issue here: each of these models was based on the concept of a group. Now, a group of participants is necessary for any social phenomena and obviously a group is made up of individual human organisms, but we don't get very far looking at the matter in this way. If you begin by conceiving of a group and then make an analysis, the first step in reduction will take you back to the individual — back to the organism-centered models that have already proved inadequate.

The Development of a Behavioral Systems Approach

In the late 1950s we at last recognized something which took us beyond these group models to the study of behavior and the current behavioral science era. The recognition was this: Although, physically speaking, a group is made up of human organisms, social organization and the processes of group are made up of behaviors; more accurately, they consist of integrations of behavior.[3]

We had already learned homologous operational truth about the organism — that the living organism is not merely a pile of organs or even an arrangement of them as it is on the anatomist's table. It is an organization of processes among organ systems, i.e., of organ behaviors.

Similarly, communication is not made up of people or even of individual expressions but of patterned relations among the behaviors of multiple people.

If we were to study communication, then, we had to retrace our steps from the high-level inferences of the psychological and social sciences and get back to the study of behavior itself. We had to examine action, describe it, analyze its form, and try to define meaning behaviorally. The psychodynamicist had to delay his inferences about personality and describe the behaviors on which he based these inferences. He had to describe what others in a transaction could see. And the sociologist had to describe the relations of behavior which brought and held people together. He could not merely classify groups and abstract qualities of relationships.

I think this realization was behind the widespread movement toward behavioral science which emerged about 1960. This movement was not merely a revival of behaviorism and neobehaviorism. Behavior has come to be observed in its own right; that is, we study its structure and do not merely make inferences about neurophysiological or cognitive processes.

When we came to recognize the significance of behavior in communication, we discovered that others had long been working in the field.

One discipline had been at work on this very problem for three decades. The structural linguists had developed methods for studying the structure of language behavior (Sapir 1921; Bloomfield 1933). In the early 1950s these methods were not widely known in the other sciences of man and had not been applied to units of behavior other than speech or to units larger than the syntactic sentence. The behavioral science era resulted in a broad dissemination of structural linguistic approaches and in their extension to behavior in general. The methodology of the research reported in this book depends upon a structural linguistic orientation, as do other new methods for the study of behavioral integration.

The methods of the structural linguists are suited to the examination of behavioral structure. In the late 1950s and the 1960s at least some principles of this method were applied to the study of behavioral integrations larger than the sentence (Z. Harris 1952; Scheflen 1966) and they were applied to behaviors other than language (Birdwhistell 1952, 1966; Pike 1954).

The study of behavioral relations requires that we emphasize operations for examining synthesis. The classical approach of analysis by reduction thus becomes one tactic in an ultimate strategy for reconstructing a view of the larger picture.

Methodologies for such synthesis which developed in the 1950s and 1960s have been described by several authors (McQuown et al. 1969; Pike 1954; Schneirla 1951; Rock 1962; Barker 1963; and Scheflen 1966). The variation of these approaches used in this research has been called variously 'linguistic-kinesic analysis' (Brosin 1967), 'communication analysis' (Scheflen 1966), and 'context analysis.'[4]

The operations for synthesis require that we not concentrate on the relations of a behavior to some conceptual system about behavior, but rather that we examine the relations of one behavior to another and these to a third until we have identified all of the behavioral elements that constitute a single defined subsystem of behavior or change.

Here is an analogy: The classical biologist would observe an animal and assign it to a class of animals in a taxonomy. The social biologist began to observe the relationships of the animal to other animals with whom it lived or related, and he visualized flocks, herds, or prides of animals. Then the behaviorally-oriented social biologist began to observe the calls, or the displays, or the aggressive rushes of animals — the behaviors rather than the animals. By observing these behaviors in relation to other behaviors, he visualized call systems, displays in a courtship dance, and mutual rushes in defense of a territory.

Since the processes of behavioral integration follow the principles of any other system, I will call this general orientation a behavioral systems view.

To study such complexity, we needed a technology. We cannot examine multiple modalities of behavior in detail at a single observation. Armed with eyes, ears, and a notebook, the observer has his hands full merely to hear the speech and to note the gross actions of one participant. The sound motion picture and, more recently, the video tape provided the needed technological means for thorough observations. Given a film record we can go over again and again the events of a transaction, systematically observing one, then another, behavioral modality and testing their various relations until we have described the synthesis of elements in the over-all picture.

The shift to a behavioral focus, the ability to study complex behavioral integrations, and the development of the new recording technologies, all occurred interdependently. None of the aspects of a behavioral systems approach would have been possible without the others, just as the computer and cybernetics could hardly be imagined as separate developments.

All of these developments are offshoots of a systems orientation shift in the subject matter of study which occurred

with the coming of the behavioral science era. Whereas researchers were excluded from many confidential activities of
society, we now seemed to be welcome and could bring cameras. In the past we had studied the people of esoteric cultures,
institutionalized deviants, and subprimates, but in the 1960s
we turned to the study of the people next door, to our own urban
cultures and middle-class institutions, and to the naturalistic
study of our nearest other-animal relatives, the primates.

The behavioral systems researchers of the early 1960s
deeply distrusted subjectivist accounts. We had never known
how to handle a subject's account systematically, so we ignored it. We looked at subjects but did not interview them. We
did not care what they had to say and did not want to hear it.
But a way of dealing with both visible behavior and subjectivist
conceptions had to evolve.

M. Harris (1964) advocated that subjects be both observed
and interviewed. Now in many projects, video recordings or
movies of behavior are made in naturalistic situations and afterward are shown to the subjects, who are then interviewed in
depth about their behavior as it appears on screen. An untra-
ditional idea has gradually emerged from the work of Bateson
(1955), Pribram (1964), and others, about the relations of
cognitive and motor behavior. These matters are discussed in
detail in Section B of this volume.

The Research Which Led to This Volume

In 1959 Dr. Birdwhistell and I established a project at
Eastern Pennsylvania Psychiatric Institute to study communication in psychotherapy and other transactions through the context analysis of motion picture films. A clinical project at
Temple University also was reorganized to study the methods
of therapists. We decided that the two projects should corrob-
orate on the analysis of a method. The Temple team, consisting
mainly of clinicians, was to make a clinical appraisal, and the
Eastern Psychiatric Institute team of Birdwhistell and Scheflen
was to make a context analysis.

Experimental sessions, in which two psychotherapists, a
schizophrenic patient, and (on two occasions) the patient's mother participated, were observed and analyzed.

The First Publications

The sessions were examined clinically by Doctors O.
Spurgeon English, Catharine Bacon, and Warren W. Hampe.
Dr. Arthur H. Auerbach made a content analysis. In the

course of the study, the method of context analysis became clearer and less unwieldy. When the results of all the studies were brought together, it was apparent that the data was of interest to two different groups: psychotherapists, who might be chiefly concerned with the clinical data and conclusions; and behavioral scientists who were interested primarily in research method. We therefore decided to publish two monographs about the study: one describing the Whitaker-Malone method by clinical constructs and content analysis, and the other illustrating the context analysis of the first session. The clinical book, edited by Dr. O. Spurgeon English, was entitled Strategy and Structure in Psychotherapy (1966). The title of the method book was Stream and Structure of Communicational Behavior (Scheflen 1965) — the book upon which this revised edition is based.

B. THE EXPERIMENTAL SESSIONS

The Procedure

We knew that the psychiatrists, Doctors Carl Whitaker and Thomas Malone, had a unique approach to the psychotherapy of schizophrenia. They agreed to become subject-therapists and accordingly spent the first two weeks of October 1959 in Philadelphia being observed and studied. In order to approximate their usual living situation, they brought their wives and younger children along. Both families lived in apartment suites in a center-city hotel. To reduce extraneous pressures, they had few social or professional engagements: each of them addressed open psychiatric meetings only once. Observation of and discussion with them was limited to the research team.

A schizophrenic patient, whom we will call Marge, was selected by the research team from a neighboring public hospital. She and her mother were told that the procedure would be experimental. The patient lived in a residential unit of the Institute for Direct Analysis during the two weeks of the observational sessions. This unit is a three-story brick row house adjacent to Temple University Hospital in an upper-class urban neighborhood. The house had been remodeled previously, with every effort made to keep the atmosphere that of a private home. (Scheflen 1961). The unit was staffed by three young people who had been trained by Dr. Rosen's direct analytic staff.

As was their usual practice, Whitaker and Malone asked that the patient's mother be present at the first two sessions. Nine thirty-five minute sessions were arranged on consecutive weekday mornings: two with the mother, seven with Marge alone.

After the ninth session, Malone elected to see the patient once
for a tenth session. All sessions were tape recorded and observed by the researchers. The first, third, and ninth sessions
were recorded on motion picture film. In order to keep some of
the variables constant, the filming was done in the same living
room of the residential unit in which the films of direct analysis
had been taken. After each session the observers met with
Whitaker and Malone for two hours to discuss the events of the
session and their theoretical premises.

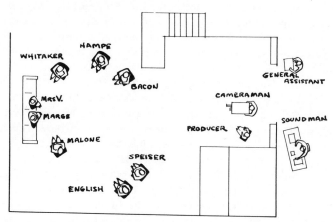

Figure 1: Seating Arrangement for the Filmed Sessions

Present at each session were Whitaker, Malone, the patient,
(and in the first two sessions) the mother, three or four observing psychoanalysts, and the project administrator.[6]

The Participants in Session I

When strangers come together for a transaction, information about them is offered to the others. They are often introduced or they introduce themselves. And whenever we give an
account of a transaction we begin with an introductory statement
about the participants. For instance, we begin a stage play or
athletic context or an account of a party by reviewing the dramat-
is personae. In these introductions something is conveyed about
each one's background, his social position, and maybe about his
personality.

Before Session I the researchers talked with Whitaker and
Malone and asked them at length about their careers, methods,
and plans for the experimental sessions. And several of us interviewed Marge and Mrs. V, obtaining their history and observing

their interview behavior. In the preliminary interviews we told each of our subjects something of what we had learned about the others — approximately the information outlined in the description below.

The patient, Marge. A 17-year-old girl of Italian extraction, Marge spoke in a soft, often childish, and barely audible voice. Her south Philadelphia idiom was immediately apparent, and her speech was colored throughout with Italian-American expressions typical of her background. In later sessions a drawl like Whitaker's was clearly detectable. Physically, Marge gave the overall impression of well-developed femininity. She was rather tall and dark complected, not pretty, though she might be considered 'kind of cute.' Her dress and grooming seemed appropriate.

Marge was the only surviving child of Italian-born parents. A brother had died in infancy. Although the mother had had hallucinations and other psychotic manifestations, the family apparently had been cohesive. The father, it was implied, was jealous and overly possessive. He died when Marge was sixteen. Following his death, Marge became sexually promiscuous, ultimately became pregnant and had an abortion. Marge had been hospitalized at another institution six months before Whitaker and Malone saw her. She had been seen frequently during this hospitalization by a psychoanalytically oriented resident physician and she seemed to be well-acquainted with the current concepts of the etiology of schizophrenia. This was evident in her many statements implying maternal deprivation, which seemed calculated to direct the psychiatrists' attention to her mother's shortcomings.

The mother, Mrs. V. At 48 years of age, heavy, stolid, and impassive, Mrs. V sat hunched forward with her knees about six inches apart and her dress pulled well down. She wore a polka dot dress, low-heeled shoes, and heavy-guage stockings. Her hair was worn straight, and she did not appear to be wearing make-up. She presented the picture of a good-natured immigrant peasant.

Mrs. V did not seem aggressive, hostile, or cold, as schizophrenogenic mothers are often considered to be. She was plain and self-contained, yet had a faint pleasant smile and occasionally displayed a hint of friendliness or coquettishness. She did not show the marked shifts in total posture that Marge did. In fact, she moved very little. Her history indicated that she had had psychotic symptoms, such as an inability to eat for months, and ideas of hallucinations about the flight from her home. Her affect during the sessions was slightly flattened. At this writing Mrs. V is a patient in a state mental hospital.

She spoke in a typical nonstandard Italian-American dialect. The history, as she presented it, seemed calculated to turn aside blame, cover the family secrets, and make psychosis seem impersonal and unrelated to their emotional lives.

Psychotherapist, Whitaker. Carl Whitaker was born in Raymondville, New York, in 1912. He trained in medicine at Syracuse University and in psychiatry at the University of Louisville in Kentucky. He was formerly Chairman of the Department of Psychiatry at Emory University, then leader of a private group practice in Atlanta, Georgia. He is currently Professor of Psychiatry at the University of Wisconsin.

Large, youthful looking, and bespectacled, Whitaker is generally serious and thoughtful. He has a droll sense of humor, a quiet amiability, and an occasional flair for the provocative and unconventional.

He spoke sixty times during the session, considerably more than Malone, and the content of his statements fell into five clearly discernible types of comments (see Section A). Whitaker spoke only to the women, and at no time did he and Malone speak to each other.

Psychotherapist, Malone. Thomas Malone was born in Mahanoy City, Pennsylvania, in 1919. In 1948 he began to assist Whitaker and subsequently decided to study medicine in order to become a psychiatrist. He graduated from the Emory University School of Medicine in 1953. Malone is currently in practice at the Atlanta Psychiatric Clinic.

Youthful, sturdily built, and good-looking, Malone was more active in general, more verbal in discussion, and more aggressive in manner than was Whitaker. Like Whitaker, he tended to be serious, introspective, and candid about himself and his work. He gave the appearance of a scholarly intellectual and was more inclined than Whitaker toward conceptualization and research interest. In Session I he was serious, untalkative, somewhat stiff, and immobile kinesically. His speech was formal when he was talking to Marge and less so when talking with Mrs. V. In later sessions he was active and informal.

The Basis for Our Study: Communicative Behavior

In communicational theory we say that the behavior of each participant is communicative; that is, it is patterned and structured according to some tradition. If so, it is potentially recognizable and meaningful. Therefore, behavior is the basis for the social processes of communication.

I do not want to suggest an old dichotomy by such a statement. I am not implying that some behavior is communicative and some is not. I do not believe it probable that anyone will behave in a nonstructured and nontraditional way. We learn to behave systematically in becoming socialized and enculturated, and it is very hard to behave in any other way. So it is redundant to speak of communicative behavior, when all behavior is apparently patterned and capable of being recognized and comprehended, i.e., communicative.

But another type of distinction is critical in communicational theory. While each participant follows some customary blueprint and agenda in guiding his contribution, a considerable range of variation is allowable. Thus a participant can modify, shape, and adapt his behavior to a given situation. Certain unit forms of behavior which are traditional on the social level were employed in Session I (discussed in Part I of this book). There were, of course, individual styles and particular management and adaptions which the participants made in accordance with their own plans, sometimes directly influenced by the special situation of Session I (Part II).

PART I

Customary Behavioral Communication
in Session I

Emphasizing traditional unit forms of behavior
employed by the participants during Session I. Section A is concerned with unit forms at the level of
positions, Section B contains analysis of these units
and their constituents, and Section C presents the
synthesis of the units in constructing an over-all
picture of Session I.

SECTION A

The Communicative Positions
in Session I

Introduction

WHERE TO BEGIN THE ANALYSIS

THE FIRST ISOLATION: FOCUSING ON THE BEHAVIOR
OF ONE PARTICIPANT AT A TIME

Our problem is how to study and describe great complexity.
We are beginning with a traditional isolation focusing on one participant — watching his behavior and analyzing it. Then we isolate the behavior of another participant and so on.

In general systems theory, such a focus holds us at the organismic level of organization (Bertalanffy 1950; Miller 1965).
Such an Einstellung is traditionally taken in classical biology,
medicine and psychiatry, and the psychological sciences. In this
focus we do not see social organization or communication, but
rather the behavioral contribution of each individual to the total
process. We must bear in mind that it is a heuristic practice to
focus on one person as if he were behaving alone, but we can
later integrate the contributions of each person by standing back
and visualizing their relations at the social level.

THE SECOND ISOLATION: DELINEATING A LEVEL

The structure of behavior is such that small activities are
successively combined into larger and larger configurations.
Words, for example, are combined with gestures and pitch patterns to form sentences. Multiple sentences are combined and,
together with postures of address, form utterances. Or we can
begin by viewing the total structure of a transaction and analyzing
this step by step to its component acts. Thus an activity is made

17

up of subactivities which are made in turn of 'sub-subactivities' to the smallest element of phonation and movement.

This kind of successive integration is called a hierarchy of levels — in this case, levels of behavioral integration, not of conceptual or physical systems (Miller 1965). In the case of behavior the integrations consist of successive patterns of movement or change.

When we study such a hierarchical integration, we must examine all of the constituent movements or else we will not be able to reconstruct the relations between them. Operationally we define these relations by continually moving our observational focus back and forth from parts to wholes, because each defines the other. Any given unit of activity is at once, depending on how we look at it, an integration of smaller acts and a unified entity that occurs in some larger configuration. So we break down activity analytically to its constituent sounds and movements in order to describe it. Then we test the relations of these constituents to make sure they go together as an entity. These operations are described in Appendix B.

SELECTING AN INITIAL LEVEL

In operations like these, where we go back and forth alternately examining the composition of an action and then its location in a larger system of activities, it does not matter where we begin. Theoretically we could start with any level. We could view first the total behavioral integration of Session I, then take an analytic direction. Thereby, we can separate successively smaller elements until we describe microunits of speech and gesture. Or we could start by examining all of the microacts and depict how they were combined in the total structure of Session I.

Actually we are going to begin in the middle. I am going to isolate a level of activity whose units I call positions. These units of activity involve the orientation and movements of the total body of a participant. They are of a duration from seconds to twenty minutes or more. Since they involve the whole body they are the smallest unit of behavior which occurs naturally at the individual or organismic level. A person can arrive at a transaction, perform one position, and leave, but he cannot be present and perform less than a position. He cannot, that is, act with only some part of his body. There is another reason to begin here. At the beginning and ending of a position, a gross shift in bodily position occurs which is easy to spot in reviewing the transaction.

Chapter 1

THE POSITIONS IN SESSION I

At the beginning of Session I each participant assumed an initial position. He sat down in a particular posture and oriented himself to the others. While holding this posture and orientation he performed a sequence of activities. When these were completed or interrupted, he shifted his posture and orientation to another configuration and began another activity. Then he went back to his original position and repeated the sequence.

Here in Chapter 1, I will describe the positions which each person took in Session I. Then in Chapter 2, I will describe the characteristics and features of any position and tell how we identify each one as a unit of activity.

THE INITIAL POSITIONS IN SESSION I

At the beginning of Session I each participant entered the room and chose a seat.

Customary conventions were observed. The men and the women were introduced to each other by the project coordinator. The men remained standing at their chairs until the women were seated. Then each participant sat down, arranged himself and his clothing, and faced the others.

The women sat on the couch and the men took one of the chairs which had already been placed at each end of this couch.

The Initial Postural Arrangements

Mrs. V. sat on the sofa, crossed her ankles, pulled down her skirt, and tucked it under her. She sat upright and forward.

19

Her torso was oriented about midway between the two men.
From this position she could traverse her head so as to face alternately either of them.

Marge positioned her body similarly, but slouched down and sat back farther on the sofa. Thus she sat lower and less forward than her mother — a position characteristic of one who is subordinate or of one who will not lead off with an active part.

Thus the women sat side-by-side on the sofa, assuming bodily orientations which allowed them to see and address the men. They would have to turn ninety degrees to face each other. Side-by-side positions like these are customary for relatives, lovers, friends, and colleagues when addressing strangers (see Chapter 7).

The men took chairs which faced each other, but they turned their bodies toward the women.

Whitaker took the chair nearer to Marge and pulled it forward to the end of the sofa. He thus placed himself near the younger woman with whom he would later side in the mother-daughter arguments. When Whitaker sat down he crossed his legs, left over right. The upper leg which projected outward was thus placed across the space between him and Malone. Since Malone did the same thing, the men erected a sort of postural barrier between the camera and the four central participants, thus defining a group separate from the observers.

This configuration is also customary for a semicircular group arrangement. Status figures or men will sit on the end chairs and mark off their group as if they were guarding an entrance.

Malone assumed a posture almost identical to Whitaker's. He sat back in his chair, folded his arms, crossed his right leg over his left leg, and took out his pipe.

Thus the postures of the two men were identical. They were mirror-imaged replications of each other. Parallel postures like side-by-side placement occur among people who are allied or will take common sides on an issue (see Chapter 7). It was not that one of the men copied the other for they both sat down at the same instant. They sat alike because each used a positioning which is characteristic for psychotherapists at the beginning of a psychotherapy session. To generalize a step further, the crossing of arms and legs is typical for strangers who have just sat down together for the first time. The postures of sitting back are used by all participants except the one who will lead off the exposition. We can infer that Mrs. V had this role by prearrangement since she alone sat forward as Session I began.

The Behavior That Occurred While These
Initial Positions Were Held

Mrs. V's Explanation

As the session began, Mrs. V, sitting erect and forward, began to tell the story of the day her daughter became psychotic. She quoted a statement that Marge had made that day, saying that Marge had asked to be helped upstairs to her room. When the movie camera was turned on, Mrs. V was in the process of quoting Marge and imitating her voice. 'Help me upstairs,' she said. Then Mrs. V added a parenthetical remark, a comment on what she had just described. Acting a little shocked and incredulous, she said, 'A young girl like her.' Then she repeated her imitation of Marge's plea, saying again, 'Help me upstairs.'

Notice that the mother has a tendency to comment disparagingly on her daughter's behavior. We will see that Marge later turned the tables and did this to her mother. In fact, through much of the session Marge's utterances and gestures consisted of disparaging and protesting commentaries on what her mother was saying. Note the relation of these two kinds of utterances. The first describes an event which occurred elsewhere; the second comments on that description. Later I will call this kind of commentary metacommunicative behavior.

Mrs. V continued by saying: 'and . . . uh . . . the next day I thought she'd get better by . . . ah . . . ah . . .. She has the doctor's prescription . . . .

I will not quote the whole of Mrs. V's statement here. All of the lexical behavior of Session I is reproduced in Appendix A, and these details appear on a transcript in Chapter 3. I would rather focus on the larger configuration. I will call this total behavior of Mrs. V's explaining. These actions — her posture orientation, and utterance, considered as an integrated entity — made up her initial position in the session. This position she repeated again and again (Figure 1-1).

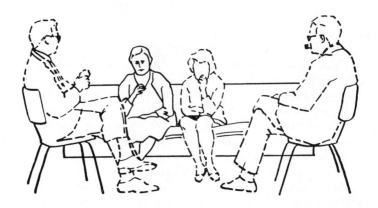

Figure 1-1: <u>Above,</u> Mrs. V explaining: Mrs. V told about Marge's psychosis and the V family history. <u>Below,</u> Whitaker explaining: Late in the session Whitaker explained the purposes and intentions of the sessions. Note that he sat forward and addressed the women.

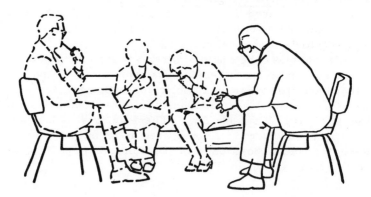

In the psychological sciences, the speech and body language which occur in a position are often called the content. So we can say that a position has or includes a content. In an explicitly conversational transaction, of which psychotherapy is a variant, we can expect the activities which occur during a position to be primarily language behavior. In fact, most psychotherapies explicitly rule out other kinds of gross behavior. But we should bear in mind that the activities of positions in other kinds of transactions might not be primarily linguistic. They might, for instance, consist of love-making, mother and daughter grooming, feeding, or cooperative product manufacture.

The Complementary Speaker: Marge

The explicit first task of Session I was the giving of a history, a history of Marge's illness and of the V family. Marge had a stake in this. As one who had something to say about the subject we would expect her to comment and add detail. Mrs. V had the lead, but her daughter sat at her side as a junior partner in the task.

Marge sat huddled up near her mother. She added statements but tended to do so disparagingly. She muttered comments under her breath about what Mrs. V said, made faces which mocked and indicated incredulity. She covertly appealed to the men for attention and created distractions by addressing the camera, sprawling on the sofa, and exhibiting her legs.

I call Marge's initial position passive protesting. I will describe the activities which gave the impression of passive protest in later chapters. Here, where we are seeking an overview of positions, I will merely diagram the position in Figure 1-2.

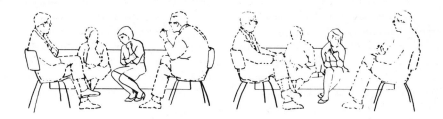

Disparaging (Marge)   Lamenting (Marge)

Figure 1-2: Activities in Marge's Position of Passive Protesting

24

The Listeners: Whitaker and Malone

Whitaker and Malone sat back looking at Mrs. V and listening.

As I said, their postures were typical for listeners who are not yet actively engaged — sitting back in their chairs, arms and legs crossed. Occasionally, they intercalated a question. More often they indicated attentiveness by keeping the eyelids slightly widened, nodding occasionally, and slightly cocking their heads (see Chapters 3 and 4).

These positions I will call listening and questioning (Figure 1-3).

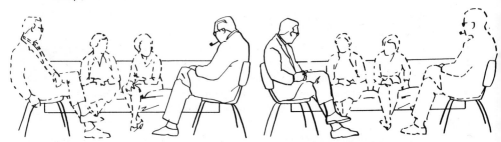

Listening (Whitaker)   Listening (Malone)

Figure 1-3: Drawings from the Position of Listening and Questioning

Markers and the Duration of a Position

The Completion of a Sequence

We can make the following generalization: A position is taken and held while some activity is carried out — explaining, passive protesting, or listening and questioning (in the case of the initial positions of Session I). We can also note that ordinarily the position is held until this activity is completed or until it is interrupted. In the case of an interruption a participant may hold the position and attempt to regain the floor. Failing this he will terminate the position and assume another one.

We confirmed this assertion by repeated observations. If a participant comes from our own cultural background, we can recognize most of the activities he will carry out in a position. They are familiar sequences which in totality produce customary Gestalten — they finish an idea or topic or accomplish a simple task. As a consequence we know from experience when they are completed.

If we do not know the configuration we have to discover it by context analysis. We have to find repeated occurrences of this type of sequence and establish that it is a regular and customary entity (see Appendix B).

Markers of the Position's Duration

When the included activities of the position have been completed, the performer will leave or else he will take another distinctly different orientation and posture and perform some other task or phase. Thus, a shift in posture which involves the total bodily orientation occurs between one position and the next. Such a shift provides a visible indication that one position has been completed and a next position is beginning. So the completion or abandonment of an activity and a shift in posture and orientation are coterminous. We identify one in terms of the other. In a formal activity like psychotherapy (especially when the participants are strangers) the posture and orientation of the position will be held stationary, fixed, relatively immobile, even rigid. (In Chapter 2, I will introduce some complications and exceptions, but I will hold here to the general principle.)

It is my belief that the postural configuration of the position is held deliberately — though not consciously — throughout the positional performance in order to indicate that the position has not been completed. It is held, I am claiming, in order to show that a position still obtains or is 'in effect.' I believe that this systematic holding and shifting behavior is an evolved dimension of communication, learned and transmitted in culture to make possible a mutual orientation in the steps of a transaction. In any event the researcher can use this behavior to identify segmentations in the stream of behavior — in this case, the positions.

At a suggestion of Birdwhistell (1963), I will call the posture which is held during a unit performance a transfix.

With the shift in posture and orientation at the completion of the position, there is also a pause in movement and speech and often a special signal of completion. Such combinations of behavioral elements that indicate completion I will call junctures. The term is borrowed from structural linguistics where it is used to describe the terminal behavior of the syntactic sentence (Z. Harris 1951; Gleason 1955).

Collectively the transfix and the juncture mark the boundaries of the position. So I will call these markings behaviors.

THE SECOND COMPLEX OF POSITIONS IN SESSION I

After about a minute some of the initial positions of Session I were changed, and a new configuration of positions appeared. I will therefore speak of the initial phase of positions as Period 1 and refer to the new or second configuration as Period 2.

Marge's Shift to the Position Contending

Marge's initial position of passive protesting ended with a dramatic postural shift. She stood up and sat down nearer to Whitaker, in a posture something like the one he was using. Thus she ended the initial posture in which she had huddled near her mother and instead sat as Whitaker did (Figure 1-4). We will see later that this change in her positioning represented a change in alliance from her mother to Whitaker. This change seemed to be fostered or invited by Whitaker's behavior: just l efore the shift occurred, Marge had mumbled inaudibly, Whitaker turned to her and said, 'Why don't you say what you wanted to say, Marge.'

Marge's second position occurred again and again. Each time it had the same characteristics. Marge began this position by crossing her legs, but she immediately uncrossed them and instead crossed her ankles. Then she stood and sat down near and like Whitaker.

With this shift Marge's behavior changed markedly. She sat forward on the sofa. She appeared alert and attentive to the others, whereas before she had seemed depressed, withdrawn, and dissociated. She brought her body into the tonus and position which courting women use. Her head was high and slightly cocked, eyes bright, chest out so that her breasts were raised and prominent.

Marge's Transitional Position
of Appealing-Lamenting

Just at the time when Marge shifted from passive protesting to the position of contending, she would turn briefly to Whitaker. She would say something to him of an appealing or lamenting nature, such as 'I'm dead' or 'She [her mother] talks crazy to me.' In speaking she would briefly hold a tête-à-tête with Whitaker. This position lasted only a few seconds. Then Marge quickly turned to her mother.

In the example above, Marge pointed to her mother and made an accusation: 'She is mentally ill' (see Figure 1-5).

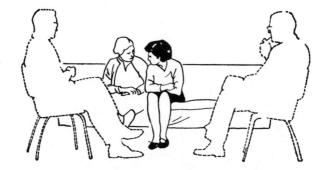

Sitting with Mother

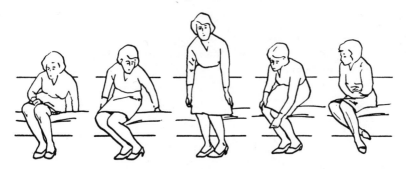

The Shift

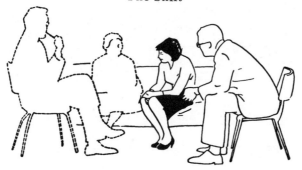

Sitting with Whitaker

Figure 1-4: Marge's Positional Juncture

On other occasions she would act courtingly to Whitaker in this transitional position by putting her hand on her hip, protruding her chest, and forming the model's position of 'cheesecake.'

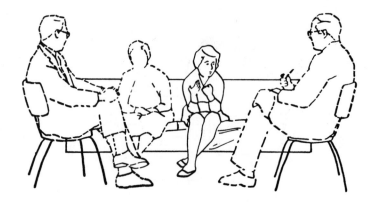

Figure 1-5: Marge's Positions. <u>Above,</u> Marge Lamenting to
Whitaker. <u>Below,</u> Marge Accusing Her Mother
Whitaker.

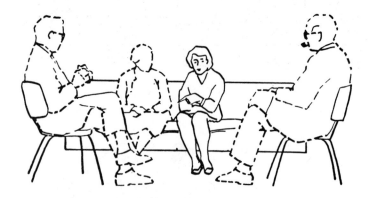

<u>Shifts in the Positions of the Other Participants</u>

With Marge's dramatic shift the others changed their behavior.

<u>Mrs. V's Adoption of the Position,</u> Defending

When Marge shifted to contending, Mrs. V uncrossed her
ankles, leaned even farther forward, stopped her narrative, and
defended her story against Marge's challenge. It looked for a
moment as though she were going to stand up. Thus Mrs. V
changed her position to a configuration I will call <u>defending</u>
(Figure 1-6).

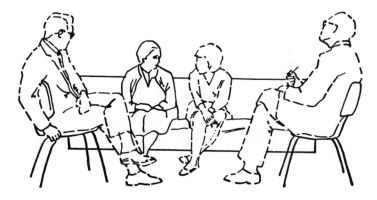

Figure 1-6: Mrs. V's Second Position, Defending

After Marge made an accusation to her mother, the two women turned to face each other and argue the allegation. Mrs. V
usually would defend her position, but sometimes she would con-
cede.

Malone's Position of Intervention

When mother and daughter turned to each other and contended,
Malone would perform a brief position of intervention, which terminated this second configuration of positions.

Malone would lean forward, unfold his arms, and grasp his
right knee with his hands. He would then rock forward in his
chair toward the women. He spoke first to Marge, directly or
indirectly scolding her; then he supported Mrs. V and invited
her to continue her narrative. This position lasted about ten
seconds or so, just long enough for Malone to say a few sentences;
then he returned to his initial baseline position of listening and
questioning. Intervention is about the simplest type of position
that we ordinarily observe in a conversation. It consists only of
a postural shift, then a brief speech and facial expression, and
then a return to the baseline posture (Figure 1-7).

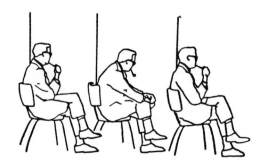

Figure 1-7: Malone's Rocking Forward in Intervention

The Termination of a Period 2

The phase of Session I in which the positions of contending and defending appeared will be called Period 2. Malone's intervention was followed by a sequence of events which ended Period 2: Whitaker turned his head away from Marge, and Marge dissociated herself from him. She looked away, acted bizarrely, and then stood up again in repetition of her previous dramatic juncture. Then she sat down near Mrs. V as she had been sitting at the beginning of the session. When Marge sat near her, huddled up to her again, and remained silent, Mrs. V crossed her ankles again and sat back in her initial posture. Then she resumed her narrative where she had left off when Whitaker and Marge had interrupted her.

The men turned back to Mrs. V and again attended her story. Thus the second constellation of positions ended with a return to almost exactly the original constellation of explaining, passive protesting, and listening and questioning.

As I will describe in Chapter 2, these two configurations called Period 1 and Period 2, recurred again and again until minute 23, after which a Period 2 arrangement persisted. Thus the positional arrangements alternated or oscillated from periods of exposition to periods of argument.

From my experience with other conversations I would speculate that the original positions would have persisted for this twenty-three-minute period without marked change if only one of the women had been present or if Marge had been in accord with the story and had accepted a secondary position in the narration. From twenty to twenty-five minutes is characteristic duration for a position of exposition in a formal conversational transaction.

OTHER POSITIONS IN SESSION I

Several other brief positions occurred in Session I.

Marge's Brief Position of Intervention

Marge sometimes attempted to interrupt her mother's explanation with a brief position of intervention. When her mother
was speaking to Malone and Whitaker, Marge would suddenly sit
well forward or even stand between them. She would assume a
facial expression of shocked indignation and say something out-
rageous such as, 'I want to be raped.' Then she would immediately return to her basic position of passive protesting.

Unlike Malone's intervention, Marge's attempt (Figure
1-8) was usually ignored. But I think these two positions belong to a common class.

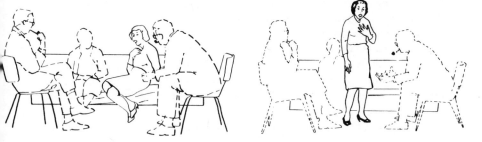

Figure 1-8: Marge's Position of Intervention in Session I

Marge's Position of Resigning

Another brief position was often enacted by Marge. She
would sprawl back on the sofa and dissociate herself from participation. I will call this position resigning (Figure 1-9). This
action seemed in some ways the inverse of interfering While the
former was an active interruption, resigning was a withdrawal.
Marge performed the position in an exhibitionistic way, and she
must have known from her previous psychotherapy that psychiatrists actively engage a patient who acts autistic or withdrawn.
So the intent of resigning may have been similar to that in interfering.

The brief positions were of a different logical type than the
more lasting positions of explaining, listening and questioning,
contending, and defending. This distinction is not based on their
brevity, but rather on their function in the transaction. They

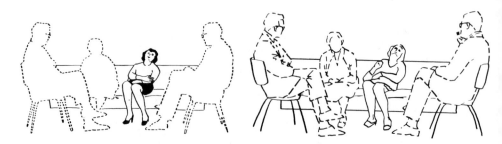

Figure 1-9: Marge's Posture in Resigning

were not informative in the customary sense of that word, but
rather they served to change and govern the relations of the session.

Another brief position of this type occurred.

During the performances of the language positions, Marge,
Whitaker, and Malone carried out well-defined sequences of
nonlanguage behaviors.

For example, Marge and Malone moved synchronously during the first five minutes of Phase I., Whitaker and Marge engaged in some tentative quasi-courting behavior. Marge carried
out elaborate sequences of Kleenex display; then Whitaker used
his hands in a similar way.

Because these behaviors did not involve the total body, they
were not positions. Hence, I will describe these activities in
Section B.

The Position, Tactile Contacting

On one occasion these sequences did escalate until they
momentarily involved the total posture and orientation of the
performer. Thus, a position occurred.

At 24 minutes Whitaker thrust his hand under Marge's nose
and asked her to smell an object which he held there, apparently
a small piece of cheese he had picked up from the floor. As
Marge was smelling it, she and Whitaker touched briefly.

Whitaker and Marge were totally oriented to each other at
that instant, turning to each other to speak and touch. So they
enacted a total, though transient, position which I will call tactile contacting. This action, although technically a position,
belongs to a more complicated sequence of nonlanguage behavior.
I will postpone describing it until Chapter 3, where nonlanguage
sequences are described.

COMMENT: THE CUSTOMARY CHARACTER
OF THESE POSITIONS

I have described a total of nine positions in Session I. All of these recurred again and again.

Five more durable positions lasted on the average from one to about four minutes. These positions feature exposition by language. They are:

> Explaining (Mrs. V, later Whitaker)
> Passive protesting (Marge, Mrs. V in Phase II)
> Listening and questioning (Whitaker, Malone,
> sometimes Marge)
> Contending (Marge, shared by Whitaker)
> Defending (Mrs. V, supported by Malone)

We can characterise some of these positions as explicitly informative. Their content consists of language and gestures which portray some distant event, or else they are reciprocal positions to such an exposition, i. e. , positions of listening and questioning for details. Mrs. V's narrative was expostulatory in this sense and the elaborations elicited by questioning and contention collectively resulted in explanations. And Whitaker's later explanation of psychotherapy was analogous, in that it was primarily informative. During positions like these the others listened, but sometimes made remarks or asked questions.

A second kind of position also was employed, a position that was directed to the relations of the transaction and not to its content. Positions of this type were:

> Interfering or intervening (Marge and Malone)
> Resigning (Marge)
> Appealing-lamenting (Marge)
> Tactile contacting (Marge and Whitaker)

I have not singled out these nine positions from a larger number. They were the only ones I could find in Session I. This I find to be usual in a conventional transaction. Each participant shows a repertoire of maybe two to four basic positions. Notice that the same basic position may be shared or used by more than one participant.

In examining other conversational transactions, one will find that most of these positions occur there as well. In fact, they are common property in Western cultures. They are traditional, culturally coded ways to behave in transactions which feature narration and argument. Each participant will have his own style of enactment and the contents can be widely varied and accommodated, but the basic positional form is dictated by custom.

Chapter 2

SYSTEMATIC VARIATIONS IN THESE POSITIONS

It is not necessary to replicate a position exactly in order that it be recognizable and communicative. It must be replicated within an allowable range of variance. This condition provides a good deal of latitude for manipulating and accommodating a unit performance.

In Session I there were obvious variations in each recurrence of each type of position. But it was possible to relate these variations to particular dimensions of the context, so we can claim that the variations were systematic and not random. In this chapter I will compare the various occurrences of each position.[1]

SYSTEMATIC VARIATIONS IN THE LARGER LANGUAGE POSITIONS

In Phase I (the first twenty-three minutes) of Session I, the more durable positions which featured language and listening recurred five times. They were from one to several minutes in duration.

Mrs. V's explaining was addressed to the men who listened to and questioned Mrs. V. Marge sat huddled up against her mother and passively protested what the older woman said. (I will call this constellation of positions Period 1.)

This Period 1 would last a minute or so and then give way to a configuration of contending and defending, which I will call Period 2. Marge would initiate a Period 2 by standing up and then sitting down close to Whitaker and challenging her mother's story. Mrs. V would defend the story. The women thus argued, but one of them usually backed down rather quickly.

Malone would rock forward and intervene. Then Marge would act bizarrely and Whitaker would turn away from her. Marge would then stand and sit down in her original position near Mrs. V. This juncture behavior ended Period 2.

A few minutes later the Period 1 constellation recurred. Thus there were five oscillating cycles of these arrangements in Phase I (Figure 2-1).

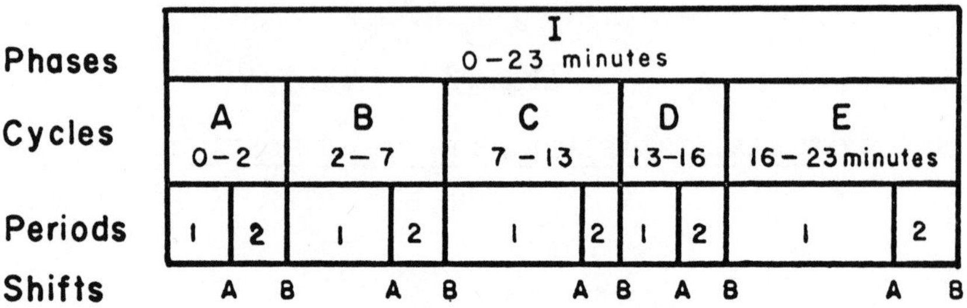

Phases	I 0 – 23 minutes				
Cycles	A 0 – 2	B 2 – 7	C 7 – 13	D 13 – 16	E 16 – 23 minutes
Periods	1 ⎮ 2	1 ⎮ 2	1 ⎮ 2	1 ⎮ 2	1 ⎮ 2
Shifts	A B	A B	A B	A B	A B

Figure 2-1: Cycles and Periods in Phase I of the Session

Regularities from Recurrence to Recurrence

The positions were recognizably the same at each recurrence.

A Period 2 first occurred at 0 minutes: 54 seconds. Since the initial minutes of Session I were not filmed, I do not know exactly how long this interval was from the first encounter. After this first occurrence the Period 2 constellation appeared about every five minutes as follows:

        5 minutes: 36 seconds
       10 minutes: 39 seconds
       14 minutes: 55 seconds
       19 minutes: 08 seconds

One can start the film at any point and immediately see whether a Period 1 or a Period 2 is in progress.

Mrs. V's Use of the Positions

Mrs. V assumed positions in each Period 1 and each Period 2 which were strikingly alike. She assumed almost exactly the same posture for her narrative, sitting erect and slightly forward, hands on her lap, ankles crossed. Her facial expressions and gestures seemed automatic. Her voice qualities varied little. The story sounded as though it had been practiced.

In defending her story she also repeated a routine. She would first look to the men and try to make light of Marge's accusations. When Marge persisted, Mrs. V would uncross her ankles, turn to Marge and argue, then rationalize her part in the difficulty.

Mrs. V would uncross her ankles and lean slightly forward each time she assumed the position of defending. She appeared about to stand up. Then when Marge would sit near her again and fall silent, she would recross her ankles and resume her narrative (Figure 2-2).

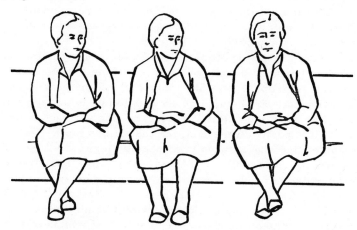

Figure 2-2: Ankle-crossing as the Marker of Mrs. V's Positional Sequence

Each time Mrs. V shifted positions she returned to the same baseline. Thus we could depict her performance as a simple oscillation from explaining to contending and back again.

But each time Mrs. V explained she spoke about a different episode in the history of Marge's illness and the V family. To do this, of course, she had to alter the language structure of her narrative. This is a common type of systematic variation. The basic narrative posture and orientation are repeated over and over and each recurrence does feature language, but the particular subunits of language are systematically varied to compose a different topic and meaning (see Chapter 4).

Marge's Use of the Positions

Marge's behavior was more complicated. She kept intercalating the brief positions of resigning and interfering in her longer positions of passive protesting and contending. In the transition between a Period 1 and 2 she intercalated an appealing position directed at Whitaker and then she and Whitaker engaged in Kleenex-play and hand-play sequences that ended in tactile contact. I will come back to these brief positions later in the chapter and confine the description here to her major narrative positions of passive protesting and contending, which oscillated with Periods 1 and 2.

Regularity in Passive Protesting and Contending

Marge addressed her passive protesting to the floor, the ceiling, and to the men. She addressed her contending to her mother. So each occurred in the same context relationship.

There was no difficulty in distinguishing passive protesting and contending on the basis of form.

In passive protesting Marge tended to look away from the others. She appeared dissociated and all of the clinicians agreed that she was schizophrenic. She mumbled and insinuated and made inferences. She held her body hypotonically and did not appear either attentive, alert, or sexual. She sat back on the sofa and held a posture near and like that of her mother's.

In contending she changed her behavior markedly. She directly addressed her mother. She appeared alert and clinicians did not consider her behavior schizophrenic. She spoke clearly and directly. And her body was hypertonic. She appeared to be in a courting state that we might expect of a young woman. She sat forward on the sofa in a posture like that of Whitaker's and as close to him as the furniture arrangement would allow.

Regularities in Marge's Juncture Behavior

One of the most remarkable and interesting repetitive sequences appeared in Marge's behavior at the shift from passive protesting to contending. The sequence provided a characteristic and recognizable juncture. As noted above, this juncture occurred five times. I will describe here only the first, second, and fourth recurrences. The third and fifth were the same basically, but they were interrupted several times, reinitiated, and therefore complicated.

At each repetition Marge performed the following sequence:

> She would first sit up and place her feet together on the floor.
> Then she would sprawl and quickly sit up again.
> Then she would wave her Kleenex or drop it.
> Then she would lift her skirt and cross her legs in the manner of 'cheesecake,' quickly uncrossing them again.
> Then she would stand up and sit down like and near Whitaker.

Then she would cross her left ankle over her right;
Then sprawl on the sofa;
Then wave her Kleenex.
Then cross her legs in a bizarre, inappropriate way;
Then sprawl again.
Then she would again stand up and this time sit down
    near and like her mother — thus ending Period 2.
Then she would cross her ankles right over left.

Notice in Table 2-1 that these behaviors are listed in the left column. In the three columns on the right are the recurrences which I am describing. The times of each recurrence are listed in seconds beginning at zero (time zero was the moment when Marge stood and shifted to the Period 2 position of sitting with Whitaker). If the behavior did not occur, a dash appears on the table.

TABLE 2-1

The time of occurrence (in seconds) of Marge's juncture behaviors on three recurrences. The times are recorded from the zero point of shifting her posture from passive protesting to contending.

	1st Occurrence	2nd Occurrence	4th Occurrence
Feet on floor	-43	-42	-45
Resigning	-53	- 2	M
Kleenex display	M	-52	-47
Cheesecake	-27	+ 3	M
Stand-up shifts to Whitaker	0	0	0
Ankle-cross left over right	+ 5	+ 2	+ 2
Resigning	+36	+49	+ 8
Handkerchief display	M	+46	+53
Improper leg cross	+58	+46	+53
Ankle-cross right over left	+71	+68	M
Resigning	+81	+92	
Stand-up shifts to Mother	+57	+81	+210

The time sequence of these behaviors is plotted in Figure 2-3. I plotted the occurrences on the magnetic board, marking the time of occurrence for each behavior with an arrow, and photographed the plot (see Appendix B). Notice that twelve successive behaviors are plotted on the rows I have included. Certain behaviors which the others performed are also plotted in order that their relation to Marge's shifting behavior can be seen. The heavy vertical bars identify the sequence as it occurred at each period shift.

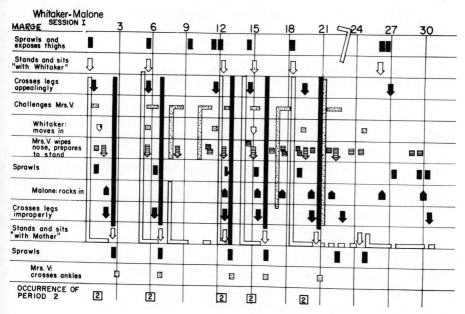

Figure 2-3: Plotting of the Juncture Behaviors which Occurred Between Period 1 and Period 2

Variation in Marge's Positional Performance

Hence, there is no doubt that each recurrence of passive protesting and contending belong to classes of positions which were repeated again and again. But there were marked variations with each replication.

Marge, like Mrs. V, verbalized a different topic in each recurrence (see Chapter 6). She also changed the qualities of performance at each replication. She spoke more and more aggressively, sat farther forward, and sat closer and closer to Whitaker each time.

The duration of each Period 2 increased:

First occurrence lasted	0 minutes:	57 seconds
Second " "	1 "	21 "
Third " "	1 "	58 "
Fourth " "	3 "	30 "
Fifth " "	5 "	27 "

It is clear that these successive variations were systematically progressive. She stepped up the tempo and frequency of contending step by step. Also she did not return, as Mrs. V did,

to her original baseline posture after Period 1 was completed.
In successive Period 1's she sat less and less close to her mother.

Variation Due to Incomplete Performance

Marge's behavior also showed a less systematic, a more
contingent variation. Depending on whether Malone intervened,
for example, and whether Whitaker lexically supported her position, Marge would vascillate in her positional performance in
either period. If Whitaker looked at her in a Period 1, for instance, she would try to initiate a position of contending. Hence,
there were abortive Period 2 behaviors in Session I.

For example, Marge would sit up and put her feet together —
the first behavior in any junctural shift to Period 2. She
would wave her Kleenex, expose her legs, and mutter a challenge.

If Whitaker took up her insinuation, she would lean closer to
him. If, however, Malone started to rock forward or Whitaker
turned away, she would sprawl back on the sofa, dissociate herself from the others, and resume passive protesting.

Similarly, when Marge was contending she would often re-
sign for a few seconds, then come back to the posture of contending, but withhold speaking. In a sense she would freeze for a
second, then go on and escalate the sequence by another challenge
to her mother.

The pattern of her behavior would thus hold and loop. She
would perform steps A-B-C, for instance, then hold at C. Or
she might backtrack and enact A-B-C, then B-C, then go on to
D. This is a common configuration of sequencing, which we can
also relate to the supporting or noncooperative behavior of others
in the transaction.

Thus we can distinguish between progressive, programmed
variation, and variation, which is contingent upon other events in
the context. If the enactment of a position is interrupted or broken off, the position will appear in an incomplete form. Thus
abortive or abbreviated positional units appeared in Session I.

In Session I Marge repeatedly tried to interrupt her mother
and gain support for contending. She would mutter an accusation,
start an appeal to Whitaker, and so forth. In many instances the
men ignored her and she sprawled or addressed the camera. On
five occasions she developed a well-advanced initiation of contending and seemed ready to stand up and sit near Whitaker, but
Malone rocked in and intervened.

Similarly, Malone did not complete some of his intervention
positions. He would start to rock in, but Marge would fall back
and turn away. We might judge that Malone did not have to complete the position, since Marge responded to his preparation.

Later in Session I, after Whitaker had explained the Session,
Malone started an explanation, but all three of the others interrupted him after a few words. He had taken the typical posture
of explaining, sitting erect and forward, and addressing Mrs. V.
There was little doubt what position he was initiating, but we did
not learn what explanation he was going to offer.

Representations of Positions

In established relations full positions may come to be re-
duced to the simplest representative abbreviations. Thus a
mother may signify a long harangue on the irresponsibility of
her children who are leaving her to her death merely by placing
her hand over her breast and sighing. This was exemplified in
Session I: When Marge misbehaved Mrs. V would uncross her
ankles and lean forward, shifting her weight to her legs. We
could guess she was taking the first steps to standing up. We
might conjecture that this is an abbreviated performance of a
longer routine in which she may have once stood and punished
Marge. Maybe in time the preparation to stand represented the
whole and served to monitor the unacceptable behavior. When
Mrs. V uncrossed her ankles, Marge would stop exhibiting her
thighs, although she did not give up her challenges.

Whitaker's Progressive Use
of Listening and Questioning

Whitaker maintained a posture of listening and questioning
throughout Phase I. At 23 minutes he took over the floor, made
an explanation, and turned to make brief physical contact with
Marge. But his position of listening was punctuated by periodic
postural shifts, each of which brought him a few inches closer to
Marge.

At his third shift he had to actually shift his body weight to
his legs, so we must consider the second and third variations of
the moving-in series as a different position. Notice that one can
lean forward with balance only so far without uncrossing his legs
and establishing a leg-buttocks tripod.

The sequential progression was effected by escalating three
dimensions of the postural orientation. First, the body was
brought successively into a vis-à-vis orientation. Thus Whitaker
and Marge started the session at right angles, but turned more
and more toward each other at each step in the progression.
Second, they moved forward and toward each other, becoming
closer at each move. Third, Whitaker progressively uncrossed
his arms and legs. He started the session with his legs and

arms crossed, then uncrossed his arms at six minutes and uncrossed his legs at 12 minutes.

At the beginning of a transaction, when the participants are
strangers, they will ordinarily keep their distance and hold their
arms and/or legs crossed. I will call such a posture closed —
a term that refers to the relative nonpreparedness for engagement. As the participants engage more and more actively they
will progressively turn to face each other, uncross their extremities, and often lean closer to each other. I will call this positional variant open (Figure 2-4). In psychotherapy this sequencing has been institutionalized for the formation of rapport (Chapter
11).

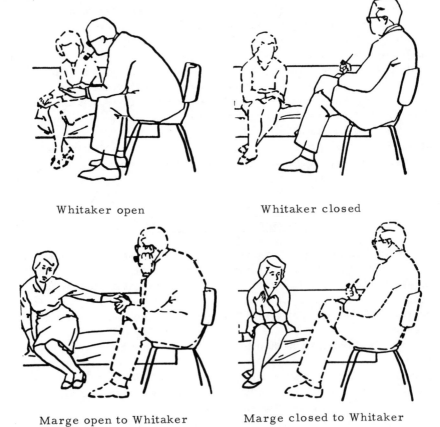

Whitaker open   Whitaker closed

Marge open to Whitaker   Marge closed to Whitaker

Figure 2-4: Open and Closed Postures in Session I

Whitaker did not gradually inch forward toward Marge. He
stayed exactly the same distance away until the sixth minute interval, at which point he made the move.

The shifts were also regular in clock time. They occurred about every six minutes as follows:

First occurrence	0 minutes:	54 seconds
Second "	5 "	36 "
Third "	10 "	43 "
Fourth "	14 "	29 "
Fifth "	19 "	06 "

Each step in the progression was associated with an increased directness in Whitaker's challenges to Mrs. V's story and in his overt support of Marge. As I will describe in Section E, the moving-in shifts corresponded to the progressive application of Whitaker's tactics of psychotherapy.

These regularities appeared also in the other sessions filmed: in the other sessions with Marge, Malone took up this same progressive sequencing. He moved in at six, twelve, eighteen, and twenty-four minutes and he established tactile contact with Marge at 12 and 24 minutes in each of these sessions. We also filmed three sessions which these men conducted with a male patient, and one therapist moved in every five minutes in these three sessions.

Another interesting regularity occurred in the Whitaker-Malone sessions at the eighteenth minute when the therapist made his third move-in shift. At this point some participants — a different one each time — told the others about a day dream he had had. When he did this he made a characteristic gesture. He held his hands together, palms up, and formed a bowl-like configuration. This gesture occurred with the 18-minute shift in all three filmed sessions and not at any other time (Scheflen 1967).

It is thus apparent that certain behaviors of Session I were highly regular in clock time. This is often the case in a transaction. For example, the duration of the classical psychotherapy session itself, like the duration of a classroom lecture, is established by custom at fifty minutes.

The duration of certain microsequences is also sometimes regular. For example, Marge, then Malone, engaged in a preening ritual at the beginning of Session IX. In each case the ritual took exactly 11.6 seconds (see Chapter 3).

On the other hand, some patterns of behavior are highly irregular in astronomical time. They take as long as is necessary for their completion and this may vary markedly depending on such contingencies as the experience of the participants.

Regularity in Malone's Behavior in Phase I

Malone's behavior, too, was strikingly repetitive in Phase I. He held the basic position of listening and questioning with remarkably little movement, except for his periodic interventions. Malone made ten such interventions and each of these was highly repetitive in form and content (see Chapter 1). Each of these positions occurred in the same context — i.e., whenever Marge contended her mother's story.

REGULARITY IN THE BRIEF INTERCALATED POSITIONS THAT MARGE PERFORMED

Marge periodically resigned by sprawling back on the sofa, and from time to time she stood up and interfered with Mrs. V's account. These behaviors appeared to occur contingently. They did not occur at regular intervals, did not vary progressively, and were intercalated both in Period 1 and in Period 2.

Resigning

Marge performed resigning eleven times in full development, and on six other occasions she performed an abortive version. She would sprawl in a characteristic context — at times when her mother indicated that Marge's psychosis was insignificant or was not Mrs. V's fault, and also in Period 2, when Mrs. V denied or rationalized an accusation or challenge that Marge had made.

Standing Shocked

On four occasions Marge stood up and made a startling statement, assuming a facial expression of shock as she did so (see Chapter 1). On seven other occasions Marge enacted this behavior without standing, so these occurrences were not positions, but a subunit performance in passive protesting or contending.

Marge performed this position in a characteristic context. She would address a number of appeals to Whitaker and a series of insinuations without response from the others. Then she would put her hand on her mother's arm and make a more direct accusation. If Mrs. V did not respond she would stand shocked. By contrasting four positions which Marge used, we can identify four degrees of activeness in her interventions:

In resigning she would sprawl back and dissociate.
In passive protesting she would sit back and protest
   indirectly.
In contending she would sit forward and directly con-
   front her mother.
In standing shocked she would actually stand between
   Mrs. V and the man Mrs. V was addressing.

INDIVIDUAL DIFFERENCES
IN POSITIONAL PERFORMANCE

In a number of cases several participants made use of the
same type of position. Whitaker and Malone, for instance, both
used a remarkably similar version of listening and questioning.
And in Phase II, Mrs. V performed a position very like passive
protesting. Obviously, each person will perform a conventional
position in the particular styles of his ethnic background, class,
gender, and so forth. And each participant can manipulate and
accommodate his performance according to his plans and the
situation. So we speak of individual differences in positional enactment. This issue will concern us in detail in Sections C and D.

The Temporal Occurrence of Positions in Session I

The temporal occurrence of many of the positions in Session
I can be visualized by examining Figure 2-5.
Notice that the arrows in row 1 show the occurrence of
Marge's leg-crossing behaviors. Roughly, the interval between
the pairs of leg crosses demarcates the appearance of Period 2.
In row 2 the occurrence of Marge's high bodily tonus also corre-
sponds to her position of contending. In rows 3 and 4 are plotted
occasions when Marge sat with Whitaker and Malone. The occur-
rence of the Kleenex- and hand-play sequences is plotted in row
5. In rows 6 and 7 certain subunit behaviors of Whitaker and
Malone are plotted for reference. At the occasions of the arrows,
Whitaker said something in support of Marge's allegations or
Malone attacked these.
The moving-in progression of Whitaker is plotted in row 8,
and Malone's interventions are plotted in line 9.

48

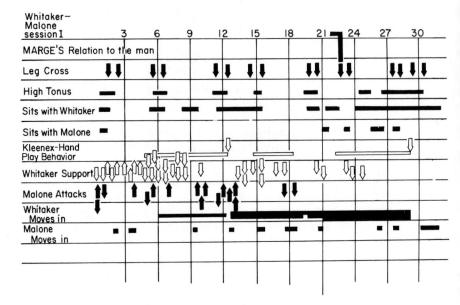

Figure 2-5: The Occurrence of Some Positional Variables in
Session I

COMMENT: THE DEFINITION OF
A BEHAVIORAL UNIT

I have been claiming that certain configurations of behavior, which I have called positions, occurred again and again in Session I. In communication, meaning depends upon the recognition of such customary unit forms of behavior, so the issue is critical and we had better take time to define the unit.

Segmentation of the Stream of Behavior

Suppose we go back for a moment to the first step in observation. When we screen the film we notice that each participant performs a stream of behavior simultaneously. In fact, he performs several streams of behavior simultaneously. He speaks, gesticulates, changes facial expression, smokes, and so on.

Each of these streams of behavior is segmented. The activity occurs in bursts. The participant speaks, then falls silent, then moves, and then is still for a time. He shifts posture, holds the new posture, then shifts to another posture. I have called these stops and shifts, junctures, and the bodily posture held between them a transfix.

The Paradigm of a Position

Consider the kinesthesiology of taking a position. The participant holds a posture of the entire body, but he moves certain bodily subregions. [2]

The total body is positioned on a substantial base which acts as a fulcrum. Either the person stands on firm ground or sits on his buttocks, though other stances occur in different cultures and in informal activities. From such a position he can move some bodily subregion, e.g., the head or upper torso and hands (or his upper leg if his legs are crossed and he is seated). He can move these bodily regions without shifting the base position of his whole body. Thus:

A. the participant stations his head, addresses
someone and speaks an utterance; and

B. he stations his torso and uses his hands to
gesticulate or carry out a physical task.

Notice that I am not describing things. I am describing relations of movement and utterance. By constructing the following paradigm of the position, we can visualize these relations. A participant takes a given posture and orientation; while holding this position, he:

1) speaks and gestures in a recognizable way
2) addresses this and other behavior to another
person; and often
3) smokes or performs other physical tasks.

Then he shifts his posture and orientation and begins other sequences of activity.

The Hierarchical Structuring of Behavior

Notice that the actions which a participant performs while holding a posture are subunits of the total position. He speaks a number of sentences and gestures which are elements or components of his total behavior in that sequence.

Actually the behaviors in a position consist of successive divisions of subunits and sub-subunits. For example, the utterance is one subunit of a position and the utterance in turn is divided into syntactic sentences, and each of these syntactic sentences are divided into words, and so on. In a systems model we speak

of such an arrangement as a hierarchy of levels of integration.
(Each component or division is said to be a 'lower' level of integration than the whole in which it occurs.) The subunit behaviors of the position will be described in Section B.

By the same token the position is but one element in some
still larger integration of behavior. Through time, for instance,
each position is one step or component in the total format of behavior which that individual uses. And at any given time the position of each participant is related to or addressed to the positions
which the other participants are using.

Note this relation as shown in Figure 2-6. If one examines
the behavior of Malone, alone, his posture can be termed a transfix — in this case the posture which marks the duration of his
rocking forward. But examined in relation to the other participants, his posture can be seen as an address or orientation. In
this case his position is addressed to Marge. Thus at the social
level of observation Malone's posture is but one element in a unit
of Marge-Malone relationship.

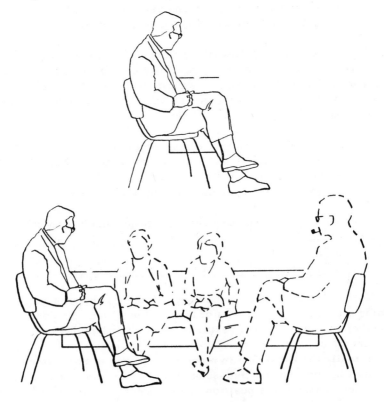

Figure 2-6: Malone's Postural Transfix in Isolation and the
Same Posture as an Orientation or Address

Unit I				Level of the Position
A	B	C	. . . N	Level of the Point Subunit
1 2 3 4 /	1 5 6 /	1 7 8 4 /		Level of the Syntactic Sentence

ADDENDUM TO SECTION I: REVIEW OF THE POSITIONS

I would like to add certain data about the positions of Session I which I omitted from the text to make it more readable. I will first review the criteria for determining that two positions are isomorphic and therefore replications of the same unit form. Then I will schematize and depict the positions which recurred again and again in Session I, so they can be reviewed at a glance. Then I will provide some simple statistics about their frequency and indicate diagrammatically their times of occurrence.

Criteria for the Isomorphism of a Position

In Appendix B I will describe the operations for identifying any behavioral unit. Here I will simply mention the criteria for deciding that certain positions are indeed replications of some customary unit.

It would not be possible to classify unit performances if the occurrences shaded into each other according to a continuum of variability. Identification depends on the occurrence of fairly clear-cut and contrastable forms. This has to be the case if communication is to occur. A given form must be recognizable and identifiable to have an assignable meaning. There are, of course, transitional forms, but a participant cannot perform many ambiguous and transitional positions if he is to engage in communication. Thus the theoretical basis for finding behavioral isomorphism is the necessity of patterned regularity in communicative behavior.

Operationally we proceed as follows: The film is screened again and again and those positions which look alike are identified tentatively and isolated by rephotographing them or splicing the film. All of the probable recurrences are then compared by description of their common features. Some of these can be measured.[6]

To explicate the criteria we make use of the schema of hierarchical structuring. Isomorphism must occur at three levels of integration, as follows:

1. The Gestalten of the form. If the posture is a familiar one we recognize it and know when it is completed. Customary positional performances are familiar in common culture. For example, when the novelist speaks of such things as a menacing posture, a compromising position, and an aggressive stance, we can picture the behavior he refers to — at least in a general way. In an analogous way I have characterized positions of explanation, contention, and so on in Session I.

2. Regularity in the type of subunit or content. If the form is unfamiliar we have to delineate it by context analysis (see Appendix B). We must show that a pause in activity, a postural shift, and a characteristic form of juncture behavior occurs.

    The subunits of a given position will be of the same logical type at each recurrence. They will consist of narration, for example. In Chapter 2, I showed that these criteria held for the nine positions which occurred in Session I.

3. Recurrence in a particular context. A given type of position will ordinarily recur each time in the same general type of context or in some limited range of different contexts. For example, Marge's passive protesting appeared whenever her mother started to explain and whenever the men listened to the older woman. And Malone interfered each time Marge contended or started to contend.

ADDENDUM TO SECTION A:
REVIEW OF THE POSITIONS

Content and
General
Characteristics:

Two participants, Mrs. V and Whitaker, gave lengthy expositions: Mrs. V explained her history and attitudes; Whitaker explained his purposes and intentions. Malone started to explain, but was interrupted. Explaining for Mrs. V consisted of sequences of recounting points, interspersed with a few maintaining points. It was, therefore, a position, while Whitaker's explaining was a unit of one point. Whitaker's explanation occurred after the minute 23 as the handplay sequence was drawing to a climax.

Constituent
Points:

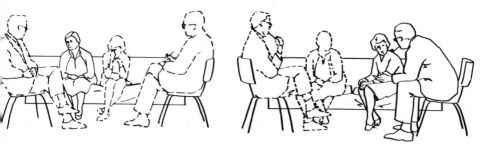

Recounting (Mrs. V)   Explaining (Whitaker)

Junctures: Leaning slightly forward or backward for
Whitaker and Malone; ankle uncrossing for
Mrs. V.

Transfix: Maintaining slight leaning-forward posture
for the men; leaning slightly backward and
ankles crossed for Mrs. V.

Context: The position, explaining, was coterminous
for Mrs. V with Marge's passive Protesting.
It was reciprocal to Malone and Whitaker's
listening and questioning.

The Position: Passive Protesting
(Marge and Mrs. V)

Content and
General
Characteristics: This position, which recurred ten times in
the session, lasted as long as five minutes.
Marge used the position before the minute
23, Mrs. V after that time. Lexically and
kinesically, Marge insinuated, disparaged
and lamented, sometimes seeking reconciliation with her mother. In Mrs. V's use of
the position, lamenting and conciliating were
more prominent.

Constituent
Points:

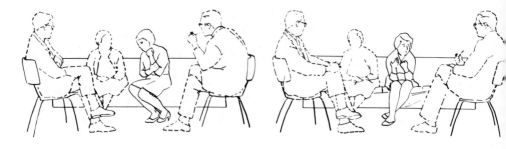

Disparaging (Marge)   Lamenting (Marge)

Markers
Standing up
(Marge)
Ankle uncrossing
(Mrs. V)
(Junctures)

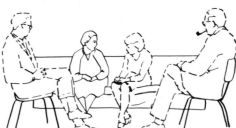

Standing up
(Marge)
 Ankle crossing
(Mrs. V)
(Junctures)

Conceding (Mrs. V)

Maintenance of upper body posture; sitting with Mother for Marge; sitting with Marge for Mrs. V.

Transfix

Context: The position generally occurred in one wo-
                        man's repertoire when the other woman was
                        engaging the attention of both other men.
                        Thus, one woman would be passively protest-
                        ing when the other was recounting or explain-
                        ing. The two women in this complementarily
                        would sit in postural parallelism.

The Position: Listening and Questioning
(Whitaker and Malone)

Content and General Characteristics:

When Mrs. V explained the men listened, occasionally asking questions. They signalled attentiveness by the usual means of nodding, head-cocking, and eyebrow-raising. Mrs. V and Malone similarly used this well-known position when Whitaker explained.

Constituent Points:

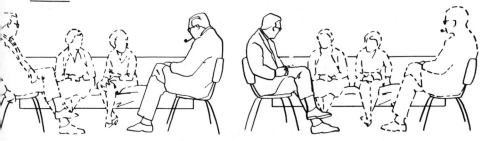

Listening (Whitaker)   Listening (Malone)

Junctures:

For the men, sitting back and inclining the head forward or tilting the head marked the beginning juncture; sitting up and moving forward marked the terminal juncture. Mrs. V sat back to explain and slightly forward to listen.

Transfix:

Maintaining the postures described above.

Context:

Listening was reciprocal to explaining; it was terminated by contending and maintaining.

The Position: Contending (Marge)

Content and General Characteristics:

This position recurred ten times, lasting about one to two minutes. Whitaker and Marge shared the position, performing it simultaneously. The content consisted of insinuations, accusations and challenges to the mother's account, which were picked up by Whitaker. Sometimes these positions

included courtship-like positions, e.g.,
tête-à-tête postures between Marge and
Whitaker. Late in the session, contend-
ing-like positions were shown by Malone
and Marge but these did not have the lexical
content of contending.

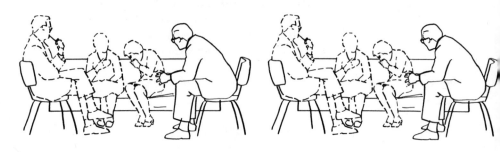

Insinuating (Whitaker)   Challenging (Whitaker)

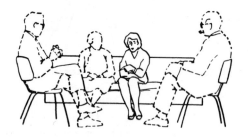

Accusing (Marge)

Junctures: Contending ended with standing up for
                          Marge; rejecting for Whitaker. Whitaker's
                          rejecting was apparently triggered by sexy
                          provocativeness or repelling on the part of
                          Marge.

The Position: Maintaining (Mrs. V)

Content and   Each time Marge and Whitaker contended
General   Mrs. V's account, she defended, rational-
Characteristics: ized, and reaffirmed. Malone supported
                          her, though sometimes ironically. One or
                          both of them criticised Marge, and Mrs. V
                          was then invited to continue her narrative
                          (usually by Malone).

<u>Constituent</u>
<u>Points</u>:

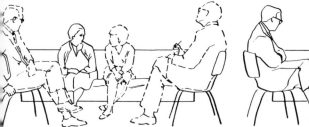
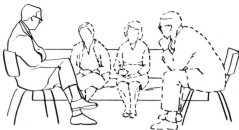

Defending (Mrs. V)   Supporting (Malone)

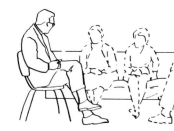

Confronting (Malone)   Restarting Mrs. V's Narrative
                                                (Malone)

<u>Junctures</u>:   Mrs. V ended the position of maintaining
after Marge had ceased contending. Mrs.
V then crossed her ankles as the terminal
juncture. Malone rocked backward from a
posture of sitting forward.

The <u>Positions</u> <u>of</u> <u>Intervention</u> <u>or</u>
<u>Interferring</u> (<u>Malone</u> <u>and</u> <u>Marge</u>)

<u>Content</u> <u>and</u>   There appeared in Session I a number of
<u>General</u>   actions that had all the characteristics of
<u>Characteristics</u>:   positions but functioned to monitor and
interrupt relationships. Like certain
points, then, positions can serve as monitors. (The fact that an action that appears
as a unit at one level reappears at a higher
level should occasion no surprise. Put
another way, a unit at one level can be

60

coterminous with one at a higher level.
An umpire's gesture in baseball may
at the same time be terminal to an out,
an inning and a game. A phoneme may
be a morpheme and even a syntactic
sentence — for example, the shout,
'Hey! '

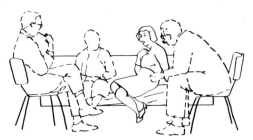

Shocking (Marge)

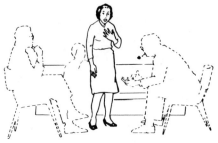

Standing Shocked (Marge
— not included among
points.)

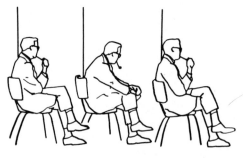

Rocking in and out
(Malone — not included
among points.)

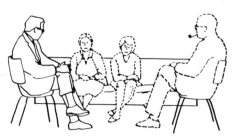

Confronting (Malone)

Transfix:

Upper body or complete postural maintenance, i.e., sitting with Whitaker for Marge:
sitting with Marge for Whitaker. High leg
tonus was maintained by Marge during contending. Often in the shared position of contending Marge and Whitaker began in tête-
à-tête postures but they themselves interrupted their relationship by repelling and
rejecting each other.

| Context: | The position was reciprocal to Mrs. V's and Malone's maintaining. The position contending appeared alternately, in Marge's presentation; i.e., she alternately contended and passively protested in her relationship to Mrs. V. |

The Position Resigning (Marge)

| Content and General Characteristics: | Resigning was similar in content, timing, and configuration to positions of interfering. Generally, however, it did not function to interrupt. The difference may be purely a matter of successfulness in this group. But the distinction was great enough to tentatively classify 'resigning' as a separate position. |

Marge often fell back on the sofa in a sprawling posture, muttering in the intrapersonal mode, sometimes crossing herself or making a self-stabbing motion. These positions were often accompanied by comments of resignation or exaggerated hopelessness or by religious appeals and by gestures indicating 'What's the use?' These positions were 'self-monitored' in that Marge snapped back to sitting erect as though the act of sprawling were unacceptable to her and in itself stirred her to come forth contentiously. The positions were probably of mock resignation rather than actual expressions of hopelessness.

Mrs. V used a similar position but infrequently and without the histrionic exaggeration. She extended her hands, palms upward, shrugged her shoulders and looked at the men with a 'What can I do?' expression.

62

Constituent
Points:

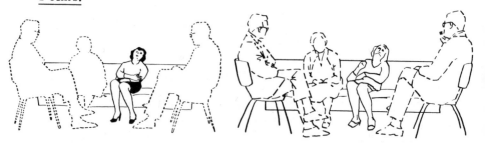

Resigning (Marge)   Sprawling and Stabbing (Marge)

Juncture: The position ended with an abrupt sitting
                 upright, bringing Marge into active rela-
                 tionships to the others.

Transfix: Marge realigned her entire bodily stance so
                 as to be physically withdrawn from the others.

Context: Resignation in one woman occurred when the
                 other woman was strongly maintaining a pos-
                 ition.

THE FREQUENCY OF POSITIONS IN SESSION I

Thus, the four participants in Session I used nine types of
positions. Actually they took a total of seventy-two positions in
the whole session. So they repeated certain positions a number
of times.

Passive protesting occurred six times (five times by Marge
and once by Mrs. V); listening and questioning was discontinued
and begun again sixteen times (once by Mrs. V); explaining occurred six times (once by Whitaker); contending occurred five
times, defending ten.

Marge performed resigning eleven times. She interferred
by standing shocked on four occasions. Malone intervened ten
times. Appealing occurred three times, and contacting twice.

These behaviors also occurred a number of other times as
subunits of a position. In these cases the entire body was not
involved, but the behaviors were performed as a subunit in some
other position. I will describe such occurrences in Section B.

There were occasions when a position occurred so trans-
iently that it was difficult to determine whether it was a position

or a subunit of a position. There were eleven such instances in Session I which I did not count as positions in the totals above.

At levels below the position the subunit forms were some-times difficult to classify. The enactment would be ambiguous, especially when Marge used the behavior in question. She would sometimes combine two different kinds of subunits, so it was not possible to distinguish the type. But this ambiguity did not characterize the positions and the problem of categorization was not very difficult.

SECTION B

Analysis of the Position in Session I

Introduction:

A. ANALYSIS WITHOUT REDUCTIONISM —
An Operational Comment

In this section I will make an analysis of the positional units. But before I begin there are two kinds of information I must provide — the principles of analysis that will be followed, and some additional data from Session I.

In the analysis, elements of the whole are isolated so they can be described and measured separately. Accordingly I will describe subunits of the positions. But there are certain principles of context analysis which govern the operations of such an analysis. If we are to see how behavioral integration is communicative we cannot destroy our view of this integration in the process of isolating and viewing the component behaviors one by one. Therefore we must avoid certain reductionistic practices that have characterized the presystems analysis of behavior.

CLASSICAL PROBLEMS IN
THE ISOLATION OF VARIABLES

If one is to conduct an analysis of a transaction which is not recorded on film or videotape, he is forced to observe selectively. He must take one or a few variables, observe and note these, and ignore the others. At a single visualization there is no way to record all of the behaviors which transpire and deal systematically with its integration. So in the past, certain reductionistic procedures have been forced on the investigator. Let's review two of these as a means of approaching the procedures we should use.

64

1. The a priori selection of certain behaviors: The remainder
being ignored. When we were limited to noting a few of many
events we had to decide in advance what behaviors we thought
were especially important or interesting. The best we could do
was watch for these. Thus only certain events were studied and
we had no way to reconstruct the integration of events. For example: Until the last decade we had a tendency to say that communicative behavior consisted of speech. And it is still common
practice to reduce the content of a transaction to a mere transcript
of the sequencing of words. In this practice other elements of the
position were ignored. Thus in psychological research the stress
and pitch patterns, the nonlanguage sounds, and vocal qualifiers
of language were neglected. The linguist ignored the postural
markers, the multiple types of bodily language behaviors, and
the physical task behavior. Such reductionism by selection is
like seeing the organism as a system of endocrines alone.

As a consequence we could not identify the behavioral basis
of the systems concept of organization (Bertalanffy 1950, 1960).
We could not describe step by step or level by level the Gestalten
of behaviors which were recognizable and communicative. We
had to act as though the whole consisted only of certain components. And sometimes we came to believe this. We made reductionistic generalizations. A table was 'nothing more than'
a collection of atoms; the organism consisted of cells; speech
was made up of words.

The fact, of course, is that speech consists of complex integrations of address, juncture, verbalization, pitch and stress
patterns, and vocal modification. And speech is integrated hierarchically — that is, the utterance is made up of integrations of
syntactic sentences and kinesic behaviors; the syntactic sentence
is an integration of pitch, stress, morphemes, junctures, and
head movements; the morpheme is an integration of vocalizations,
stops, and head-eye movements; and so forth (Chapter 4). So
we avoid the practice of reductionism without regard to intermediate levels in present attempts to study the communicative structure of behavior.

2. The reliance on abstractions about behavior. We could take
cognizance of complexity without film recordings if we gave up
the hope of describing the constituent elements of behavior and
instead merely abstracted their properties or qualities. Then
we could scan a complicated action and generalize, for instance,
that it was sadistic or masochistic, aggressive or passive, attentive or autistic, communicative or incomprehensible. We
could then take these abstracted, mentalistic ideas which we
formed about the behavior in progress and deal with them as variables for quantification or correlation.   —

But the results were not very satisfactory. The next investigator would abstract a different set of qualities and, lacking a precise notation of the events which occurred, we could not compare notes. Often we ended up with a set of artificial abstractions which did not accord with the behavioral forms and segments which naturally occur in a transaction.

The classical dichotomy between verbal and nonverbal behavior is a prime example of such an artificial, conceptual dichotomy which does not fit the naturalistic integration of units in human discourse.

There are certain nonverbal acts which invariably accompany verbalization, e.g., stress and pitch changes. There are verbal sounds which are not part of language proper — sighs, sobs, and ahems, for example. And there are classes of non-speech behavior which have no regular association with each other and, therefore, do not constitute any kind of functional entity which we can lump as 'nonverbal.'

If we are to see how behavior is communicative we must identify the customary Gestalten or configurations which are recognizable among participants — those to which meaning is customarily ascribed.

In English language, for instance, we have a morpheme 'dog' and another 'god,' but we do not have a form, 'og.' We would not segment a 'no smoking' sign into 'nosmo' and 'king.' The half inning in baseball consists of three putouts. We cannot understand the game if we think that two or four putouts are naturally occurring subunits. Similarly the gesture, palm-on-chest, consists of raising the palm to the chest, placing it, and returning it to baseline. There is no point in subdividing the usual performance into hand-raising and hand-lowering, nor would we gain anything by including foot waggling in this gestural configuration just because it happened to co-occur.

In context analysis the subunits of a unit are determined by systematic observation by a methodology I describe in Appendix B. We determine which actions regularly occur together and pass as recognized Gestalten in a transaction.

By the same token we do not want to describe units of behavior as combinations of events which are of various logical types. The behavioral unit which can be seen in communication consists of sounds and movements. Items of the physical ecology may be used in the performance of a unit, but these items are of a different logical type. Also we can abstract qualities and make judgments about behavior, but these judgments constitute behaviors of a different logical type. Because they are not in the behavioral unit, the unit does not contain goodness, masochism, or recognizability, and we must distinguish between what occurred

in the participant's actions and the inferences which he or
we made about them. So the descriptive adjectives like social,
psychological, or environmental are not elements of the behavioral unit, but belong rather to the mentalistic operations which
accompany visible behavior. These, too, are important in communicational processes (see Chapter 8), but we do not want to
mingle them willy-nilly with our descriptions of visible behavior.
So the position may consist of speech, smiling, and smoking. It
does not consist of words, friendliness, and a pipe.

ANALYSIS OF THE POSITIONS IN SESSION I

To fulfill the criteria of context analysis, then, I have to
study and describe all of the behavioral elements which occurred.
This is nearly possible because I can go over the film again and
again until I have described all of the movements, sounds, and
holds which are captured on the moving picture. We can hold to
the operational principle that all participants are doing 'something' at all times, for even silence and immobility are meaningful. So I cannot have gaps in the chronology of the analysis.

I must examine the relations of each behavioral item to find
out which sets or clusters occur together regularly. These make
up the traditional, customary, or naturally occurring units which
are communicative (see Appendix B). Then I have to determine
the contextual location of each subunit. I have to be able to assign
it to the larger unit of behavior in which it occurs. Eventually I
reconstruct the schema of integration level by level — from positions to microacts and from integrations of micoacts back to
positions. This I have done for Session I.

PRESENTING THE DATA IN THIS VOLUME

In order to present the analysis in this volume, then, I
should take each position one by one and present the details of
its composition. I should show the exact behavioral relations of
the speech, gestures, postures, and other subunit components
for explaining, passive protesting, contending, and other positions. But no reader would wade through such endless detail.
To make this volume readable I must jump to certain abstractions and present some measure of generalization.

Here are the steps I will follow in presenting the analysis.

First, I will isolate certain subunit behaviors of the position and indicate their level. Some of these I will catalogue as
completely as I can. For example, I will try to describe all of
the gestures, tasks, representational and juncture behaviors
which occurred, because these kinesic units are not well known

and need to be characterized. But in the case of the speech units I will simply illustrate some of these in order to review their structure. The remainder will merely be reproduced in Appendix A as a traditional transcript or orthography of speech content.

Second, I will classify the various subunits of behavior according to logical type schemas which have already been advanced by other authors. Miller (1965) has distinguished systems of three logical types: physical, behavioral, and conceptual. I will begin by converting the phenomena of Session I into the logical type of behavioral systems. (Later I will move into a discussion of the invisible behaviors of cognition.) M. Harris (1964) has distinguished between actonic and communicative behaviors, and Bateson (1955) has distinguished between communicative and metacommunicative behaviors. Having studied the appearances of the subunits of Session I in larger units, I can abstract what each one appeared to do in the larger context. I will use these abstractions of function as a basis for assigning the various subunits to one of the logical type categories which Harris and Bateson have distinguished.

Then, I will present a description of each of three logical types of behavior in each of the three chapters of Section B: Chapter 3: Point Units Which Serviced and Related the Participants; Chapter 4: The Language Points of Explaining and Listening; and Chapter 5: The Metacommunicative Points of Session I.

Thirdly, I will add an addendum to Section B to review the units of Session I at the level of the point — a level just below that of the position. Then the reader who is interested in detail can refer back to Section I and get an idea of how the subunits were integrated into the positions of the session.

B. THE MULTIMODALITY TRANSCRIPT

To depict more of the details of the positions, I prepared a multimodality transcript of Session I and will produce the first five and one-half minutes of this transcript in the fold-out sheets to follow. The transcript depicts the lexical behavior of each participant through the first cycle, cycle A, and the second Period 1 of cycle B. It also depicts certain postural configurations and body movements for each participant. Unfortunately a detailed linguistic and paralinguistic analysis was not made of Session I, so I can only report the speech orthography and mention certain linguistic and paralinguistic features.

I hope the reader will follow this transcript as he reads the text of the chapters to come. See the foldout following page 80.

Chapter 3

POINT UNITS THAT SERVICED AND RELATED THE PARTICIPANTS

He that has eyes to see and ears to hear may con-
vince himself that no mortal can keep a secret. If
his lips are silent, he chatters with his finger-tips;
betrayal oozes out of him at every pore.
— Sigmund Freud. Collected Papers, 3,
London: Hogarth, 1949, 94.

Ordinarily an account of a communicational event would begin
with a description of the language behavior. But I will begin instead with a description of certain nonlanguage activities which
appeared to service the participants and the relationships thus
maintaining and developing participation and interrelationship.

Some of these behaviors were simple physical tasks at their
inception but they quickly came to be used as signaling devices
or sequences of representative activity which were shared among
members of the group. So I will first distinguish simple ecological acts or <u>actonic</u> behavior and then describe a class of representational behaviors, i.e., behaviors that represented more
complex social activities like courtship and maybe play.

THE PHYSICAL TASK OR ACTONIC POINT UNIT

If we had film recorded the hour or so before Session I and
the hour afterwards we would have observed a good deal of physical task behavior which prepared for the main event. Cameras
were set up and the furniture was arranged. Marge was dressed

for the occasion by the clinical assistants and after the session the two therapists and the observers were served luncheon.

M. Harris (1964) has described sequences of task behavior like this and termed them 'actones.' And some of Pike's 'behavioremes' are physical tasks of this nature — eating breakfast, for instance (Pike 1954). Such behaviors are addressed to props or other things, but the objects of address can be other people in activities like feeding, love-making, and grooming, and the object of such behavior may be the self.

I am going to consider such behaviors as members of a common class, suggesting that they service the site, the participants, and the relationships of the transaction. Such activities thus maintain a transaction, but they can also be used to change it.

In some transactions actonic behavior is featured. People come together in order to manufacture a product, to feed, to groom each other, or to prepare a site for a later transaction. In transactions that are explicitly conversational such actones are intercalated in the stream of language behavior. So people may munch a candy bar, smoke, adjust the lights or furniture while they are speaking or listening.

In Sessions III and IX complicated servicing behavior was introduced at 12 and at 24 minutes. In Session III, for instance, Malone combed Marge's hair and got her to comb his.

Actonic Acts in Session I

Actonic and servicing behavior was less conspicuous in Session I. Behaviors of this type occurred as follows:

1. Pipe lighting. Whitaker took out his tobacco, filled his pipe, and lit it. It is noteworthy that he did this about a minute before he shifted his position and moved in closer to the women at 18 minutes. He moved back to his original position at 29 minutes.

Malone also filled and lit his pipe. He did so in each instance just after Whitaker had done so. In fact, we will see, Whitaker did not make the moving-in behavior until Malone had lit up or at least until he had shown that his pipe was lit by tamping it and blowing a conspicuous puff of smoke through the bowl.

The pipe lighting act, then, was an actone, but the smoking behavior which followed constituted some kind of signal system (see Chapter 12).

2. Nose blowing. At 4 minutes: 45 seconds, Marge took a Kleenex from her skirt and blew her nose. Immediately afterwards Malone took a handkerchief from his pocket and blew his nose.

Malone put his handkerchief away, but Marge continued to hold her Kleenex. She waved it around and then dropped it near Whitaker.

3. Picking up. At 12 minutes Marge dropped Kleenex on the sofa near Whitaker. He moved forward, uncrossed his legs, and rested his weight on his legs. Then he picked up the Kleenex and handed it to Marge. This act was the occasion, then, of Whitaker's second moving-in shift.

At 22 minutes Whitaker leaned forward and picked up a minute object from the floor. He played with this in his hand for the next few minutes, then put it under Marge's nose and ordered her to smell it.

Notice again that the picking-up act was not simply an element of housekeeping. The object which was picked up was used for a number of minutes in a kind of playing and signaling behavior and these sequences terminated in a brief physical contact between Whitaker and the girl.

4. Contacting. We can conceive of the tactile acts in contacting as actonic behaviors which connected two participants. McBride (1966) calls this kind of behavior bond servicing.

5. Clothing adjustment. From time to time the men adjusted their coats. When Marge sat down near Mrs. V, the mother tucked her skirt under her legs as if to separate herself and define her territory. When Marge would change her leg positioning she would rearrange her skirt. As is usual in such behavior, she lifted her skirt slightly before pulling it down, thus giving the men a lady-like peek at her legs.

On other occasions, however, Marge exhibited her thighs by allowing her skirts to ride up. Then she would pull her clothing down when she stood up.

These behaviors, too, were elements in more complex sequences. Some of them were constituents of preening routines that I will describe later. The exhibitionistic leg behavior served to turn the men away from Marge (point 4, repelling: see Addendum to Section B). This is usually the case. The myth is, that a woman is seductive if she exhibits thighs beyond the mode of an era or lets her knees drift apart, but observations in any mixed company will show that this behavior regularly causes men to cover their eyes, avert their faces, move back, and turn to someone else for conversation. On the contrary, preening behaviors such as the brief skirt lifting, pressing the calves together, and showing a little thigh will bring attention to a woman.

6. Stroking. Marge would stroke her lower thighs with a slow, rhythmical movement. When she did this Malone would stroke the seat of his chair in the same movement.

This behavior is depicted on page two of the fold-out multi-modality transcript. The significance of synchronous movement between two participants will concern us later.

Formation of the Actonic Point: Modalities of Behavior

Notice that two of these behaviors constituted a brief intercalated position. Whitaker turned his whole body to Marge at the second contacting and spoke to her as he put his palm under her nose. And he used his whole body in picking up the object from the floor. But the others are actions which involve a single bodily region. They are carried out with torso and hands while the participant is also speaking or listening.

In other words the participants use their bodies differentially. They perform one set of behaviors in one relationship and another set in some other relationship at the same time. For instance, Whitaker picked up Marge's Kleenex, handed it to her and brushed her hand, without taking his face and eyes away from Mrs. V. This was the case in each of the other actonic acts I have described. The men lit their pipes without watching what they were doing. They kept listening to Mrs. V as they did so. And Marge did not stop her passive protests or contentions to exhibit her thighs or wave her Kleenex. In the case of the stroking behavior the lower half of the body was involved, while Marge simultaneously directed her upper body to Malone or the camera, and turned her head to address Whitaker.

Thus the body is differentiated in its communicative usage. The head, face, and vocal apparatus are used in one relationship, the upper torso and hands in another, and sometimes the lower body and legs are employed in yet a third relationship.[1] Notice, too, that the activities of these regions are of different logical types: i.e., the activities of the head region involve facial expressions and language, which are symbolic actions; the activities of the body and hands can be symbolic when gestures are used, but these actonic behaviors alone are not symbolic. These differential activities have led communication theorists to distinguish modalities of communication or channels of communication at the social level. Thus human communication is multi-channeled (Birdwhistell 1965) (Table 3-1).

TABLE 3-1: A Listing of Behavioral Modalities in Communication

LANGUAGE MODALITIES

Linguistic

Lexical or Verbal Forms	Sapir, 1921; Bloomfield, 1933; Pike, 1954
Stress, Pitch and Junctures	Sapir, 1921; Joos, 1950; Harris, 1951; Pike, 1954; Austen, 1962

Paralinguistic

Nonlanguage Sounds	Trager and Smith, 1956; Trager, 1958; Pittenger & Smith, 1957; Eldred & Price, 1958
Vocal Modifiers	Pittenger, Hockett & Dehany, 1960; Duncan, 1966

COMMUNICATIVE BODILY MODALITIES

Kinesic* and Postural Forms (including movement, facial expression, tonus, positioning, and so on)	Darwin, 1955; Effron, 1941; Deutsch, 1951, 1952; Birdwhistell, 1952, 58, 60, 61, 63, 65, 66, 67, 69; Goffman, 1955, 1961; Scheflen, 1963, 64, 65A, 65B, 67, 68; Ekman, 1964, 1967; Hall, 1959; Condon and Ogston, 1966, 67; Charny, 1966; Kendon, 1967, 1969 A, 1969B; Ekline, 1963
Parakinesic and Postural 1962	Birdwhistell, 1969; Mahl, Danet & Norton, 1959; Berger, 1958; Howes, 1955, 1957; Dittman, 1962; Ekman, 1965; Haggard and Isaacs, 1966
Tactile Forms	Frank, 1960

ARTIFACTUAL BEHAVIOR
(Including dress, cosmetics, insignia,
use of props, and bodily noise)

* Birdwhistell has called units of body motion which have a communicative function, 'kinesic' behaviors. They appear to have a morphology analogous to that of language; i. e. , small elements of movement are successively integrated into larger units (Birdwhistell 1952, 1960, 1965).

I use these regional differentiations as the first of two bases for distinguishing the subunits of the position. The behavior of the upper or lower body or the head region constitutes one division of positional behavior. And the participant who directs his head to one vis-à-vis and his body to another and performs a different kind of sequence in each of these relations is evidencing multiple simultaneous actions in a position. The basic bodily posture of the position is maintained during these differential activities so the constituent modalities collectively belong to one position. Mechanically, the participant positions his body, balances on his buttocks (or on his buttocks and legs), then directs his head toward one relation and his body toward the other.

Notice that these regional activities are addressed to someone; the bodily region is oriented to someone, and the activities are pitched or directed to this person.

Sometimes different logical types of activities are addressed to the same person. Marge, for example, would look at Whitaker and speak to him. Simultaneously she would turn her body to him and act courtingly.

In this case, however, the two behavior sequences thus addressed differed markedly in the significance of their content. Marge acted sexily, but she spoke a lament, saying she was dead (multimodality transcript and points 8 and 14, Addendum to Section B). In this case we can say that the addresses are co-oriented but the messages are different and actually antithetical. This kind of behavior is one form of 'double binding' (Bateson et al. 1956). Bateson and others have attributed double binding to schizophrenia, but we see it in many transactions where the participants are not known deviants.

Sequences of Point Behavior: Point Units

Actonic sequences within a position are often addressed to one person after the other. Marge, for example, would address a Kleenex display to Malone, then to Whitaker, then back to Malone.

So the behavior of a bodily address and modality is often segmented into sequences of actonic behavior. These constitute separate subunits of behavior. So the position is subdivided according to two kinds of dimensions: by bodily region and by successive segmentations of any of these. We will see in Chapters 4 and 5 that speaking behavior is also segmented in this way. So a model of positional divisions might look like the following:

	Constellation 1	Constellation 2	. . . N
Head-Language Performance	Address of topic to one person, then	Address of another topic to another person	. . . N
Torso-Actonic	Torso address and actonic sequence in one relationship	Torso address to another relationship with another kind of actonic behavior	. . . N

Each of these subunits of behavior has the characteristics of a unit as I described them in Chapter 2. I will call them point units because they roughly correspond to a point that a participant may make in a transaction, i. e. , one idea, actonic task, or representation (Chapter 5). I will describe point units that featured language and gestures in the next two chapters.

Types of Actonic Points

The simple actonic or physical task units seemed to be used in three types of point performances:

Type A — Merely maintained the performer's orientation in the group.
Type B — Seemed to signal to other participants.
Type C — Were representational acts that suggested more complicated activities.

Type A: 'Contentless' Points That Maintained Orientation

Often a participant will orient his body toward others in the basic posture of a position, then turn his head and address some particular member or some person who has not been included in his basic postural orientation. In such cases he may not perform any activity with his body and hands, but rather hold these regions motionless. Sometimes the converse relation is seen. The body is addressed and a sequence of nonlanguage behavior is directed to another person. Meanwhile, the head is addressed to some other person but the face is held 'dead pan' without expression or speaking.

This kind of behavior seems to do several things which we can abstract as a single function. First it does offer distracting and invitational behavior to those addressed. It does not comment on what is occurring in the active modalities. It therefore directs attention elsewhere to some principal activity — speaking, for example. Thus the 'contentless' point can maintain orientation in a relationship which is at the moment 'inactive.'

Type B: Actonic Points Used as Signals

We might not ordinarily think of actonic task behaviors as communicative. They do not stand for or symbolize distant things or events. But they are communicative, whatever their purpose or intent.

The actonic sequence is a customary sequence of action. It is therefore recognizable and meaningful to anyone who observes its occurrence. The observer can know what is going on and often he can name the sequence and gain information about the context from seeing it occur. He can also join in the performance; he can 'commune' with what is going on.

Thus the actonic sequence is as important in maintaining social organization as is language and gestural communication. The actonic point can also be used to signal. It can be used to direct or pace or represent some other behavior. An infant, we would say, does not at first cough in order to solicit his mother's attention, but he can soon learn that the cough has this consequence and he can later learn to use the cough accordingly. In the psychological sciences we have often acted as though any behavior that is not intended to provide information is not communicative. If we take this position, either we overlook a great deal of significant activity in communication or else we have to use what Kubie calls the teleological fallacy, and attribute some specific motive to every act (Kubie 1964). So a behavior is communicative if it is customarily patterned, regardless of the performer's intent.

The Pipe-Smoking Signals

As I have described, Whitaker lit his pipe before making his 18-minute shifts toward the women. And Malone 'answered' by lighting his pipe.

Only when Malone had responded did Whitaker make the postural shift. So the pipe lighting seemed to be a signal.

This hunch — that smoking behavior was a coordinative signal — was borne out by the analysis of smoking behavior in Sessions III and IX. In these sessions Malone was the active therapist who moved in toward Marge, and Whitaker stayed back in

his original closed posture until after minute 24 of the session.
In these two sessions Malone first lit his pipe, then when
Whitaker did so, Malone made the move-in shift.

In Session IX, when Malone was the initiator, he once started to move in toward Marge without waiting for Whitaker to light
his pipe. But he never completed the move-in, returning instead
to his original position. Then, several minutes later when
Whitaker did light up, Malone completed his moving-in shift
(Scheflen 1967).

The pipes were used as signals in another way. The active
therapist smoked right handed until after 24 minutes in each
session. The less active therapist smoked left handed until his
move-in at 20 minutes. Thus the specific handedness in smoking
reliably indicated who was the active therapist in the moving-in
progression.

Mrs. V seemed to crack this code rather quickly. Whenever
Whitaker would light up he would soon thereafter form a coalition
with Marge and she would act sexy and begin contending. Mrs. V
at first made the nose-wiping signal or warning when Marge got
sexy, but after the first two repetitions of this sequence she
started monitoring when Whitaker lit his pipe. Later still, she
monitored when Whitaker took out his pipe.

The Kleenex and Hand-Playing Sequences

The 'housekeeping' activities of nose blowing and picking up
an object from the floor were similarly used in a signaling activity (Figure 3-1). After Marge blew her nose, she kept the
Kleenex in her hand. She shook it and waved it in a way that I
think was a signal to the men. She would shake it toward Whitaker
when addressing him. And she waved it back and forth between
the men when she was seeking to speak to both of them. Just
before 12 minutes, as I have said, she dropped it near Whitaker.
In retrieving it he moved into his second progressive posture
and touched Marge. Marge again dropped her Kleenex near
Whitaker at 18 minutes and immediately afterward he began his
third moving-in shift. Whitaker behaved analogously in the second half of Phase I.

You will recall from Chapter 2 that he picked up the object
at about 23 minutes and played with it for the next two minutes.
He held it in his left palm and rolled it around with his right
index finger. Marge watched this behavior, enthralled as though
hypnotized. Then at 24 minutes Whitaker held it under her nose.

The function of Whitaker's behavior is puzzling. It occurred
only once so there was no way to make a context analysis of it. [2]

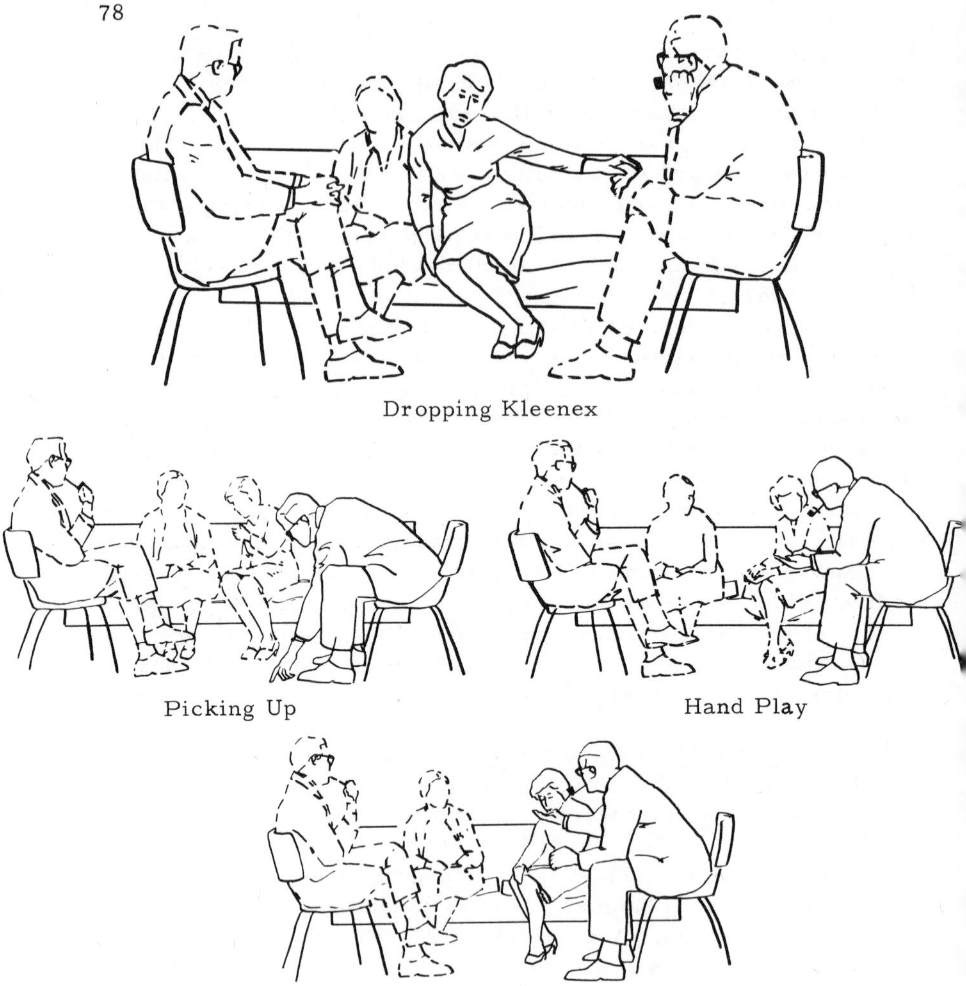

Dropping Kleenex

Picking Up   Hand Play

Contacting

Figure 3-1: The Kleenex and Hand-Play Sequences

Type C: Representational Points

Defining Representational Behavior. I have already indicated that the actonic points, like nose blowing and clothing arrangement, were single units in larger sequences of activity. The remainder of these sequences consisted of point units that were not directed to physical tasks, but rather seemed to be representative elements in bond-servicing activities like courtship and mutual play.

Such behaviors look like acts that would be found in courtship or fighting or feeding if the participants in such activities

TIME: (In minutes and seconds) ⟶   ⟶ 10 seconds ⟶   ⟶ 20 seconds   5 sec. pause

MRS. V: . . . . Help me upstairs, a young girl like her, help me upstairs, and, uh — the next day I thought she'd — get better by, ah, ah — she has the doctor's prescription — am, am — Did I say anything wrong, dear?
                                                                        TURNS APPEALINGLY TO MARGE

MARGE: Mrs. V Recounting – Point 6   Whitaker Listening – Point 2   SMILING, SHAKING HEAD IN EXAGGERATED MOCKING OF HER MOTHER   Listen . . . TO MRS. V   You said I ought to have a good sleep and eat. WHISPERS TO HER MOTHER

WHITAKER: Well, why don't you say what it is you wanted to say now, Marge?

MALONE:

BASIC POSITIONS:
  8. Explaining (Mrs. V)
  1. Passive Protesting (Marge)
  9. Listening (Whitaker, Malone)

Malone Listening – Point 2

Marge: Sitting with Mother

TIME: 30 seconds   40 seconds   PERIOD 1 ends   PERIOD 2 begins
                                                                            50 sec.

MRS. V: Well, the next day she —   ha-ha. The next day she —   Yeah, I don't care what you said . . . TURNS TO MARGE PATRONIZINGLY   You stopped what?   You stopped getting angry.   At me, at me - I remember I usta get

MARGE: Gonna go to hell. CROSSES LEGS IN LADYLIKE MANNER R over L KNEE   Yes, I did.   I did.   I did stop it, I did. LOOKING COY, HEAD TILTED, BABY TALK   Gettin' angry.   You know, you know, mother, you know who. LOOKS AT MOTHER, SMILES, TOUCHES HER ARM, GOES INTO POSTURAL SHIFT

WHITAKER: Appealing – Point 14   Was that what you started to say before when mother — sorta stopped you or you stopped yourself?

MALONE: MALONE MOVES HIS LEG IN PERFECT SYNCHRONY WITH MARGE'S   Getting angry at whom, Marge?

RESEARCH OBSERVER CROSSES LEGS IN SAME MANNER. THUS, AT 3-SECOND INTERVALS THREE PEOPLE CARRY OUT SAME ACTION.

Sitting with mother   Postural shift   Sitting with Whitaker

TIME: 1:00 min.   1 min: 10 sec.

MRS. V: angry, everybody gets angry   Well, everybody gets angry, I usta get angry at my mother. SMILES AND LOOKS TO MALONE IN MANNER OF ONE WHO HUMORS A CHILD   Yes, I want to tell you

MARGE: . . . . or somethin'   When did I sta –, start, or stop – gettin' angry?   Mother – tell me somethin' (. . . .)

WHITAKER: Conciliating – Point 1   When did – when did you stop getting angry at mother, Marge?   When did ya stop getting angry?

MALONE:

BASIC POSITIONS:
  2. Contending (Whitaker, Marge)
  3. Maintaining (Mrs. V, Malone)

Marge: Sitting with Whitaker

Selective Listening – Point 2*
(Whitaker to Marge)

a

TIME: (In minutes and seconds) ——————————→ ——————————→ 1:20 ——————————→ ——————————→ 1:30

MRS. V: anything I can tell ya.   No. I, I, wouldn't do da things I do do if I hated you – I'd just stay home and – wouldn't care whether – I heard from you.
LAUGHS EMBARRASSEDLY. SQUIRMS.   LAUGHS   No, you're, uh, not getting angry, everybody gets

MARGE: (......) these people. Do you hate me?   Me? You're watching me get angry with my mother.   TURNS AWAY FROM   STROKES HER OWN KNEES
LOOKING IMPISHLY, WATCHING MEN'S   GESTURES TO WHITAKER IN   THE MEN.   SENSUOUSLY, EXHIBITION-
REACTION TO HER TRICK QUESTION   FASHION OF "WHAT DO YOU   ANGRY AND   ISTICALLY.
THINK OF THAT STATEMENT?"   AGITATED.

WHITAKER:

Defending – Point 7*   What did ya say, I didn't hear ya?   Repelling Begins – Point 4*
(Mrs. V)   (Marge)
MALONE: Pictured later

BASIC POSITIONS:
2. Contending (Marge, Whitaker)   MALONE AND MARGE SHOW
3. Maintaining (Mrs. V)   SYNCHRONOUS SLOW WRITHING
MOVEMENTS OF THEIR RIGHT HANDS.

Selective Listening (to Marge) – Point 2

TIME: 1:40   1:50

MRS. V: angry – I'm nervous too. I have a reason to – (don't ya think?)   Marge, don't talk like that. You'll be gettin' home....   You're just goofy now. If you'll just . . . .

MARGE: What do ya think I am, an animal or somethin?   I don't know what you're talking about – waddya mean, feel like an
GASPS   REBUFFED, SHIFTS AWAY FROM WHITAKER

WHITAKER: Sometimes I feel like an animal – don't you feel like an animal sometimes?
SUDDENLY AND MARKEDLY
TURNS HEAD AWAY FROM MARGE

Really?

MALONE: It would be sa–fer for someone to watch you.
MALONE STROKES CHAIR IN SAME RHYTHM AND TIMING
AS MARGE STROKES HER LEG

SECOND INSTANCE OF
PARALLEL SYNCHRONOUS   Confronting – Point 9*
MOVEMENTS OF MALONE   (Malone)
AND MARGE.   Rejecting – Point 3

TIME: END OF PERIOD 2 | PERIOD 1 BEGINS AGAIN   2:00   2:10   3 sec. pause

MRS. V: **B** Oh, Marge.   He died. It'll be a year this December 3rd.   December 3rd, it'll be a year.   3rd.
WIPES HER NOSE

MARGE: animal? . . . Sexy, you mean? Oh boy.   Don't say that word, you know don't say that word, sexy.   He's dead with myself, I get sexy with myself, you know what I mean? I was dead.   Real dead
COVERS MOUTH – IMPROPER LEG CROSS   IMITATING HER MOTHER   GESTURE LIKE CROSSING HERSELF

WHITAKER: Or mad

MALONE: Where is your husband?

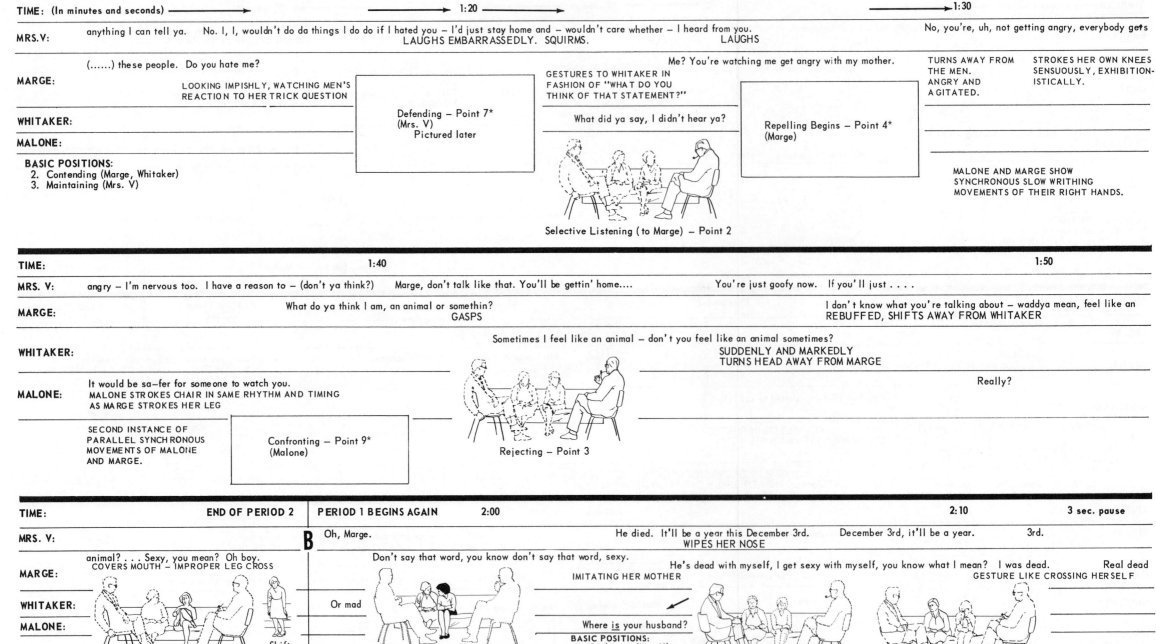

Repelling – Point 4   Shift   Marge Returns to Sitting with Mother   BASIC POSITIONS: Confronting – Point 9   Recounting – Point 6
8. Explaining (Mrs. V)
9. Listening & Questioning
(Whitaker and Malone)
1. Passive Protesting
(Marge)

* The drawings were done from the film at the most significant or clear-cut occurrence of a particular point, though it must be remembered that
they recur over and over. The points will be pictured only once or twice; the other occurrences are marked with an asterisk (*).
b

were actually standing or sitting together in tactile contiguity.
Imagine, for example, two lovers who are sitting across the
room from each other. If they were sitting together they would
hold hands, but across the room each person holds one hand
as he would in hand-holding. Or a person may hold out his
arms as if to embrace another, or a person may make sucking
or eating movements as though he were being fed. Such acts
refer to and suggest the larger sequences in which they normally
occur but they are not symbolic in the sense that words are.
They look like the larger behaviors they represent. So I will
class them as iconic behaviors and call them representational
acts. Since they were point units in Session I, I will call
them, representation points.[3]

Representational Point Sequences in Session I. There were
isolated representational acts from feeding, e. g. , sucking and
chewing acts, but the usual repetitive sequences in Session I
were of three kinds: (1) dominance-submission sequences,
(2) quasi-courting activities, and (3) the sequencial manipulation of objects in the hand that I have already described, hesitantly characterized as play.

Dominance-Submission Displays. Territorial size and dominance
are interdependent among animals (McBride 1964, 1969), and
man is no exception. Those of highest status have the largest
offices in a company, and the higher social classes have larger
properties. The rule also holds in a transaction. So larger
territories or locations were afforded to Whitaker and to Mrs.
V, the older, in the session. Mrs. V and Whitaker maintained
positions of sitting forward and erect when they explained. They
also commanded the space in front of their eyes and Malone and
Marge ordinarily did not stare into this space, except when they
made an active intervention and interrupted the narratives.
    Actually, dominance displays characteristically occur when
someone begins to interrupt and this occurred regularly in Session I. When Whitaker asked a question he would sit taller, protrude his head, and jut his jaw. Such kinesic behavior characterizes a question which we would interpret lexically as a demand
for reply. When Malone interrupted Marge, he would rock forward as I described in Chapter 1. He would also jut his face,
hold it higher than usual, and keep his head erect. He placed
primary stresses on his utterance and he articulated clearly in
a steady, slightly slowed pace as is often done in command
(see Chapter 5).
    A striking thing about Session I, as compared to other trans-
actions I have studied, was the lack of dominance displays between

the men. Only in Session IX did such behavior occur when they differed about their strategies. Ordinarily males in a transaction will periodically exchange flurries of head raising, chest protrusion, jaw jutting, fist-doubling, staring, hooking the thumbs in the belt, and raising the voice.

But Marge and Mrs. V engaged in many periodic dominance displays toward each other and Marge sometimes directed these toward Malone. In contending Marge would sit up, very erectly, face her mother, meet her gaze, and raise her eyelids. She would, for a moment, speak loudly and sometimes take her mother's arm — a tactile act that usually holds a relationship and silences the addressee.

In answering, Mrs. V would at first show classical submission behavior. She would lower her head, lower her eyelids, [4] and cock her head — a head position we often characterize as downcast.

But Mrs. V would soon reassert herself as she countered Marge's accusations. She would display the dominance behavior I have already described and Marge would fall into submissive behavior, gradually retreating from her contention. Marge showed similar submissive behavior toward Malone when he rocked forward and confronted her. And Mrs. V did so when Whitaker accused her or made an insinuation.

It is difficult, I think, for a Western woman to maintain dominance against a male display. If she does she will probably be accused either of masculine or of seductive behavior.

I would warn the reader against generalizing that dominance or submissive behavior is merely a personality trait which labels its performer. To be sure, some people usually maintain dominance and others usually are submissive, but exchanges of such behavior regulate the interaction. Ordinarily they do so in an automatic way that is not obtrusive or interruptive. They indicate, for instance, who will speak and who will listen at any moment. And a submissive display does not necessarily indicate a weak character. It may prevent a disruptive escalation of competitiveness and make possible the ordinary give and take of the transaction.

Quasi-Courting points. Much of the representational behavior in Session I was made up of elements from customary courtship behavior. In another publication I have shown that this behavior occurs in psychotherapy when rapport is being formed and it does not lead to seduction (Scheflen 1965). So I will call it quasi-courting. I assume it is akin to, or a form of, flirtation behavior.

The representational acts of quasi-courting include micro-sequences of eye brightness, eyelid lowering, head cocking, smiling, stroking the legs with the hands, and exhibiting the palm or wrist (an intimate act for women).

In normal courtships these microacts accompany an increasing body tonus. Women bring up the head, protrude the chest so that the breasts are displayed, and bring up the legs into the tonus we see in a model's 'cheesecake' position. In males the abdomen is drawn in and the chest protruded.

Women may add to this complex a series of more overtly seductive acts like placing the hand on the hip, crossing the legs and displaying the thighs, and preening, e.g. making-up the face, brushing the hair back with the hand, opening a sweater or coat, or so forth. Males will also brush their hair back, re-arrange their coats to square the shoulders, pull up the tile, and pull up their socks (Birdwhistell 1963).

In Session I Mrs. V occasionally showed attenuated and abbreviated quasi-courting behavior to the men. And Malone evidenced this behavior in relation to Marge during the early minutes of Session I. Whitaker displayed subtle quasi-courting to Marge through much of the session. He began with little behavior of this kind and increased the frequency as he and Marge progressively strengthened their coalition and challenged Mrs. V's story.

Malone quasi-courted Marge from minute 23 on and in subsequent sessions. In later sessions he did so consciously and deliberately to interest Marge and teach her to distinguish this behavior from seduction. (Marge had been a prostitute and had been unable to relate to men without having sexual intercourse.)

But Marge's quasi-courting was overt, obvious, and exhibitionistic. Just before any Period 2 she would begin to escalate the representative acts and courting tonus. At the beginning of a Period 2 she would cross legs and exhibit the total seduction routine as she made a sexy comment. During Period 2s she would retain the courting tonus, then end the period with a bizarre caricature of sexiness. She would exhibit her thighs grossly and make a silly imitation of sexiness. Whitaker would then break off his relationship with her and a Period 1 would recur.

Thus Marge would escalate a subtle point performance of quasi-courting in which she used only her body to a full and ostentive display.

Some of these behaviors are depicted in Figure 3-2.

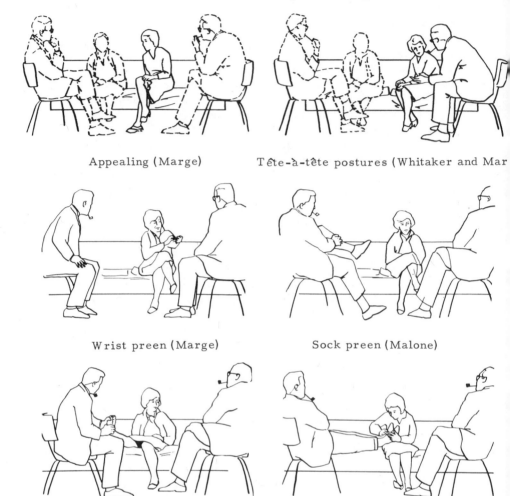

Appealing (Marge)   Tête-à-tête postures (Whitaker and Mar

Wrist preen (Marge)   Sock preen (Malone)

Exchange of foot-rubbing (Marge and Malone)

Figure 3-2: Quasi-courting Behavior in Session I and IX

Other Nonlanguage Behavior in Communication. Dress and
style. Dress, cosmetics, insignia, and the qualities of style are
also communicative. I will describe these in detail in Chapter 6.

Odor, body noise, and the like. We can point to other classes
of nonlanguage behavior which undoubtedly have a communicative
function. Odors are emitted and perceived, but these behaviors

are not recorded on motion picture film so I have no analytic experience with them. I also do not know of any research literature on the function of odor in human communication. Audible peristalsis, purposive joint cracking, denture noise, feet shuffling, and so forth have been studied (Watson 1962). These behaviors did not appear in Session I.

COMMENT: THE FUNCTION OF ACTONIC AND REPRESENTATIONAL BEHAVIOR

We can advocate the idea that a task behavior and a representational behavior maintain and develop relationships. Time and again in Session I a representational sequence would occur between two people, who would soon afterwards turn and speak to each other. And later I will claim that the quasi-courting sequences are one tactical behavior for making rapport with a psychotherapy patient (Part II).

If we are to have communication, two conditions must be met: first the participants have to behave communicatively, and second they have to be in attentive relationships to each other and can perceive the communicative behavior that each one performs. So the necessary contribution of a participant involves coded, meaningful behavior which is related to others.

We want to avoid dichotomizing these aspects. As a transaction proceeds, a meaningful behavior may develop a relationship within which some next phase of communicative behavior can occur. A recognizable meaningful language performance is just as likely to develop a relationship as is a set of physical contacting and quasi-courting behavior; so all of these dimensions maintain social organization. Similarly we can speak of physical task behavior but we do not want to dichotomize physical task and communicative behavior. The physical task behavior may maintain the communicational process as well as the spoken content. In fact speaking is the explicit task in a conversational transaction. So the task is to behave meaningfully while maintaining the relationships and holding the situation in a state favorable to the process.

We do best to hold that people have a number of different modalities and bodily regions to work with in maintaining the communicational process. They use each of these in a multichanneled system and features of each modality are integrated in a communicative unit like the position. And multiple simultaneous communicational relationships collectively maintain the group and constitute the social organization.

Chapter 4

THE LANGUAGE POINTS OF EXPLAINING
AND LISTENING

During most of the time in Session I some participant, usually Mrs. V, was engaged in narrative or explanation. In narrative the behavioral units feature language. Syntactic structures
which have meaning are articulated, i.e., they refer to events
which took place in remote contexts. Maybe forty per cent of the
point units of language which occurred in Session I were informative in this sense.

The utterance consists of a sequence of point units. These
are marked by address of the head and eyes and by voice projection. The face and sometimes the hands supplement the articulation. The language component consists of one or more syntactic
sentences or the reciprocal behaviors of listening, questioning,
and providing comprehension signals. Meanwhile, the remainder of the body may be engaged in some other relationship and
some other kind of activity.

The units I am calling language points seem to correspond
to what others have called 'an utterance' (Z. Harris 1951; Jaffe,
Feldstein, and Cassota 1956).

THE COMPOSITION OF EXPLAINING

As we have noticed, Mrs. V offered an explanation in every
cycle. At 23 minutes Whitaker explained the purposes and plans
of the session. Malone started an explanation in Phase II but
was interrupted. Marge made some brief statements of narrative, but almost all of the girl's utterances were comments
about what Mrs. V said or else about her own feelings and state
(see Chapter 5).

84

I will define narrative as a series of declarative statements about events which have taken place elsewhere. The explanation is a more comprehensive activity which involves one or more narrative sequences and some elaboration of these in response to questioning, challenges or noncomprehension. Mrs. V, for instance, would narrate in each Period 1 and defend or rationalize her account in each Period 2.

Mrs. V's Narrative

Mrs. V's narrative at the beginning of the session was typical of her later narrative behavior, and, in fact, of narration in general. We can observe many of its features at the beginning of the multimodality transcript. The lexical data of the entire session is reproduced in Appendix A.

The camera crew had technical difficulties and did not record the first minute or so of Session I. Before the film began the participants were introduced, they took chairs, and Mrs. V was invited to begin the narrative with an account of Marge's original illness. She started by telling of a morning, a year before, when Marge would not walk upstairs. At the beginning of the transcript Mrs. V quoted Marge as asking, 'Help me upstairs.' Then Mrs. V commented on her daughter's behavior with a tone of mock incredulity and disparagement: 'A young girl like that.'

Then Mrs. V repeated her quotation: 'Help me upstairs.'

Mrs. V now had enacted three point units. She made two kinds of statements (and repeated one of these) — each having the configuration of head-eye positioning which demarcates it as a point unit.

Mrs. V was looking at Malone during these comments. Next she paused, saying: 'and . . . ah . . .' as she turned her head and eyes to Whitaker. These kinds of nonlanguage sounds are usual in a narrative. Technically they are components of paralanguage (Trager 1958; Trager and Smith 1956).

Maybe they are abortive statements that never proceed to utterance. Maybe they fill time and hold the floor until a speaker decides what to say next. In some cases they complete a measure in the meter of speaking. In any event Mrs. V used these nonlanguage utterances while she was shifting her orientation to Whitaker. A period of transition between units produces a movement that Pike (1954) called a 'slur.' Between very small units the transitional period may last for a large percentage of the unit duration and thus constitute a relatively conspicuous feature of the performance.

Facing Whitaker, Mrs. V articulated a next idea in her narrative: 'The next day I thought she'd . . . get better by, ah, — she has the doctor's prescription.' Meanwhile Marge had whispered something in her mother's ear; so Mrs. V turned to her daughter and said: 'Did I say anything wrong, dear?' Then Mrs. V turned back to Whitaker and went on with her narrative.

Notice the features of this sequence. A series of utterances are made, each of which deals with some idea — some phase or episode — and each is addressed to a different listener. Thus the total utterance is punctuated by a shift in the head-eye orientation.

The head, eye, face, and vocal-respiratory apparatus are involved in such a performance. The remainder of the body is held as a positional transfix oriented to the audience as a whole. The whole body is not turned from listener to listener nor was it turned to one listener as it would be in a one-to-one conversation.

Mrs. V's narrative was short this first Period 1. But after the second minute she resumed, and longer stretches of recounting occurred. The reader is invited to follow these on pages three and four of the foldout. The same configuration obtained. She addressed an utterance to Malone, then to Whitaker, and sometimes she swept her head slowly back and forth from one of them to the other. But her basic postural orientation was not altered. She faced the observers sitting upright, ankles crossed, her hands on her lap. Occasionally she faced Marge and responded to one of the girl's comments. Occasionally she raised her hands and gesticulated.

Whitaker's Explaining

At about 24 minutes Whitaker raised his head and faced an area between the two women. He said: 'We're doctors of people's feelings — and we want to see if we can help ya — with some of these feelings you've been talking about.' Marge commented and Whitaker addressed her for a moment, replying: 'Crazyness, you know — that's right, emotions.'

At this point Whitaker and Marge made the tactile contact I described in earlier chapters. Then Whitaker turned to Mrs. V and continued his explanation: 'We wanted to talk to you, and then we're going to see Marge every day — except over the weekend — and so forth.'

The complete text is reproduced in Appendix A.

As I said in Chapter 3 the bodily regions are often used differentially in speaking. Whitaker's behavior exemplified this as he spoke or listened to Mrs. V, while he engaged in hand activity with Marge.

Mrs. V did not do this very often. She sometimes gesticulated with her hands, but ordinarily she kept her body motionless
and addressed the men. Thus she maintained an orientation to
a point midway between the two men. Whitaker did this too, but
only his lower body was used in stationary orientation.

Whitaker oriented his pelvis and pointed his feet in such a
way as to include both Malone and Mrs. V. It is a regular

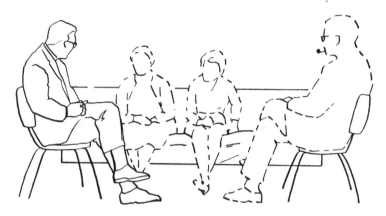

Figure 4-1: Multiple Simultaneous Point Performances. Above,
Malone is speaking to Mrs. V and facing her, but
his body is oriented to Whitaker and the two men
are using the same posture and moving synchronously (see Section C). Below, Whitaker speaking
to Mrs. V, moving his hands in relation to Marge
and orienting his body to a point between Malone
and Mrs. V.

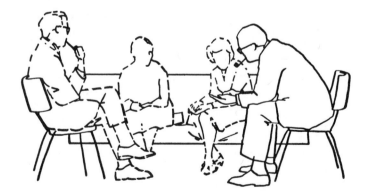

behavior in any group for standing members to point their feet in such a way as to include all other group members (Goffman 1963). When sitting they address their torsos to each other. If, however, they turn their upper body to some one person they usually maintain an orientation to the others by lower body placement, as Whitaker did in Session I.

So Whitaker sometimes maintained three simultaneous relations and concurrently performed three point units; i.e., speaking to Mrs. V, hand-playing toward Marge, and orienting his body to Malone and Mrs. V, thereby dividing his position into three modalities (Figure 4-1).[1]

BEHAVIORS THAT MARK AND ADDRESS
THE LANGUAGE POINT

In performing a language point, the head and usually the eyes are held in a given position until the utterance is completed. The face is pointed to a listener and the voice is projected for his audition. As in the case of a position, then the same behavior which marks the point's duration also addresses it to a vis-à-vis. Therefore, I will speak of the marking behavior as the behavior of address.

The Head-Eye Address in Narrative

The head is ordinarily held erect, forward, and slightly elevated in the address of a narrative. In middle-class Americans, at least, the face is directed to the auditor.

In face-to-face conversations, the orientation of the Western subjects I have studied, is rarely eye to eye. Each fixates his vision just out of range for eye-to-eye gaze holding — approximately at a spot between the cheek and shoulder of the other fellow. A direct gaze holding orientation is generally seen in a seduction or a dominance battle. In fact, the dominant participant usually commands an imaginary area in front of his eyes and face. Subordinates keep their gaze out of this area unless they are to make a direct confrontation. When central vision is focused on the cheek-shoulder area of a vis-à-vis, the remainder of his upper body will be visible in peripheral vision at the usual conversational distance. When movement occurs elsewhere in the body it will trigger an orienting reflex. Focal vision is shifted briefly to observe the moving part.

There is another convention of orientation in a conversation. It is impolite to look at listeners. One is to look at the speaker of the moment.

Thus, either sustained avoidance or maintained gaze holding
may be an affront with relative strangers. As a consequence we
rarely get to observe the behavior of listeners and we do not ordinarily see the total bodily behavior of others in conversation.

The accuracy of an orientation is also worthy of comment.
In an audience of, say, forty or fifty people a speaker can
'point' his head and eye convergence with sufficient accuracy to
single out one auditor. This object of attention usually is aware
that he is being addressed. Similarly we can project our voices
accurately enough to evoke a response from some one person in
a group — sometimes even if this person is behind us. With
reasonably high resolution, motion pictures, and a little practice,
an observer can tell which participants are addressing each other
at any time.

The interested reader should become acquainted with the
careful experimental studies of Kendon (1965) on gaze in interaction.

The head is not always held rigidly during the point performance. If the speaker is addressing several listeners whom he
regards as a unit, he may sweep the head laterally, back and
forth from one listener to the next. But the movement is regular
and oscillatory and the head is held in the same vertical plane.
Or the speaker may nod at one listener and thus oscillate the
head in a vertical plane. Sometimes the speaker advances his
head progressively higher and higher or farther and farther
forward with each point as he develops a theme. In any case
the regularities of head posture during a point are recognizable. [2]

Supplementary Transfix Behavior in the Point

Head and eye position are not the only features of the point
transfix. The utterance is made in a voice projection appropriate to the distance between the speaker and his listeners. He
usually holds this projection until the end of the point.

Some quality of language, some paralanguage form usually
accompanies the point utterance. Such a paralinguistic feature
may be customary for addressing that kind of listener, e. g. ,
baby talk, formal tones, contempt, or the like, and each utterance in that point may be marked with that voice quality.

If the hands are used in a point utterance, they are often
positioned for the duration of the point.

Marge sometimes placed a tactile hold on her mother while
making a point. Whitaker would take his pipe out of his mouth
and hold it in the air until he finished a point.

Sometimes the hands are simply held in the air until a point
is completed.

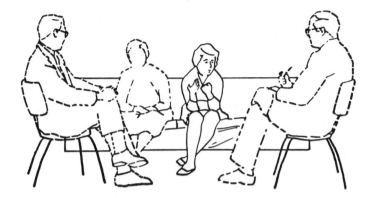

Figure 4-2: Supplementary Transfixes of the Point. <u>Above</u>, Marge kept her arm upright toward her face throughout a segment of lamenting behavior. <u>Below</u>, Whitaker would suspend his hand play with point utterances of his explanation.

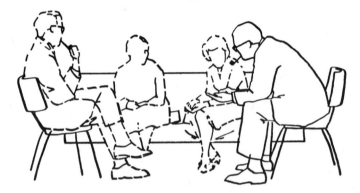

On occasions a speaker or listener will hold a foot in the air or point a toe until the completion of a point unit. Sometimes point units are marked by cocking the head to one side during these utterances.

Junctures of the Language Point

When a speaker has completed his point unit or given up the prospect of doing so, he will shift his head position. Ordinarily he will lower the head and eyes for a moment and he may bring down his hands or fold them on his lap. If his head has been cocked, he may bring it erect. In short he discontinues the transfix behavior which he held during the point performance. He may, then, remount the address to make another point, shift the address to another listener, or himself become a listener.

As we will see, a characteristic linguistic juncture also occurs at the end of the last sentence of a point utterance. A supplementary juncture may also occur (Figure 4-3).

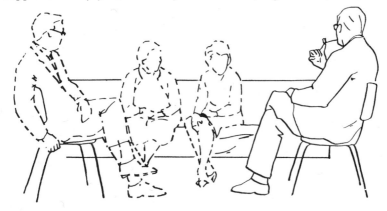

Figure 4-3: Supplementary Juncture Behavior. At the end of any utterance the speaker will turn his eyes or face away from the addressee or lower them. Whitaker often turned his head far away from Marge when he finished an utterance.

THE CONTENT OF THE POINT UTTERANCE

Markers of the Syntactic Sentence

Technically speaking, the point utterance consists of one or more syntactic sentences and associated kinesic elements. Normally these constituent subunits produce a recognizable and meaningful Gestalten of language, which are often called the 'content.'

Each syntactic sentence of the point is a behavioral unit which is also marked.

In a sequence of syntactic sentences, each will be separated by a brief pause in articulation, and pitch will be held constant at this juncture. So will the head, the eyelids, and brows (Birdwhistell 1963). Such a 'single-bar' juncture indicates that the utterance is incomplete and the speaker will continue (Z. Harris 1951; Gleason 1955).

The last syntactic sentence of the point, however, will have a special, terminal juncture: a change in pitch and a stop in vocalization. This change is usually a fall in pitch in the case of a declarative. If the point ends with a question, however, the pitch will rise and the questioner may hold his address until he receives an answer (or gives up the expectation).

92

This terminal linguistic juncture is accompanied by a terminal kinesic or body-motion signal (Birdwhistell 1963). The head and eyelids (or sometimes the hand) are slightly lowered with the pitch fall of a declarative and raised with the pitch rise of a question. These syntactic junctures occur at the completion of speech even if the head-eye orientation is maintained beyond this time (Figure 4-4).

Head Movements as Markers

I'm going to go downtown . . . . and then I'm going over to Bill's. . . .

. . . Then I'm going home. . . . . What are you going to do?

Eyelids as Markers

. . . Then I'm going home. . . . . What are you going to do?

Hand Movements as Markers

. . . Then I'm going home. . . . What are you going to do?

Figure 4-4: Some Postural Kinesic Markers of American Syntactic Sentences [Courtesy of R. L. Birdwhistell. Drawings reproduced from the author's article in Psychiatry (Scheflen 1964).]

These linguistic and kinesic junctures indicate the completion of the point utterance. But they also provide additional signals about the expected response. Thus a rise in pitch (terminating a question in grammar) demands a verbal reply, while a pitch fall (with a declarative) does not.

The Lexical Structure of
the Syntactic Sentence

Sometimes the point consists of a single syntactic sentence as in the case of Mrs. V's opening narrative which is described above. This is often the case as well with questions and commands (see Chapter 5) and the syntactic sentence may contain but a word or two. Thus a participant may hold a head-eye address and occasionally interject a single syntactic sentence, or he may form a point address or even a total position for a single utterance, saying, 'No,' or, 'I agree.'

Syntactic Order in the Sentence

The tradition of sequencing (which we can abstract as syntax) requires that the first words of the syntactic sentences belong to a class known as the subject and the second to a class known as the predicate. The predicate consists of a verb and usually an object. So the syntactic sentence generally presents a proposition, e.g., a noun (subject) is depicted as taking an action (verb) upon another noun (object) (Whorf 1956; Chomsky 1957).

Morphemic Subunits

Notice that the syntactic sentence is itself composed of subunits of even smaller behavior — units of pitch and stress change and units of vocalization. The lexication of the syntactic sentence consists of phrases and words (which I will not here differentiate). Some words are morphemes and others are made up of morphemes.

The morpheme is an utterance which is shorter than the word. In grammar the morphene is classed as a stem-form, a prefix, or a suffix. These are combined to form words.

A great many combinations of phonemes can occur in the morphemic sequence, but there are rules which constrain the types of combination. There are no 'xz,' 'cz,' or 'qa' sequences in English, for example, but sequences of consonants followed by vowels are common. By the same token, sequences of prefix-stem-suffix are established by cultural tradition, so we have forms such as 'child,' where the morpheme is a word in itself, and combinations such as 'children' and 'childish.' But we do not have the forms, 'prochild' or 'childious.'

We can abstract rules from these observations. A good many kinds of sequential order are allowed by the customs of language, but the number is limited. The orders and combinations are determined by syntactic rules which have evolved in common culture (Spair 1921; Chomsky 1957, 1966; Sebeok, Hayes, and Bateson 1964. This lawfulness applies at all levels of integration from the morpheme to the whole transaction and probably to even high levels of integration.)

The lexical behavior of Session I consisted of the customary combinations of morphemes, each of which were more or less standard in their morphology. About 7,000 morphemes were uttered in Session I and maybe 5,000 words. Virtually all of these were standard English forms, which the researchers and all of the participants, as far as we could tell, understood. There were a few unusual forms. Marge and Mrs. V called day dreams or hallucinations, 'mind-pictures.' And two Italian forms appeared — 'fungoo ala madre' and 'Maria.' Thus with few exceptions all participants used the same basic system of lexical forms — they all spoke English.

Even units as small as a word appear to have markers. Condon and Ogston (1967), using very fast filming techniques, have shown a microeyeblink at the beginnings and ends of certain morphemes or words. Phrases also are often marked by head nods.

Birdwhistell (1966) has shown that a lateral microsweep of the head is made over compound words which would be hyphenated in written English. These begin exactly at the start of the first word and end with completion of the last. Presumably the head sweep indicates that the two lexical forms are to be seen as a unit.

Phonemes

Each morpheme is composed, in turn, of a sequence of elemental sounds whose forms are also patterned so that they are recognizable. Their sequencing is structured to produce given morphemes.

A speaker manipulates the vibrating column of respiratory air by placement of his larynx, glottis, tongue, teeth, and lips (McQuown 1964). Of an estimated 100,000 possible sounds or phonemes that can be made in this way, each culture uses some fifteen or more, which are the distinctive elementary units of its language. In English most linguists distinguish forty-three such basic elements of language which are called phonemes.

This sketchy account does not do justice to what is known about language, but we have to cover thirty minutes of behavior, so we cannot focus on the small behaviors of a single modality. The reader is, therefore, urged to consult the comprehensive

works of such structural linguists as Sapir (1921, 1956),
Bloomfield (1933), Z. Harris (1951), Hockett (1958), Chomsky
(1966), and Gleason (1955).

Notice also the number of levels of behavioral integration
we must deal with in a transaction — at least eight are identifiable from the phoneme to the cycle. Each has recognizable
structure and marking indicators.

Kinesic Microacts with Morphemes and Phrases

Kinesic indicators occur with these subunits of speech as
well as with the junctures of the syntactic sentence.

There are also, at all levels, microacts which Birdswhistell
(1963, 1969) has called 'referencing signals.' Pronouns and pre-
positions are often ambiguous in their reference. Participants
using these classes of morphemes generally point with their faces, eyes, or hands to the referents. In using 'we' a head sweep
is often employed to demarcate a subgroup (Birdwhistell 1966).
In using phrases like 'up and down' or 'over there' a sweep of
the head is employed to indicate some special area (Birdwhistell
1966). Some physical feature like an item of decor or a picture
that symbolically represents relevant context may be referred
to by pointing with the head.

A speaker may use his hands to draw a figure in the air
and thus try to picture something he is describing. Mrs. V
often did this. Birdwhistell calls such behaviors 'demonstratives' (Birdwhistell 1969).

Ordinarily particular facial configuration occurs with each
point unit and often a gesture of the hands. I will describe these
behaviors in the next chapter.

Paralinguistic Forms

I have already mentioned paralanguage sounds. In addition
an utterance at any level will have a pattern of vocal qualifiers.
Usually these are specific for a given syntactic sentence and
point, and thereby both mark the unit and qualify it (see Chapter 7).

POINT UNITS IN LISTENING
AND QUESTIONING

Listeners ordinarily address the speaker and perform point
units of head and eye address that are reciprocal to and synchronous with those of the speaker. They may sometimes lexicate in these point units, questioning or commenting, for example. But in either event they use the same address system

and ordinarily they will change point orientation with the speaker. In rapport and other qualities of coordinate relationship the participants will nod, sweep their heads, and move their hands in microsynchrony at speeds of about one forty-eighth of a second (Condon and Ogston 1966; Condon 1968), and sometimes this synchrony of movement is gross and readily visible without special filming techniques (Scheflen 1966; Kendon 1968). Thus, as Condon says, the participants dance together.

Psychotherapists tend to use a minimum of activity in listening. They keep 'dead-pan' expressions and comprehension signals, for example. Whitaker and Malone did this, but not as markedly as some therapists do (see Chapter 11). In their positions of listening and questioning they performed the following three types of customary point units.

Attending. They cocked their heads slightly and addressed Mrs. V. They suppressed virtually all body movement and facial expression in the dead-pan face that psychotherapists deliberately use to minimize influence on the speaker. They would occasionally signal attentiveness: leaning the head forward, cocking it, turning the ear, and using an overwide position of the eyelids.

Questioning. Whitaker repeatedly asked questions in Session I. He would extend his neck so that his head was high, jutted forward, and slightly cocked. He would direct his face, gaze, and convergence to the addressee — Marge or Mrs. V — take his pipe out of his mouth and hold it forward. He would then articulate the question. After speaking, he would raise his head still farther, jut his jaw slightly, and raise his eyebrows until an answer was begun. Then he would lower and retract his head, and return his pipe to his mouth (Figure 4-5).

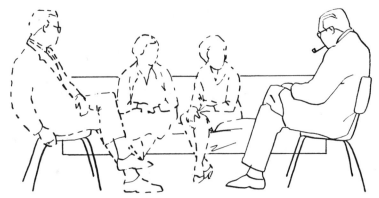

Figure 4-5: Head Protrusion by Whitaker on Asking a Question

Commenting. All the auditors of Mrs. V's narrative offered comments about what she said. These point units will concern
us in the next chapter.

COMMENT: LANGUAGE UNITS THAT ARE
'SUFFICIENTLY' MEANINGFUL

The Sufficient Depiction of an Idea

In conversational activities where narration or description
is used, it is unusual for a participant to speak a single syntactic sentence and then relinquish the floor. Usually a succession of such segments are necessary to portray an experience.
A single idea might leave so much ambiguity as to give the utterance little specific meaning. In other words, it might have so
many possible meanings that it would have little meaning.

One might conceive the task in lexical activities as the adequate representation of a referent or context not immediately
perceivable. The necessary behavior for such representation
must be coded in the sense that a kinesic or lexical unit must
be employed which has an agreed-upon relation to the object or
event of reference. Some sketch of the referent must be drawn
with icons or symbols or both. When the referent is symbolized
by nouns and verbs, these may have to be supplemented with
qualifying adjectives, phrases, demonstratives, and gestures.

Some lexical morphs refer to more highly specific referents
known to almost everyone. Phrases like 'the Statue of Liberty,'
'the U.S. Senate,' or 'the Crucifix' are examples, but ordinarily
words can have multiple referents. Words like 'set' or 'put,'
for example, have dozens of lexographic definitions. Kinesic
behavior may be even more ambiguous. Gestures or facial expressions of disapproval may give no indication of just what is
being disapproved.

Bateson (1969) has said that the meaning of a behavior is
inversely proportional to its ambiguity. We then achieve a
greater meaning by acquiring more information and thus reduc-
ing this ambiguity. We progressively eliminate alternative
possibilities. So in practice the meaning of an act will be specified by the addition of more and more behavior which supplies
information about the reference and referent. The behavior
necessary to communicate about abstract and personal matters
is likely to be complex and highly integrated.

In Session I complex positions were assembled to carry the
narrative, and multiple cyclic repetitions occurred to elucidate
the family's history. Similarly in the nonlexical channels elaborate quasi-courting and tactile routines were used — apparently

to develop a relationship. While it was clear that Marge was
ironically representing sexual behavior, it was not clear what
the implications were. To determine whether she was seeking
intercourse or attention or merely teasing we would have to
know much more about her, about Italian-American courtship
behavior, and so on (English et al. 1965).

Assembling Higher and Higher
Integrations of Behavior

Consider, then, an operational postulate. The particular
sequences or units that a participant enacts in a transaction are
those that are usually sufficient in his experience to get the job
done.[3]

In a conversational transaction the speaker must progressively build an unambiguous utterance. If a syntactic sentence is in-
sufficient, a point and perhaps a position or a sequence of positions will be used. We thus can think of the participant's task as
the assemblage of units in a hierarchy of levels.

It is as though the participant were a builder. He knows
how to form with his body a number of building blocks of sound
and movement. He puts these together according to some cognitive map into recognizable and traditional Gestalten of greater
and greater complexity.

He can assemble customary forms of movement and sound
in several directions. He can order more and more symbolic
units until he forms a communicative Gestalt. He can use different regions of his body to qualify the statement, to gain attention to it, and to minimize interference. And he can orient
each of these actions and solicit mutual participation to build
the relational structures of communication.

Cognitive Images of Behavioral Form

People must maintain some cognitive image of the behavior
they perform. They have learned certain patterns of behavior
and they can recall and re-enact these when they find themselves
in an appropriate context.

If a participant is to produce a sufficiently meaningful unit
of language behavior, he must have in mind an image of the remote event or contexts he is to depict; also he must be a cognitive blueprint of the order of speech behavior which he will have
to follow to represent the image adequately for others. And he
must hold an image of the contexts in which this particular behavior is appropriate.

The cognitive blueprint, then, must be more than a simple map of the conventional performance. It must be representation of complicated hierarchies of behavioral integration.

These ideas have already been developed by Miller, Galanter, and Pribram (1960). These men have hypothesized that cognitive images of performances and situations are maintained, which are hierarchically structured and they may be enacted as plans and recalibrated with feedback information in the situation (see Chapter 8). Pribram has postulated that such images may be maintained in circuits which involved oligodendroglia, since these proliferate with learning (Pribram 1966). Thus Tolman's idea of cognitive maps (1948, 1951) has been considerably developed. One can think about such representations in a temporal perspective. Any larger unit or context in a hierarchy extends backward in time from immediate behavior and it appears to extend forward in time when it is replicated in memory. Thus one can visualize the next events in a pattern. He can imagine and anticipate usual consequences. He can have expectancies (Tolman 1932; Lewin 1951; Rotter 1954); that is, he can imagine goals and behaviors necessary to achieve these.

Chapter 5

THE METACOMMUNICATIVE POINTS IN SESSION I

In the case of explaining, the language content referred to events at a distance — things that had happened in the V family. And Whitaker's explanation referred to events that were planned. But only Mrs. V consistently used language this way in Session I.

Marge's language behavior referred to what her mother was saying. Statements made by Malone or Whitaker tended to be confrontations and instructions. Thus language behavior was used to comment on and regulate other behavior. Often, for instance, Mrs. V would tell of an incident, Marge would comment on it, and then Malone would act in reference to Marge's behavior.

Bateson (1955) has used the term, 'metacommunication,' for behavior which seems analogous to this. He derived the idea from a question about animal play. Dogs, he observed, may rush at each other and then either romp off together playfully or fight to the finish. He suggested there was a signal, unrecognized by man, by which the dogs communicated to each other for either fight or play. Subsequently, such signals have been discovered for several species (Kaufman and Rosenblum 1966; Altman 1966).

The simplest kind of metasignals appear to specify a type of meaning or qualify the literality of an act. Smiling, for instance, may metacommunicate that a certain aggressive act is to be taken as friendly and competitive rather than attacking behavior. Certain metabehaviors appear with quasi-courting which indicates that seduction is not intended (Scheflen 1965).

100

In such instances, self-referenced metabehaviors qualify and specify alternatives, and thereby help to reduce ambiguity in a performance. But is is also evident that one can 'metabehave' to someone else's behavior and thereby alter or influence it. Furthermore it seems that behavioral units at all levels of integration may be metacommunicative. Here in Chapter 5, I will describe some behaviors of this type which occurred at the level of the point.

METACOMMUNICATIVE LANGUAGE
POINTS IN SESSION I

The metacommunicative point contains language and/or gestures and it may contain representational behavior, so there is nothing structurally distinctive about the subunit form. What distinguished the metacommunicative unit is its contextual location, its form of address, and certain qualities of its performance. I will abstract some of these features after I have described the metacommunicative language points in Session I.

Mrs. V's Metacommunicative Point Usage

I have already described Mrs. V's initial point units in Session I. The reader will remember that she intercalated the comment about Marge's behavior as she described Marge's requests to be helped upstairs. Mrs. V paused in her utterance, cocked her head slightly, lowered her eyes, and used paralanguage which indicated incredulity and disapproval. Then she said: 'A young girl like her.' Then she straightened her head, looked back at Malone, and continued her narrative.

In Period 2s when Mrs. V's account was called to question she used metacommunicative points about her own behavior. These sometimes were conciliatory toward Marge or they offered a concession. Sometimes these point units rationalized her own behavior. At 5 minutes: 05 seconds for instance, Mrs. V said 'Well, I am, I call myself mental.' (Marge had just accused her of being mentally ill.) In saying this, she looked down at the floor, put her finger tips on her chest, and used an overhigh paralanguage with laughter — a configuration we interpret as embarrassment (point 12, Addendum to this section).

Some Metacommunicative Language Points
Used by Marge

Self-references

Virtually none of Marge's utterances were narrative. Many
were performative statements about her own state of mind. The
later type of statement is illustrated in the diagram of point 8,
lamenting, which is reproduced in the Addendum to this section.
At 11 minutes: 25 seconds she said plaintively, 'Remember it
was hard for me . . . to breast feed me?' This point is diagrammed at point 14, Addendum to Section B. I wish to mention these
points but it is not clear that they were metacommunicative. It
would be my guess that they were — that they were references
to Mrs. V's mothering, but I do want to press the issue. There
are more obvious examples of her disparaging metabehavior.
In either case, Marge's self-references were metacommunicative. They described either her own state or repeated her
mother's past comments.

The Disparaging Comments in Passive Protesting

Nearly all of Marge's language points in her initial position
of passive protesting were disparaging or insinuating. As I
described above many of these were not verbalized. Some were
muttered as can be seen on the multimodality transcript.

At 10 seconds Marge mocked her mother's behavior in a
nonvocal point. At 18 seconds she whispered in a stage whisper
with mocking paralanguage: 'You said I ought to have a good
sleep and eat.' At 24 seconds she said sarcastically: 'Gonna go
to hell.' At 31 seconds she used baby talk in a mocking way. At
49 seconds she insinuated: 'You know who, Mother, you know
who.' This statement too was said with a mocking smile.

At 8 minutes: 20 seconds Marge performed a more spectacular form of indirect disparagement. She sat upright and said
'fungoo la madre' making the classical obscene southern Italian
gesture of raising her right fist and grasping her right elbow
with her left hand. She accompanied this point with a look of exaggerated shock, which presumably mimicked her mother's expected response.

Marge would make such disparaging metacommunicative
points when her mother denied or rationalized a challenge or
accusation (point 13, Addendum to this section).

Repelling

At 1:50 Marge performed a point that was at least partly metacommunicative. This point can be seen in context on the multimodality transcript. She crossed her legs improperly and said: 'Sexy, you mean, oh boy.' This remark was addressed in a mode Birdwhistell calls 'extrapersonal' — it was addressed over the heads of the others to the world at large.[1]

The referent was a remark that Whitaker had just made. At that point in the session all of the participants seemed to be making metacommunicative remarks about each other's performance:

> Mrs. V to Marge:
> 'You're just goofy now.'
> Whitaker: 'Sometimes I feel like an animal. Don't you feel like an animal sometimes?'
> Marge: 'I don't know what you're talking about.'
> Malone, with mock incredulity:
> 'Really?'

'Shocking' Point

When Marge performed her position of interfering (see Chapter 1) she would say something shocking in an apparent effort to shock her mother and disturb the mother's conversation with the men. But she herself would use a shocked, outraged facial expression that I presume was a mocking imitation of her mother's past behavior. I postulate, then, that Marge's shocking behavior was a kind of dramatized commentary on behaviors that occurred in her home and hence a behavior intermediate between direct commentary and narration.

Whitaker's Metacommunicative Behavior

Sometimes Whitaker asked simple questions, but ordinarily his comments and questions were loaded with innuendo or then amounted to confrontations. This kind of metacommunicative behavior, typical of psychotherapy, will be described in Chapter 11, where the tactics of psychotherapy are discussed.

Malone's Use of Ironic Supporting

Innuendo was used by both Malone and Marge. Both had a way of varying stress and adding vocal qualities that loaded syntactic sentences with innuendo. They also tended to use a syntactic variant that is formally known as a question but in fact is a command that implies an accusation. Note the following examples.

Marge:

<u>Was</u> I baptized <u>Did</u> I cry <u>Did</u> I get scared	(With the primary stress and pitch rise on the first morpheme, and a pitch fall on the last)

Malone:

How long <u>can</u> you remember Did you <u>warm</u> the milk Like a <u>baby</u> wasn't it Where <u>is</u> your husband	(With a primary stress and pitch rise on the morph underlined and also a pitch fall on the terminal)

But Malone used a distinctive variety of metabehavior. He would make a statement that lexically was a simple affirmation or support of Mrs. V's story, but he employed paralanguage that suggested something quite different (see Chapter 11).

STRUCTURAL FEATURES OF THE METACOMMUNICATIVE POINT

Types of Metacommunicative Address

In simple narrative and questioning, the address is direct, eye to face, or intrapersonal in Birdwhistell's terms (see footnote 1, this chapter). In metacommunicative behavior the address is directed almost anywhere else.

Intrapersonal Address

The address may be directed to oneself. The metacommunicative speaker looks down at his own hands or body or legs. This is especially likely when he is commenting on his own behavior. We often see this arrangement in confessions of shame or guilt.

Extrapersonal Address

The metacommunicative address may be directed to the ceiling or to the world at large. In this case a subtle reference to

someone present may be inferred, and if the shoe fits the referent can put it on.

The extrapersonal address may also be aimed at a vacant
chair or a space which is not occupied. In such cases we can
often infer that some absent member is being addressed, or else
some figure of the past — an introject in psychoanalytic terms
(Freud 1949; Abraham 1949).

Marge used this form of address a great deal. I think it is
quite characteristic for schizophrenic patients to do so. Such
patients will often 'detach' a bodily part, functionally speaking,
and hold it out of participation. This body part will move at
different rhythms from those of the rest of the body and from
the movements of the other participants. It is writhed and moved or held dead, as if it lacked relation to the present. Instead,
the movement seemed related to some other transaction. Marge
performed a variant of this behavior at times in Session I (see
Chapter 8). She also addressed remarks 'meta to' her mother's
behavior in the intrapersonal mode, as one would ordinarily do
in making a self-reference.

The 'Eyeball-to-Eyeball' Address

In direct command, challenge, and confrontation, the usual
address is direct eye-to-eye confrontation. Malone, Whitaker,
and Mrs. V used this mode with Marge.

Other Features of the Metacommunicative Point

The metacommunicative point, then, is often addressed at
the behavior it refers to, or in the direct form, to the maker of
that behavior. But it is also temporarily located in the context
of that behavior referred to. It is performed just after the behavior it modifies or is intercalated in the unit itself.

The metacommunicative unit also makes use of some particular paralinguistic or parakinesic quality. These qualities
are abstracted as affects in psychiatry and generally interpreted
as shame, guilt, anger, ridicule, and so on. In semantics we
would view them as innuendos or connotations.

But an operational point must be made here — a metacommunicative point about metacommunicative points, so to speak.
A unit of behavior is not clearly metacommunicative or clearly
not metacommunicative. Any utterance, for example, occurs in
a tone of voice which is metacommunicative and each gesture
and facial expression is also metacommunicative (see the discussion of the gesture, below). So all units have metacommunicative features. When a point is obviously directed at an

ongoing behavior or is heavily loaded with metacommunicative elements I have classed it as metacommunicative. But more accurately we have to generalize as follows: Any unit of behavior contains subunits or elements which are metacommunicative to the larger unit. So the metacommunicative point unit is the subunit in some larger position or period to which it supplies a metabehavioral function.

GESTURES: COMMENT BY GESTURE

We speak of the noun or verb as a symbolic behavior, by which we mean that it has a conventional referent conjured in our cognition by the appearance of that word. Thus some morphemes stand for things in remote contexts, but they do not look like the things they stand for. In contrast are other behaviors which do look like the referents they represent: diagrams, photographs, sketches, and the demonstratives I mentioned in the last chapter, i.e., shapes drawn in the air to represent abstract concepts that the speaker is trying to explain. Such replicative behavior is often called 'iconic.'

There is a class of communicative body movements of which some members are vaguely iconic, but most are symbolic. Maybe these forms are transitory forms in cultural evolution. These behaviors are of about the same complexity as morphemes or simple syntactic sentences and they almost invariably accompany these speech units. Although they have conventional meanings, these acts are often not conscious in common culture. They are formed by the hands, the face, and sometimes by the feet or the body as a whole. I will use Birdwhistell's nomenclature and call these acts gestures. Notice, however, the term applies to these particular acts and not to the microbehaviors of body movement in general, as is the case in some usages.

The Gestural Points in Session I

The gesture is a small point unit. A bodily region is positioned and addressed, the face or hands are then moved to the customary configuration of that gesture, held for a second or so, then altered or discontinued. And these point units are metacommunicative. Either they occur with a language point, qualifying the speech content, or else they occur without lexication but are referenced to the speech (or sometimes to the other behavior) of some other participant.

Mrs. V's Gestures

Mrs. V used the gesture as a metacommunicative qualifier of her statements. When her story was challenged she would reaffirm her veracity. While doing so she would place her right palm over her heart. This gesture is used typically in such contexts and is generally recognized, even when it occurs without comment, as an indicator of sincerity.

She also used a common gesture which I call nose-wiping. This gesture served as a monitor to Marge's behavior (Scheflen 1969).

Nose-wiping. The back of the index finger is brought laterally across the nostrils and upper lip. This behavior characteristically appears when a speaker lies or exaggerates or when some deviance in nonlexical behavior occurs such as sitting too close, exposing the legs, or being too informal.

Marge's Gestures

Marge once sat bolt upright, raised her left arm, flexed it at the elbow, and struck her antecubital space with her right hand. She muttered 'fungoo ala madre' with this gesture, then sat back. We recognize this gesture as a costumary Italian obscenity and Marge verbalized the usual phrase which accompanies it. But later she made the gesture in less spectacular form without verbalization. She enacted this point not in reference to her own statements, for she had not been speaking. It related instead to an assertion her mother made.

Similarly, Marge would address the camera or one of the men and make a facial grimace. These facial configurations can also be considered gestures. They often represent the expressions of ridicule, mock incredulity, anger, love, mock terror, and so forth. Presumably the facial appearance in affective states is known in common culture and can be replicated as a deliberate commentary on what is happening.

A good many of Marge's gestures were characteristically Catholic. She sometimes made the sign of the cross and another gesture of stabbing herself (reminiscent of supplicant gestures in religious ceremonies). Once she shook her hand from side to side, as if shaking off a contaminant. Marge also used the palm on chest gesture and two others that commonly appear in conversation.

1. Mouth covering. The participant may place his hand over his mouth. This gesture can occur when a speaker has

been told to be quiet or when he has just uttered a prohibited or embarrasing comment.

2. Hands outstretched, palms up. The participant extends his lower arms and turns his palms upward. (In Eastern European Jewish culture shoulder shrugging is often added.) This gesture occurred with Marge's statement of helplessness or resignation.

Gestures of the Men

As I said in Chapter 2, Mrs. V used nose-wiping whenever Marge acted sexy and allied with Whitaker. Whitaker would regularly light his pipe before supporting Marge, and after a few repetitions of this sequencing Mrs. V began to wipe her nose whenever Whitaker started to light his pipe. After the first few minutes Malone, too, wiped his nose when Marge acted sexy. On a half-dozen occasions, then, Malone and Mrs. V performed the nose-wiping point at exactly the same time.

Three of the participants make the bowl-point at 18 minutes; Marge in Session I, Whitaker in Session III, and Malone in Session IX.

The bowl. Both hands are brought together in the lap and cupped so that the hands form the configuration of a bowl. This gesture ordinarily appears when a speaker is relating a dream or phantasy (English et al. 1965).

The men used four other gestures which are characteristics of psychotherapists.

1. Eye-covering. A hand is placed, palm inward, over one eye. This microbehavior tends to appear in two related contexts: (1) men tend to cover their eyes when a woman exhibits her legs and (2) someone will cover his eyes when trying to comprehend an elusive idea or insight.

2. Eye-pointing. A participant will point to his own eye with his index finger or place the finger on the eye. This act often accompanies demands to pay attention or recognize an idea.

3. Lint-picking. The men occasionally looked down at their clothing and picked up a fragment of lint with their thumb and index finger, then reached over and shook it off on the floor. Lint-picking often occurs when a patient has said something that normally would elicit censure, but the therapist, trained not to criticize, seems to pick lint instead. Whitaker did this after he lit his pipe, presumably to rid his hand of tobacco fragments, but he did this so ostentatiously that I often thought it was an unconscious signal of some kind. At 18 minutes he picked up an invisible object from the floor and played with it for about six minutes before he offered it to Marge to smell. I will describe this kind of behavior in Chapter 8.

4. Looking up. Many therapists show a characteristic non-lexical point just before they make an interpretation to a patient (Whitaker and Malone did this). They look up to the ceiling, then down at the patient, and begin their utterance.

COMMANDS, DIRECTIVES, AND CONFRONTATIONS

Some point-unit commentaries were direct orders and instructions. The characteristics of such points usually are: (1) the use of direct eye-to-eye address, while leaning toward the addressee; (2) emphasis on the terminal juncture, e.g., bringing the head down sharply or bringing the hand down forcibly, (3) the syntactic form of the declarative on many morphemes with the use of primary stresses, loudness, and head nods.

Malone's Confrontations

In Session I Malone's units were mainly of this type. In fact his position, interfering, (position 4, Appendix A, and Chapter 1) consisted of rocking forward and performing three successive directive points. He performed this position ten times — each time that Marge contended. From his initial position of listening and questioning Malone would rock forward and confront Marge with an eye-to-eye address:

> He would address Marge and scold her for confronting (point 9, Appendix A).
> Then he would address Mrs. V, and direct her to continue her narrative (restarting, point 5, Appendix to Section B).
> And sometimes he would make a statement in apparent support of Mrs. V (ironic supporting, point 15).

In the two minutes reproduced on the multimodality transcript (Section B), Malone had not yet performed these behaviors in full development, so they are not well portrayed here. But notice that Malone began to make remarks which insinuated and indicated irony at about 3 minutes. Then at 3:35 he rocked forward, and coughed but did not yet speak. At 4:10 he wiped his index finger under his nostrils, a gesture of censure or disapproval.

Marge's Confrontations

On occasion Marge also made direct confrontations. The first was directed to the men (it appears on page two of the multi-modality transcript at 1:24). With mixed vocal qualifiers of anger and lament, she said, 'Me? You're watching me get angry at my mother.' This metacommunicative unit is at once lament, accusation, and comment on the men's behavior. Transitional metacommunicative units like this confirm our hunch that such diverse acts as insinuation and command can be classed together.

On occasion Marge also directly confronted her mother (point 11, Appendix to Section B).

COMMENT: BEHAVIOR AND CONCEPTIONS ABOUT BEHAVIOR

The Coding of Behavior

It is often said that human behavior is communicative because it is coded. This is a useful idea that summarizes much of what has been said about behavioral units and patternment. Now that we have added the idea of metabehavior, we can say how behavior can be described as being coded (Sebeok 1963).

A code must have the following characteristics:

1. A set of distinctive elements, each differentiable from the others.
2. An order to their occurrence, or combinations such that certain configurations or patterns occur (usually in the same contexts or specific environments).
3. Conventional meta-elements — signals of instruction like stop, repeat, cancel, and so forth.

Imagine how these features might be built in to a contrived code. Types of items would have to be designated as the elements of the code: colored pennants, marks on paper, electronic signals of varying duration or pitch, hand signals, etc.[2] Exact shapes and color intensities for each item would have to be selected to make them contrast obviously. There would have to be an agreement about what each item represented. There would also have to be metacommunicational elements or instructional signals equivalent to stop, repeat, end of message, cancel last element, and so on. To give the code a meaning there would have to be a syntax.

The structure of human behavior has these very characteristics. The units of behavior serve as the elements, and the hierarchical structuring provides the syntax.[3] Of course, these characteristics of coding do not have to be contrived. In the case of humans they have evolved (Sebeok 1965; McBride 1968).

Contrary to myth, these behaviors are not coded genetically. They are not species specific behavior for man, but are instead culturally relative. If one is French, he not only speaks French, but uses French kinesics, French systems of address, and so forth. Thus the forms of address and the gestures I have described in Session I are in some cases southern Italian and in other American, but they are not universal. In Black American lower class subjects, the address forms described here are not usually seen. In fact eye-to-eye behavior is rare and is distinguished in Negro culture by a special phrase which I borrowed above, 'eyeball to eyeball.' So these behaviors are culturally transmitted. In psychological language, they are learned.

Cognition and Metabehavior

By the same token we must assume that metacommunicative behavior is learned and represented cognitively.

The simplest metabehaviors have been out of awareness in common culture; many were not known until Birdwhistell and others began to research kinesic behavior in the 1950s. Consequently a participant cannot tell us about them.

For example, the nose-wiping is a common metasignal of monitoring. It appeared twenty-eight times in Session I. Each time Marge exhibited herself, for instance, her mother performed this signal, Malone often did so as well, and sometimes Whitaker did. This metasignal can be seen in any transaction when someone behaves deviantly — when a woman's dress rides up, when someone is approached too closely, when someone lies or exaggerates, or passes flatus. Often the person who commits the deviance nose-wipes himself (Scheflen 1963).

But this behavior is performed unconsciously and its significance is not known in common culture (Freud 1959). If you interview subjects about its meaning they are surprised. They did not know they performed the act, though they may be aware that they felt disapproval. They hasten to explain the monitor by saying that their nose must have itched. In other cases, however, the behavior is known, but there is a myth about its meaning. In rural New Jersey, for example, the occurrence of nose-itching and nose-wiping means 'company is coming.'

We must assume, then, that people learn the basic formats of both behaving and metabehaving by some unconscious process of identification. They visualize and metacommunicate about others enacting these parts, and they replicate these behaviors by imitation. [4]

Conceptions About Behavioral Forms

People also learn about their behaviors. In many cases the formats of a traditional performance have already been abstracted and these are explicitly taught and written about.

Traditional Conceptions of Behavioral Formats

The recipe of a national dish calls for certain ingredients to be added in a certain order. The liturgy of church services calls for precisely performed acts. The rules of the game prescribe the periods, plays, formations, and so forth. The score of the symphony and the script of the play prescribe the order of passages and scenes. In America there are a great many how-to-do-it books for the various tasks of the culture.

In the case of other traditional behaviors little is known about the formats. This lack of knowledge may not be a simple consequence of nonattention, but a conformity to a deeply entrenched Western ideal of spontaneous and individualistic performance. It would be vigorously denied that customary or prescribed steps occur in such behavior. [5] Only in the last decade have we examined behaviors like this with filmed recording and systematic observational techniques.

In activities like baby care, courtship, and holding a party, the participants would not realize and might deny emphatically that they were following a format. But each performance of these activities is so alike (in single tradition) that one has to conclude that some common traditional agenda or format must be in use.

As a consequence, we have little information but a plethora of myths about such activities. But whatever ideas, knowledge, or myth, which have developed about the formats of human behavior, these, too, have been learned by the members of common culture. These ideas about behavior also, must be cognitively represented. Thus when we ask a participant about his behavior he will produce for us a culturally traditional myth about the behavior, which is not ordinarily corrected by any systematic observations on his own part. And correspondingly he may enact this myth in language or iconic representation when he explains what he is doing, teaches it, or speaks about behaving while he is behaving.

Complex conceptions have evolved in any culture about the value, propriety, morality, and significance of any behavior we can think of. These metacommunicative systems about behavior are also learned and handed down as part of the cultural

heritage. The metabehavior of a transaction has reference to
these metaconceptual systems, which we must view as an infra-
system of thought, interrelated to but not identical with the
cognitive infrasystems for performing the behavior.

Thus when we take part in a transaction, we perform in
two infrasystems. We enact the behaviors elicited in that context, and we say, think, and feel that we have learned we are
supposed to say, think, and feel about a performance.[6] We
would be naive to think that the metaconceptual behavior simply describes what is otherwise in progress when it is likely
to make the behavior of transaction palatable and seemingly
rational. It is likely to dramatize, idealize, or even conceal
the other behaviors in progress.

The Disparity Between Behavior and Metaconceptions

So the child or novitiate in a social organization must learn
not only how to behave but also how to think and talk about behaving. And there can be considerable disparity between the in-
formational context of these two infrasystems. For example,
a child learns to speak the language of his cultural grouping in
early childhood. He learns a limited vocabulary, syntax and
the markers, transfixes, and junctures of his social group. He
also learns the posturology, representational behavior, styles
and demeanors, of his dialectic group. Then years later he
goes to school and learns grammar, that is, he learns how he
ought to speak (by Edwardian standards) and how language is
supposed to be structured (by Latin standards). He can produce either of those behavioral variants on demand. He can
even pass a test on Latin grammar using an American dialect.
(He can, that is, if he is properly middle-class.)

As a consequence a participant can enact a format according to the customary structure and separately metacommunicate
about the process.

1. He may, for instance, perform as culturally prescribed while he verbalizes or thinks about the
   usual metaconceptions about behavior.
2. Or he can exercise a kind of metacommunicative
   option. He can speak about his or someone's performance instead of behaving it. And he can, of
   course, also think or feel about it.

And some participants become accomplished in manipulating these relations to conceal or exploit the performances in a

transaction. We might guess that whatever a participant performs visibly in a given context, that he cannot not perform. He can only suppress the majority of the visible performance features.

The Methodological Significance
of the Discrepancy

If a person has private myths about his own behavior we can speak of mechanisms of defense, as is the practice in psychoanalysis (A. Freud 1946). But in the case of a conception shared by all members of an institution or culture, a discrepancy is not seen and the members of that group speak of truth and see the metacommunicative system as identical with the behavior performed.

But in both of these cases we cannot assume that the disparity between behavior and language about behavior is simply a matter of ignorance. Individuals and organizations of individuals have an entrenched stake in their metaconceptions. Their repetition of metaconceptions may make anything possible from drumming up the sun to being able to enact the roles of everyday life without loss of self-esteem, loss of job, or loss of interest. We must agree that the natural function of language is not to analyze behavior either for science, insight, or the writing of how-to-do-it books. This is a special use of metacommunication which we have recently made language serve.

A traditional psychological myth therefore comes under scrutiny. In the classical Platonic mode we regard feeling as the cause of behavior. It would be as correct to say that motor behavior causes thoughts and feelings. At best we can hold that behavior is sometimes planned and in such cases thoughts or feelings may be a cause of a performance. So we need to avoid chicken or egg positions. We would rather say that a given context triggers a specific format enactment. This enactment includes both visible (and audible) behavior and invisible cognitive behavior.

I think the disparity between metabehavior and less conscious other behavior is what the psychoanalysts have abstracted as 'the unconscious' (Freud 1953) and constructs like 'id,' unconscious motivation and the like appear to refer to behavior not countenanced in traditional explicit metasystems.

The considerations redefine fields like semantics (Korzybski 1948; Hayakawa 1941), classical semiotics (Carnap 1947), and pragmatics (Watzlawick, Beavin, and Jackson 1967).

Since subjects cannot tell us their meaning, modern semiotic studies have turned to a behavioral systems orientation

(Sebeok, Hayes, and M. C. Bateson 1964). In such a view all
modalities of behavior are examined in the study of communications and the significance of any given unit is analyzed by observing multiple occurrences in context (Bateson 1962, 1969;
Scheflen 1966). Whenever a given unit regularly is followed by
a given change in context, i.e., whenever it regularly elicits a
given corresponding behavior in other people, we can assume
that communication has occurred — even when the participants
are not aware of the fact and cannot tell us about the processes
(see Section C).

Distrust of subjectivism seems to be a factor in the present
tendency to rely on direct observation in the study of behavior.
But because metabehavior is also behavior, we will need to study
both the observable behavior and the beliefs about this behavior.

ADDENDUM TO SECTION B:
REVIEW OF THE POINT UNITS

In this addendum each type of point for Session I is illustrated
with a specific example.

In each illustration the point junctures are described at the
right and left upper corners of the picture. On top of the picture
(which shows the transfix of that point) is the mode. Below the
picture is the lexical content of that point and the time from the
beginning of the Session at which this illustrative point occurred
(see transcript, Appendix B). Next appear any metacommunicational behaviors of that point. Finally the context in which this
type of point occurred is characterized.

Note that the figure of the person carrying out the point in
question is drawn in a heavy line, while the others are in dotted-
line only.

POINT 1: Conciliating (Mrs. V; sometimes Marge)

| Mrs. V turns head from Malone to Marge (Juncture) ⟶ | Addresses Marge in interpersonal mode (TRANSFIX) ⟶ | Turns head from Marge to Whitaker on completion (Juncture) |

Conciliatory statements in this case:

Content:
0:40

'I remember I usta' get angry. Everybody gets angry.'

Metacommunication:

Smile; oversoft paralanguage

Context:

Occurs in situations when Marge and Whitaker have been contending the history and Mrs. V has been defending it. After a sharp exchange conciliating appeared.

POINT 2: Attending (Whitaker, Malone)

| (Whitaker in this case) Bends head forward, tilting it to the left, peering at Marge. (Juncture) ⟶ | listens (to Marge) (TRANSFIX) ⟶ ↓ | Turns back to Mrs. V (Juncture) |

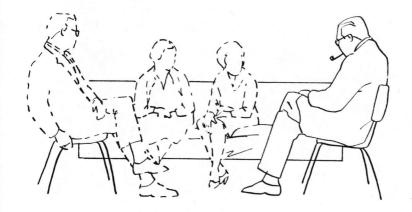

Content:
1:25

Mostly nonlexical with occasional questioning; e.g., 'What did you say? I didn't hear you.'

Metacommun-
ication:

Slightly raised eyebrows, probably overwide eye opening, indicating attentiveness.

Context:

Whitaker turns alternately to one woman, then the other, listening actively to each. In this example, he had been listening to Mrs. V, when Marge mumbled something under her breath.

118

POINT 3: Rejecting (Whitaker)

Lowers head
turns to Marge
(Juncture) ──────▶

Extrapersonal
mode, apparently
vis-à-vis Marge
(TRANSFIX) ──────▶

Turns head ab-
ruptly and far to
right away from
Marge
(Juncture)

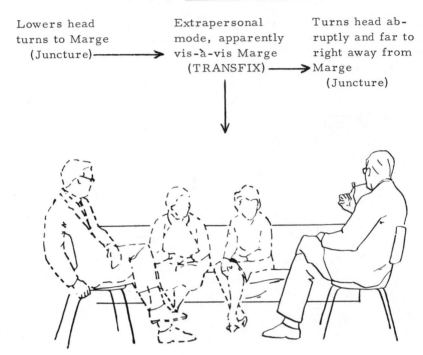

Content:
1:30

Ambiguous, vaguely critical comments to
Marge; in this case: 'Sometimes I feel like
an animal. Don't you feel like an animal
sometimes?' (This point would not be evident
from the lexical content alone. But his kinesics and the response of the other person
clearly indicate rejection.)

Metacommun-
ication:

Overfast with pipe in mouth and muttered as
though he did not definitely want to be heard.

Context:

Occurred in situations where he and Marge
had contended with Mrs. V and Mrs. V had
defended or conciliated. Malone then would
confront Marge and instruct Mrs. V to resume her narrative. Whitaker then would reject Marge.

POINT 4: <u>Repelling</u> (<u>Marge</u>)

Head and body
turned away
from Whitaker
(or Malone)
(Juncture) ———→

Extrapersonal
mode directed to
camera
(TRANSFIX) ———→

Turns and speaks
to her mother
(Juncture)

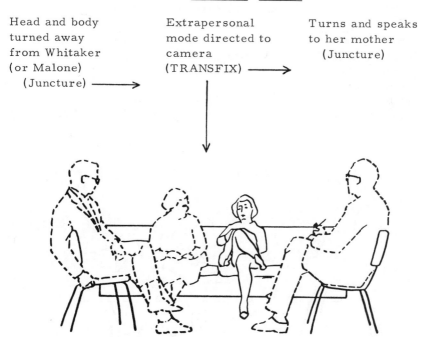

Content:
1:50

Sexually provocative statements; in this case:
'Sexy, you mean. O boy! ' Bizarre or improper
leg-crossing accompanied these utterances.

Metacommun-
ication:

Overloud with flippant, defiant facial expression.

Context:

Occurred in association with Whitaker's rejecting, which ended alliances of Marge and
Whitaker.

POINT 5: Restarting Mrs. V's Narrative
(Malone; occasionally Whitaker)

Turns away from Marge to Mrs. V and rocks in slightly (Juncture) ⟶	Interpersonal mode to Mrs. V (Rocks in toward Mrs. V) (TRANSFIX) ⟶	Rocks out, sits back and listens to Mrs. V (Juncture)

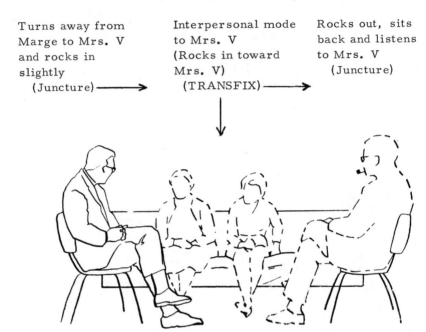

Content: 1:85	Questions directed to Mrs. V, in this case: 'Where is your husband?' (Malone's usual practice of confronting Marge, silencing her and bidding Mrs. V to resume were, in this instance, combined in a single point and sentence)
Metacommun- ication:	Overloud. Formal, authoritarian paralanguage as in a command.
Context:	In general, restarting occurred after Mrs. V defended herself against Marge's and Whitaker's challenges and at the point that Marge repelled Whitaker and he turned from her.

POINT 6: <u>Recounting</u> (<u>Mrs. V</u>)

| Turns from Marge to Malone (Juncture) ⟶ | Interpersonal mode to Marge (TRANSFIX) ⟶ | Turns to Whitaker in response to his question (Juncture) |

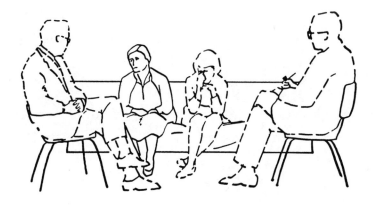

<u>Content:</u>	Statements of her history, in this case: 'He died. It'll be a year this December 3rd. December 3rd it will be a year.'
<u>Metacommunication:</u>	Expression and paralanguage of brave martyrdom.
<u>Context:</u>	Mrs. V began recounting usually after being restarted by Malone's instruction and continued until interrupted.

POINT 7: Defending (Mrs. V)

Turns from Whitaker to Marge (Juncture) ⟶ Interpersonal mode to Marge (TRANSFIX) ⟶ Looks back to Whitaker in Appeal (Juncture)

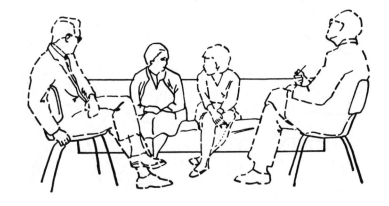

Content: 3:15	Mrs. V rationalized her past actions when challenged; in this case she does so by trying to cast doubt in Marge's memory. 'When he died I laughed, Marge? I laughed? Marge, did I laugh when he died?'
Metacommunication:	Expression and paralanguage of shocked, innocent incredulousness, implying that Marge could not be serious.
Context:	In general, defending occurred in complementary relation to Malone's ironic supporting of the mother, and in opposition to Marge's insinuations and Whitaker's challenges. Defending usually preceded Marge's backing down and Whitaker's repelling of Marge.

POINT 8: <u>Lamenting</u> (<u>Marge</u>, <u>occasionally</u> <u>Mrs. V</u>)

<table>
<tr><td>Turns to Whitaker
(Juncture) ——————→</td><td>Interpersonal mode
to Whitaker
(TRANSFIX) ——————→</td><td>Turns to Malone
(Juncture)</td></tr>
</table>

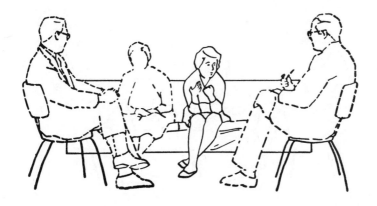

<u>Message:</u>   'I'm dead. I am dead, dead.'
3:40

<u>Metamessage:</u>   High-pitched, wailing, seemingly pleading that
                 she be taken seriously.

<u>Context:</u>   Lamenting appeared briefly, but often, during
                 Mrs. V's narrative. It seemed aimed at di-
                 verting the men's attention from Mrs. V to
                 Marge, but rarely succeeded. When it did
                 succeed, it often evoked a comment or con-
                 frontation from Malone or Whitaker, as it did
                 in this instance.

POINT 9: <u>Confronting</u> (<u>Malone</u>, <u>occasionally</u> <u>Whitaker</u>)

Malone turns to　　　Interpersonal mode　　Turns back to
Marge from listen-　　to Marge　　　　　　Mrs. V
ing to her mother　　　(TRANSFIX) ⟶　(Juncture)
　　(Juncture) ⟶

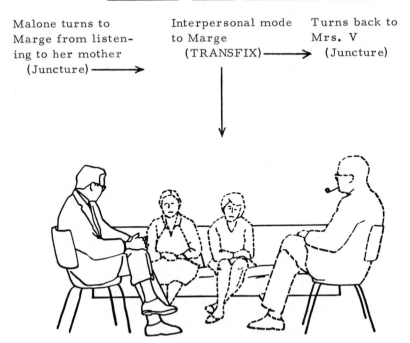

Content:　　　A confrontation often of a critical or sarcastic
3:45　　　nature, which seemed aimed at forcing Marge
to remain quiet and stop being disruptive; in
this case: 'You're the most alive dead person
I've ever met!' Marge had been interrupting
with an assertion that she was dead.

Context:　　　Malone's confronting was immediately followed
by his restarting of Mrs. V's recounting. His
confronting appeared as an interruption in the
mother-daughter disagreements when Marge
was especially histrionic.

POINT 10: Challenging (Whitaker)

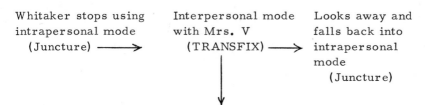

Whitaker stops using   Interpersonal mode   Looks away and
intrapersonal mode   with Mrs. V   falls back into
(Juncture) ——⟶   (TRANSFIX) ——⟶   intrapersonal
                                                          mode
                                                          (Juncture)

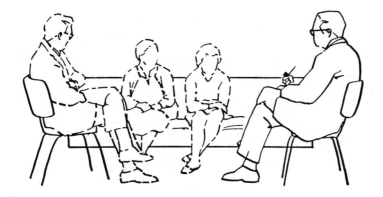

Content: 4:15	A question is asked which implies a challenge to Mrs. V's statement, in this case: 'What do you think she (Marge) meant when she said she was dead?' (Later in the session Whitaker challenged Mrs. V's assertions much more directly.)
Metacommunication:	Whitaker indicated by his clipped abrupt manner that he was not simply asking a question. The challenging character of his point was largely conveyed in the paralanguage.
Context:	Whitaker usually challenged Mrs. V at the same point that Marge accused her and turned appealingly to him. In this instance, Marge had interrupted the narrative with an insinuation: 'Remember I usta get sick to my stomach, remember that?'

POINT 11: <u>Accusing</u> (<u>Marge,</u> occasionally <u>Whitaker</u>)

Marge turns from
listening to Mrs. V
to looking at camera
   (Juncture) ⟶

Extrapersonal
  (TRANSFIX) ⟶

She turns to Malone
  (Juncture)

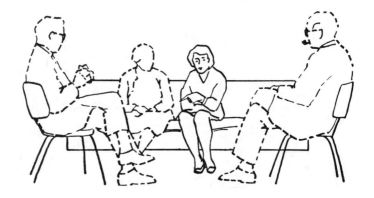

<table>
<tr><td><u>Content:</u>
  4:50</td><td>Marge directly accuses her mother of neglect, mental symptoms, etc. 'She is mentally ill!' (points to her mother)</td></tr>
<tr><td><u>Context:</u></td><td>Marge generally accused her mother at times when Whitaker challenged Mrs. V and when she and Whitaker were sitting in alliance. On this occasion, Mrs. V had been describing Marge's illness and how nervous it made her. Whitaker asked Mrs. V, 'You ever been nervous before?'</td></tr>
</table>

POINT 12: Conceding (Mrs. V; occasionally Marge)

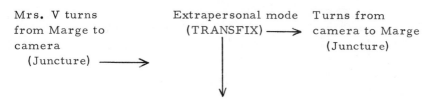

Mrs. V turns   Extrapersonal mode   Turns from
from Marge to   (TRANSFIX) ⟶ camera to Marge
camera   (Juncture)
  (Juncture) ⟶

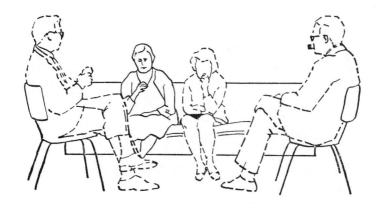

Content: 5:05	Sometimes Mrs. V did not defend but partially agreed to Marge's accusations, in this case: 'Well, I am. I call myself mental. These things make me — the whole world makes me nervous.'
Metacommun- ication:	Overhigh, with laughter, indicating embarrassment and possibly that her concessions are not to be taken literally but are to humor Marge. Note that she addressed the camera.
Context:	When both Marge and Whitaker pressed their challenges to Mrs. V's story, she at times backed down and admitted symptoms or difficulties. In this occurrence, Marge had accused her of being mentally ill.

POINT 13: <u>Disparaging</u> (<u>Marge</u>)

Marge turns away   Intrapersonal mode   Turns to Whitaker
from her mother,   (TRANSFIX) ⟶   (Juncture)
looking into space
    (Juncture) ⟶

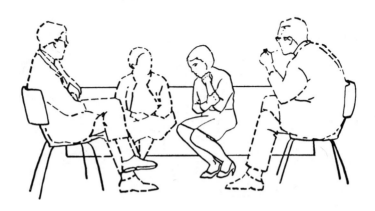

Content: A religious or vulgar epithet, such as 'Maria'
  8:20   or 'fungoo la madre' and a representative or
                    equivalent gesture. With this occurred a look
                    of mock-incredulity.

Context: Disparaging occurred when Mrs. V denied one
                    of Marge's challenges. Its effect seemed to
                    indicate that the denial was unbelievable and
                    Mrs. V's defense was thereby disparaged.

POINT 14: Appealing for Empathy (Marge)

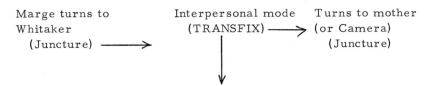

Marge turns to
Whitaker
(Juncture) ———>

Interpersonal mode
(TRANSFIX) ———> (or Camera)

Turns to mother
(Juncture)

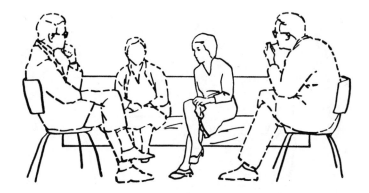

Content: 11:25	Marge turns to Whitaker with appealing or flirtatious behavior, properly crossing her legs or subtly exposing them on occasion. She would say something likely to catch the ear of a psychiatrist sympathetic about maternal deprivation, in this case: 'Remember it was hard for me . . . to breast feed me?'
Metacommun- ication:	Breaking, hesitancy and coyness, indicating that appealing to the men rather than accusation was primary function.
Context:	Appealing occurred at points of making an alliance with Whitaker — replacing, or occurring in addition to, accusing. In this occurrence Whitaker and Mrs. V have been talking about Mrs. V's other child, who died of pneumonia when he was a few weeks old. Whitaker had asked Mrs. V if she thought the child had been taken good care of.

POINT 15: <u>Ironically Supporting Mrs. V</u> (Malone)

Malone turns from
Marge to Mrs. V
  (Juncture) ⟶

Interpersonal to
Mrs. V
  (TRANSFIX) ⟶

From Mrs. V to
Marge
  (Juncture)

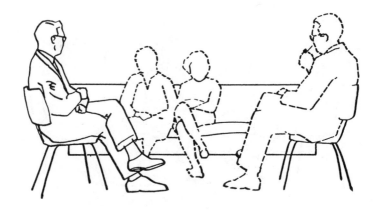

<u>Content:</u>
14:10

Statements seemed to support Mrs. V's position. 'You'd do almost <u>anything</u> for her, wouldn't you?'

<u>Metacommun-</u>
<u>ication:</u>

Heavy primary stress on word <u>anything</u> cues that Malone is not to be taken literally in his exaggerated endorsement of Mrs. V. The comments at first glance seemed supportive, but the linguistic and paralinguistic forms were those characteristic of irony.

<u>Context:</u>

Sometimes when Mrs. V was recounting and no one interrupted, it was Malone, diverging from his usual role of preventing interruption, who interrupted.

POINT 16: <u>Insinuating</u> (<u>Whitaker</u>, <u>Marge</u>)

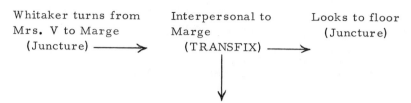

Whitaker turns from
Mrs. V to Marge
(Juncture) ⟶

Interpersonal to
Marge
(TRANSFIX) ⟶

Looks to floor
(Juncture)

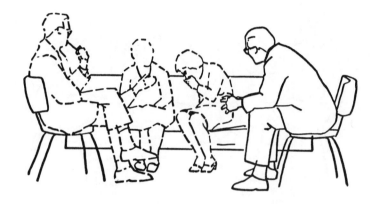

<u>Content:</u>
21:35

Like Marge, Whitaker sometimes made insinuations about Mrs. V but he made them in asides
to Marge, in this case: 'Didn't you know Mother
had wanted you dead.'

<u>Content:</u>

Mrs. V had said that she once told her husband,
'Frank, if she has to go through the eight years
I've gone through, I hope she dies right after
communion.' At times in Mrs. V's account
when Marge was silent and did not insinuate,
accuse or appeal for empathy, Whitaker would
make such insinuations which Marge would pick
up and state as an accusation to her mother.
In this way Whitaker could prompt the alliance
with Marge in which contending occurred.

POINT 17: <u>Shocking</u> (<u>Marge</u>)

Marge turns from vis-à-vis with Whitaker (Juncture) ———→	Intrapersonal mode, looking between Malone and the camera (TRANSFIX) ———→	Turns to Malone (Juncture)

<u>Content:</u>
27:45

When Mrs. V was recounting and both men were attending her account, Marge would often make a very provocative or shocking statement. In this case: 'You wanna see my sin? I won't tell. I <u>will</u> not tell. I did something to my soul. There's not a soul down there.'

<u>Context:</u>

These statements brought the attention of the men to Marge. They were particularly likely to occur if Mrs. V spoke of Marge in an impersonal way. The example above was exceptional in that Marge was already talking to Whitaker but he was being somewhat sarcastic and inattentive to her.

POINT 18: Explaining (Whitaker)

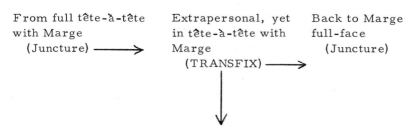

| From full tête-à-tête with Marge (Juncture) ⟶ | Extrapersonal, yet in tête-à-tête with Marge (TRANSFIX) ⟶ | Back to Marge full-face (Juncture) |

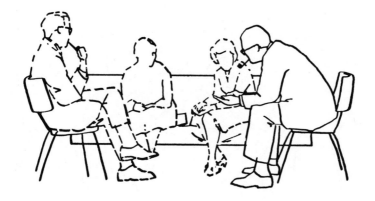

Content:
24:25

Whitaker explained something to the women, beginning as follows: 'Well, we'd like to tell you something of what you're here for.'

Context:

The women had been giving a lengthy account of an incident involving the police and a threat with a knife — Whitaker was engaged in a kinesic preoccupation with an object he had picked up from the floor. This complex shift to explaining is described in Chapter 3.

POINT 19: Contacting (Whitaker and Marge)

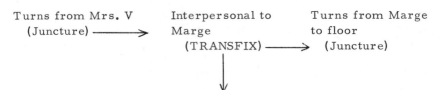

Turns from Mrs. V   Interpersonal to   Turns from Marge
  (Juncture) ————>   Marge   to floor
                                    (TRANSFIX) ————>   (Juncture)

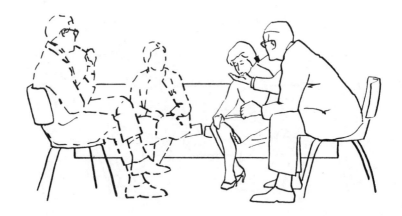

Content: 24:25	'Smell it. Smell it. What does it smell like? It's good parmesian cheese.' Physical contact with Marge.
Context:	The two occasions when Whitaker made physical contact with Marge were not so much related to the lexical account as they were to completion of kinesic series, explained in Chapter 3. Here, Whitaker seemed involved in explaining the purposes of the sessions, when he suddenly put his hand under Marge's nose and requested her to smell his hand.

135

POINT 20: <u>Kleenex Play</u> (<u>Marge</u>, once <u>Malone</u>)

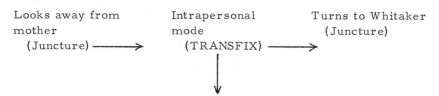

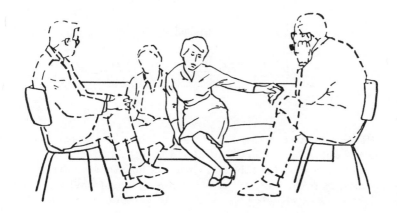

Content: These points were usually nonlexical, consisting
of displays of a Kleenex. In the occurrence
shown above, Marge dropped the Kleenex on the
sofa near Whitaker and said, 'I didn't go through
purgatory.'

Context: Kleenex play occurred when the men ignored
Marge. It ultimately brought both men into relationship with her. In this instance, Mrs. V
had been describing Marge's vomiting attack at
the onset of her psychosis.

SECTION C

Syntheses of the Positions:
Communication in Session I

Introduction:

SYNTHESIS AND THE SOCIAL
LEVEL OF OBSERVATION

Having described the constituent positional units in Section
A and the subunits (at the level of the point) in Section B, we
now tackle the job of synthesis. We ask how these units were
integrated to form the total transaction. Operationally the process consists of showing how each unit was related to the others,
but we will do this level by level.

We quickly see that each unit in Session I occurred in two
kinds of relations.

1. It had a place in a sequence of units which that
    participant performed. It was therefore a step
    in a format for that person's part or role.
2. It had simultaneous relations to the enactments
    of the other participants. The unit was addressed
    to someone and referred to someone. It was per-
    formed with and in accommodation to the unit per-
    formances of the others.

We have, therefore, options of procedure in describing the
synthesis. We can start with sequencing of points and positions
through time and describe the total performance of each participant. Then we can go back and describe how each unit step
was related to the unit performances of the other participants.
Or else we could describe the simultaneous relations of each
point as we go along and then describe the sequences in which
the relations appeared (see Addendum, Section C).

136

I will do both, level by level. In Chapter 6 I will describe both the sequential and interpersonal relations of points in a position and cycle. Then in Chapter 7 I will describe the relations of positions in the phases of Session I. As I describe the behavioral integration here in Section C, I will emphasize the behavioral features which would ordinarily appear in any transaction of the conversational and narrative type. Then, in the subsequent sections of Part II I will retrace my steps and describe features which relate to the cultural background of the women to schizophrenia and to the tactics and strategies of psychotherapy.

When we examine relations between the behavior of various participants, we are making observations at the social level of organization (Redfield 1942; Bertalanffy 1950, 1960; Miller 1965). To do so we must simultaneously watch multiple people, instead of watching one person at a time as we do at the organismic level. It takes some practice to do this. We are used to looking only at the upper body of the main speaker. But the skill can be acquired with conscious effort and the film makes it possible to go over and over the events looking at each participant's contribution.

Relations at the social level are characterized by the same regularities of form which we observed in the less complex units of behavior, because relations, too, are traditional and the agenda of psychotherapy is institutionalized. So the larger integration of behavior is governed by conventions that we can abstract as rules of technique, ettiquette, and ethics comparable to the rules of syntax at the level of the sentence.

As a consequence we cannot explain behavior in a transaction with simplistic conceptions of expression or response alone. A participant does react to others and he does behave metacommunicatively but he also goes on with the enactment of some customary format prescribed for his part in the transaction.

Chapter 6

FORMATS AND RELATIONS AT
THE LEVEL OF THE POSITION

By describing the sequential relation of point units which occurred again and again throughout Session I and demonstrating how these were integrated into positions and relations, I can show the origin of the positions described in Section A. Then we can go on to the two major types of relations, which I will term complementary and reciprocal.

THE REPETITIVE CYCLING OF
POINT UNITS IN SESSION I

As described in Chapter 4, Mrs. V began the session by recounting an episode about the day Marge became psychotic. You will recall the steps in this account:

1. Mrs. V addressed a recounting point to Malone. She quoted Marge as asking to be helped upstairs. Then she intercalated a comment about her daughter: 'A young girl like that.'
2. Then Mrs. V addressed Whitaker and said: 'The next day I thought she'd get better. She has a doctor's prescription.'
3. Then, Mrs. V turned to Marge, who had muttered a comment, and said: 'Did I say anything wrong, dear?'
4. Mrs. V tried to continue her narrative, but Marge mumbled something and Whitaker invited the girl to speak up.

When Marge did speak up, the Period 2 constellation appeared. These steps followed:

5. Marge asked her mother, challengingly: 'Do you hate me?' Mrs. V dismissed the comment.
6. Then Marge and Whitaker broke off their alliance.
7. Malone asked Mrs. V a question, thus restarting her narrative.

Subsequent Repetitions of the Point Sequence

This sequence of point units recurred again and again throughout the session. There were variations at each recurrence. Sometimes, for example, Mrs. V completed a much longer series of recounting points before she was interrupted. Marge's challenges became more and more direct and sometimes Whitaker initiated the first challenge. But the variations did not alter the basic features of these cyclic recurrences. In short, this first cycle was a prototype for point sequences which recurred throughout the entire session.

Consider, for example, the second repetition, which is depicted in the multimodality transcript beginning at 2 minutes:

> In response to Malone's question, Mrs. V recounted her husband's death. She addressed her comments to Malone at first. Marge, as usual, lamented and disparaged.

> At 2 minutes: 20 seconds, Whitaker asked Mrs. V a question and the older woman turned to him and recounted a rather long series of point units.

> At 2 minutes: 45 seconds, Marge lamented to Whitaker, then insinuated that her mother laughed when her husband had died.

The men did not support Marge this time. Instead, Whitaker addressed another question to Mrs. V. At 2 minutes and twenty seconds and at 3 minutes and 12 seconds Whitaker turned away from Marge in a repetition of his point, rejecting. Marge went ahead and challenged her mother without Whitaker's support, but she quickly trailed off and conceded. Malone started to rock forward, so Marge did not shift position and escalate a Period 2 activity. It appeared that an active period of contending was warded off.

At 3 minutes and 40 seconds another repetition of this point sequence began, (I class the sequence as a continuation of Period 1 since the full shift to a Period 2 did not occur):

> Mrs. V again recounted and Marge lamented and disparaged. Mrs. V dismissed the girl's comments. Marge appealed to Whitaker, but the men each performed the nose-wiping monitor and Whitaker turned his head away. He asked Mrs. V another question instead of picking up Marge's insinuation.

Again a Period 2 did not occur. But the point cycle immediately began again and this time did eventuate in a full Period 2.

There is no point in describing subsequent point cycles one after the other. They followed this same basic pattern of sequence throughout the session — even in Phase II when the relationships and roles changed. So it will be more economical to abstract the pattern and generalize about it, as I have in previous chapters.

Notice that the behaviors of each participant influence the others' sequence. Their actions bring about some modification or the use of an alternative performance. But in each case the format was ultimately adhered to. The performer got back in some measure to his original part. His previous position was resumed, though modified.

Point Cycles in the Position

The reader already knows that these sequences of points were integrated into one or more positions in the performance of each individual. Each person performed one or more positions in each period and there were two fully developed periods to a cycle (I will simply remind you of the positional cycles in each performance).

Mrs. V's Format of Positions in a Cycle

Mrs. V performed two positions in each cycle as follows:

A. Explaining which consisted of a sequence of recounting points, in which defending and disparaging points were sometimes intercalated. The sequence was addressed from a spot next to Marge toward Malone, then toward Whitaker.

B. Maintaining which consisted of a sequence of defending points, often ending with conciliating or conceding, and sometimes interspersed with points more typical for other participants; e. g. , ironic supporting, confronting, insinuating, disparaging, and questioning. This sequence was addressed to Marge.

Marge's Format of Positions in a Cycle

Marge carried off two well-developed and lasting positions in each cycle:

A. Passive protesting which consisted of a sequence of disparaging and lamenting points, to which she added insinuations. This position was addressed to the men, the camera, and to the floor.
B. Contending which consisted of a sequence of challenging, accusing, and insinuating points, usually followed by conciliating and/or conceding.

Marge tried to escalate challenging point units to a position of contending while she was in the position of passive protesting. These did not come off, but she did intercalate a number of brief positions in each cycle.

C. In transition between passive protesting and contending, Marge intercalated a point of appealing and sometimes a position of appealing and lamenting, which was addressed to Whitaker. At the end of a Period 2, she would again turn to Whitaker and enact the point, repelling. Through the entire cycle Marge was likely to enact an escalating sequence of nonlanguage point units, quasi-courting and Kleenex play.
D. In either phase of this cycle Marge might intercalate the brief positions, interfering or resigning.

Whitaker's Positional Format

A. Whitaker maintained a position of listening and questioning. In Period 1 he would question Mrs. V, but he would tend to pick up Marge's insinuations and challenges as Period 1 progressed. When Marge enacted repelling or when Malone intervened, Whitaker would use the point rejecting to break off the relation with Marge and the cycle would then terminate.

Malone's Positional Format

    A. Malone maintained a position of listening and questioning. He would primarily attend to Mrs. V in a Period 1, then shift to Marge in a Period 2.

    B. Then he would intervene, confront Marge, and restart Mrs. V's narrative, thus ending a Period 2 or warding off its occurrence.

    C. In the first 5 and the last 12 minutes Malone moved in synchrony with Marge, a behavior which I will later claim indicated some covert alliance between them.

The repetition of these periods and cycles produced a structure which is diagrammed in Figure 6-1.

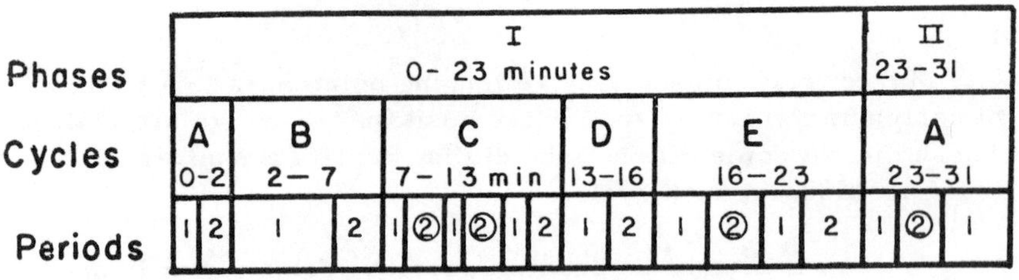

Phases	I — 0-23 minutes					II — 23-31
Cycles	A (0-2)	B (2-7)	C (7-13 min)	D (13-16)	E (16-23)	A (23-31)
Periods	1 2	1 2	1 ② 1 ② 1 2	1 2	1 ② 1 2	1 ② 1

Figure 6-1: Diagram of the Structure of Session I

THE COMPLEMENTARY RELATIONS OF POSITIONS

At any moment of time, of course, each participant was engaged in some one of these point performances and the behaviors of each point were interrelated. A number of types of such relations occurred. Consider first two such types which had a common quality.

Complementary Sequences of Language

In each Period 1 of these cycles Marge and her mother repeatedly performed in a collaborative way and addressed the behavior to the men. Just before and early in any Period 2, Marge and Whitaker showed a conjoint enactment of a similar type.

The Complementary Sequence Between Mrs. V and Marge

As Mrs. V recounted, Marge would disparage or make an insinuation about what her mother was saying. Often Marge would match one such point with each of Mrs. V's recounting points. Here is an example which began at 2 minutes: 40 seconds:

Mrs. V:	'He [her husband] had to go back to the hospital — un he died.'
Marge:	'I died!'
Mrs. V:	'But nobody could stop his death.'
Marge:	'Yep. I died. (to Whitaker) . . . Did you? (to her mother)'
Mrs. V:	'How could I stop the . . . .'
Marge:	'I cried. You laughed.'

Often the parallel metacommunicative points of disparagement that Marge used were kinesic — a look of mock incredulity, a shrug of the shoulders and upright palm gesture (which seemed to indicate: 'What can one do about a comment like that'), or a mocking imitation.

Notice the character of this relation: a metacommunicative reaction was made to a communicative utterance. Both points were ordinarily addressed to the men.

The point performances of Marge in the sequence quoted above had an additional quality of lamenting. Sometimes this quality was pronounced. Marge would match every comment her mother made with a lament parallel to her mother's recounting point in address and duration.

The Complementary Sequences Between Marge and Whitaker

Marge would make an insinuation about her mother or maybe an insinuation combined with a lament. She might repeat this several times in various forms. Then Whitaker would sometimes pick up the idea and reformulate it as a challenging question to Mrs. V. When Whitaker picked up the challenge in this manner, Marge would shift to contending and a Period 2 constellation would be initiated.

The sequence quoted below led to the first occurrence of Period 2. Notice that Mrs. V and Malone also participated in this first occurrence.

At 20 seconds Marge whispered something.

Whitaker:	'Why don't you say what you wanted to say now, Marge.'
Marge:	'Gonna go to hell.'
Whitaker:	'What was that you started to say before when Mother sort of stopped you or you sorta stopped yourself.'
Marge:	'Yes I did stop it. I did.'
Mrs. V:	'You stopped what?'
Marge:	'Getting angry.'
Malone:	'Getting angry at whom, Marge?'
Mrs. V:	'You stopped getting angry?'

If the members of an alliance carry out the same type of behaviors one after another, Birdwhistell (1967) calls it tandemic sequencing. These sequences ended up with one person (usually Whitaker or Marge) addressing a remark about another person to a third person. Thus Marge, for instance, commented on what her mother said: 'She is mentally ill.' She pointed to her mother, but addressed the remark to Whitaker. At the end of another such sequence Whitaker said to Marge: 'She [Mrs. V] is saying the devil was your father.'

As we will see, the metacommunicative comment can be addressed to someone, as the men tended to do, or it can be made about someone, but addressed to someone else. Ordinarily we would call this configuration, 'talking about someone.'

The Side-by-Side Relation

These complementary relations were almost invariably performed by people who sat side by side. Marge sat near and like her mother, when she commented on Mrs. V's account. When Whitaker took up Marge's insinuations and restated them, Marge got up and sat nearer to him and in the posture he was using.

Side-by-side positioning in a group is an indication of corroboration such as would be expected in an established relationship. It ordinarily occurs between relatives, spouses, colleagues, or allies.[1] Thus Marge sat side by side with her mother in any Period 1. But she shifted to sitting as close to a side-by-side position with Whitaker as she could whenever he supported her and allied with her against Mrs. V.

In a side-by-side relationship the partners address in common a mutual task or a third party (or parties). Thus Mrs. V and Marge, when side by side, addressed the men. But in Period 2 when Marge was, in effect, side by side with Whitaker, she came into a face-to-face address with Mrs. V.

Congruent Postures an Interactional Synchrony

Two or more members of a side-by-side complementarity[2] will probably be in the same posture. Not only will they be oriented in the same direction but at least half their bodies will show a postural isomorphism. For example, each member will have his arms crossed, his left leg crossed over his right, and each will be leaning to his left. Another subgrouping of participants may be present who share a different postural set; for instance they may all have their feet together on the floor, their hands clasped on their laps, and their heads cocked to the same side.[3] These postural isomorphisms, direct or mirror-imaged, I call parallelism (Scheflen 1964). Charny (1966), describing the same phenomena, used the term, 'postural congruence.' In any period Marge and Mrs. V showed such parallelism. But in Period 2, Marge would sit as Whitaker did (Figure 6-2).

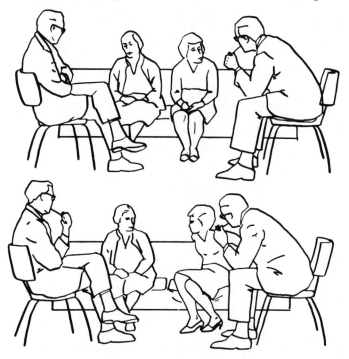

Figure 6-2: Marge in Complementarity With Her Mother; Then With Whitaker

Participants in parallel postures are likely to show synchronous movement; they puff on their cigarettes at the same

time, use similar facial expressions, direct their gazes coor-
dinatively, sometimes say the same things, and gesture alike.
Condon and Ogston (1966, 1967), using high-speed filming,
have shown that people in established relations also show synchrony of micromovements at a 'beat' of about a forty-eighth of
a second.

In general, people in parallelism and synchrony are acting
as a social unit.[4] In psychoanalytic terms, they are said to be
'identified.' But they may be following a common traditional program and need not be copying each other.

Dissociation

It is apparent that Marge was not an agreeable and cooperative partner in the mother-daughter side-by-side relation. She
indicated this in speech and gesture, as I have described. She
also indicated this by intervals of dissociation. She would sprawl
back on the sofa in the position of 'resigning.' For a few seconds
she would not engage in the activities of the session. She would
turn her head away from the others, fall into a marked hypotonus,
and appear depressed and apathetic. In these periods she did not
sit near or like her mother.

At other times Marge would partially dissociate. She would
not sprawl, but she would look down, cover her face, and seem
not to be interested in the behavior of the others. But she would
maintain her parallelism of posture and she would make comments under her breath. When we could hear these, it was evident that they were relevant to the immediate account her mother
was providing. She only appeared to be dissociated or, one
might say, her address was discontinued (Figure 6-3).

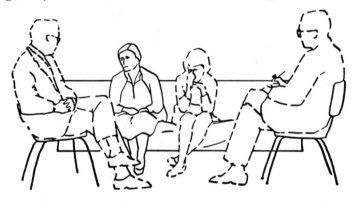

Figure 6-3: Marge Dissociated in All Modalities Except Speech

Such dissociation can be emphasized or exaggerated. A participant can make a point of not agreeing or not participating in an alliance or side-by-side relation. I think this is what Marge was doing.
Whitaker acted similarly in turning his head away from Marge.

Defining a Complementarity

So the basic feature of a complementarity is not a 'felt' affiliation or agreement. The basic characteristic seems to be the shared enactment of a single role or part. The partners share in a
division of labor — something that one of them could do alone. So
Mrs. V and Marge were to present a history that Mrs. V could
have provided without Marge. And Marge and Whitaker came into
a side-by-side relationship in a shared confrontation with Mrs. V.

In formal ritualized activities like group dancing and singing,
the partners in a side-by-side relation may perform exactly the
same way synchronously and in unison.

RECIPROCAL RELATIONS IN SESSION I

Vis-à-vis Configurations in Periods 1 and 2

In any Period 1 the two women sat side by side with each other
and faced the men vis-à-vis (Figure 6-4). At the level of the position, this constellation can be diagrammed as follows:

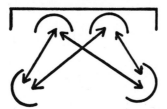

Sometimes Marge would dissociate herself, looking down or
away, and Mrs. V would face the men alone.

In any Period 2 Marge and Mrs. V came into a well-developed
vis-à-vis relationship with each other. (In a Period 1 when Marge
contended with her mother, but did not stand up and turn her
whole body, she came into a partial vis-à-vis relation with her
mother.) The Period 2 constellation could be diagrammed as
follows:

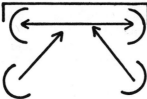

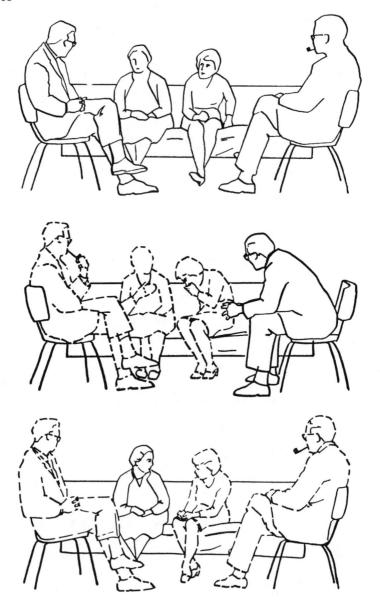

Figure 6-4: The Major Vis-à-vis Relations of Session I.
Top: In recounting, the two women face the men,
turning from one man to the other. Middle:
When Marge dissociated, Mrs. V turned alternately to Malone and Whitaker. Bottom: In
contending and maintaining the women faced each
other.

The Transitional Vis-à-Vis

Just before Marge shifted to the Period 2 arrangement for confronting her mother, she would come briefly into a vis-à-vis with Whitaker. As she returned to sitting with her mother at the end of a Period 2, she would also face Whitaker for a few seconds as they repelled and rejected each other. In these instances Mrs. V would turn and address Malone. As a consequence the group briefly broke down into two separate twosomes (Figure 6-5).

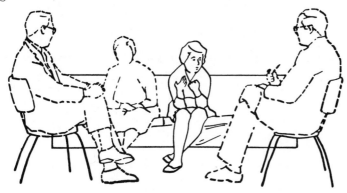

Figure 6-5: The Brief Transitional Twosomes of Session I.
Above: Before contending Marge lamented or appealed to Whitaker. Two dissociated reciprocals then occurred. Below: Before she returned to sitting with mother Marge would turn back to Whitaker and act 'repellingly.' (In the motion picture frame traced above she was captured turning from Whitaker while exhibiting her legs)

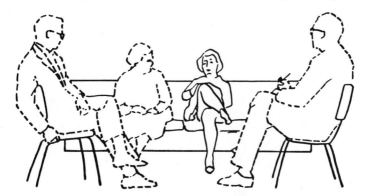

Chronologically, then, the vis-à-vis configurations appeared in each full or abortive cycle in the following order:

In a Period 1:   The women and men were face to face
                 (except that Marge was sometimes
                 dissociated). Then two twosomes
                 appeared temporarily as Marge and
                 Whitaker faced each other and Mrs.
                 V concentrated on Malone.

In a Period 2:   The women came into a vis-à-vis
                 while the men watched. Then Marge
                 and Whitaker turned to each other to
                 break off their alliance.

People who are related in a vis-à-vis orientation characteristically interact or reciprocate with each other. They so something to each other; feed each other, or court or groom or mate or else inform each other.[5]   If people are to carry out such reciprocation they will ordinarily stand or sit down facing each other. If they are not facing they will turn to each other when they begin to interact. If people find themselves in a face-to-face relation, they are more or less constrained to reciprocal behaviors, and they may have to actively inhibit such behavior if for some reason they are not to engage in it. In situations like Session I, in which two people in complementarity do not agree, they will characteristically turn to each other and try to recalibrate their relationship.

Thus Mrs. V and Marge often turned face to face for a brief argument followed by an attempt at reconciliation. Whitaker and Malone only exchanged glances once in the entire session. (This was when Marge lamented that they were watching her get angry at her mother.) I will describe the complementary relation of the men's behavior in Section E.

The behaviors among participants in a vis-à-vis relation is basically different than the complementary relation in a side-by-side arrangement. It takes at least two people to behave reciprocally.

The sequencing of reciprocal behavior may consist of simple action-reaction or interactional sequences, or such sequences may escalate or progress. Both of these types often occurred in the vis-à-vis relations of Session I as I will now illustrate.

Simple Reactive Sequences

In the simplest case one participant will ask a question and the other will answer him. But often, especially in psychotherapy,

the response is not a simple question. A communicative
action triggers a metacommunicative response.

Question and Answer Sequences

Ordinarily, for instance, a speaker makes a statement to
which someone responds with a question. This question is followed by a reply which may elicit a further question. Such
sequencing often is called interaction. For example, just after
five minutes in Session I, Mrs. V admitted she had mind pictures (hallucinations):

> Whitaker: 'What kind of mind pictures are they,
> Mother?'
> Mrs. V: 'I don t know, sort of things that come
> to my mind and . . .'
> Whitaker: 'Can you give us an example?'
> Mrs. V: 'Like I never studied in school . . . on
> account of those French people . . . .'

Communicative-Metacommunicative Sequences

But Whitaker's questions were not usually simple requests
for detail. As the session proceeded he loaded his questions
with suggestive paralanguage and they took on the quality of confrontations. For example, at 14 minutes: 41 seconds Mrs. V
denied that she had ever been sick, but Whitaker said, 'Can you
tell us about the last time you were sick?'
Psychotherapists will recognize this type of questioning.
The question constitutes an indirect challenge to the metaconceptions of the patient. It may be framed gingerly and ambiguously
so the patient can ignore the implication and answer literally if
he is unable or unwilling to pursue the matter (see Chapter 11).

Programmed Reciprocation

Interviewing

Such sequences are likely to be escalated. A progressive
series of alternative behaviors follow a tact or move toward a
focus. In the sequence below Whitaker interviews Marge, leading her toward a more specific statement.

> Whitaker: 'Do you think you understand her [Mrs. V]
> any better than you did before you collapsed?'
> Marge: 'Whew: What? . . . Oh . . . I don't under-
> stand that kind of talk.'

Whitaker:	'Can you tell us about some of that. How . . . how she talks crazy to you.'
Marge:	'I'm dead.'
Whitaker:	'You're dead.'
Marge:	'I'm dead somewhere. I'm dead. Dead I am. I can't control myself anymore. I can't control myself. I can't even mortal sin.'
Whitaker:	'Your mother control you? Do you think mother can control you?'
Marge:	'You know . . . Yes.'
Whitaker:	'Has she always controlled you?'
Marge:	'Yes. You know what I did to myself. She knows. She knows.'

The Quasi-Courting and Kleenex Play Reciprocals

The nonlexical sequences also tended to be escalated according to a pattern. Thus on two occasions Marge took out a Kleenex, blew her nose, then waved the Kleenex about, and finally plopped it down on the sofa near Whitaker. On one of these occasions Whitaker picked it up and handed it to her, thus initiating the first tactile contact. And Whitaker's hand-play sequence also built up to a tactile contact.

The same escalation occurred with the quasi-courting behavior. Marge would begin a sequence by sitting up and daintily crossing her ankles. She would then cock her head, put her hand on her hip, smile, and become increasingly coquettish. Then she would either cross her legs or exhibit her thighs. As she did this she and Whitaker would exchange glances. She would 'point' her courtship-like behavior to him and address appeals. Finally on some occasions he would move in toward her and face her so the transitional tête-à-tête configurations would occur (Figure 6-6).

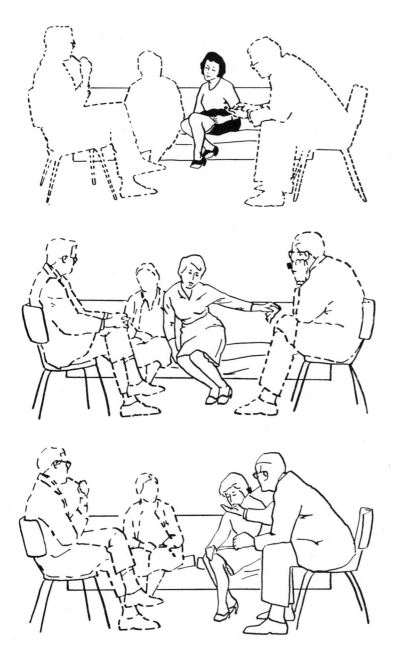

Figure 6-6: Behaviors in Formation of the Whitaker-Marge
Relationship

The Alliance-Breaking Reciprocals

The sequence of mutual rejection between Marge and Whitaker at the end of a Period 2 also escalated in a regular pattern: Marge would sprawl, then cross her legs in a bizarre caricature of sexy behavior (Figure 6-7), making a sexy, provocative comment as she crossed her legs. Whitaker would then turn his head away from her. Marge would then look away from Whitaker. She would lower her head, appear dejected, and look to Malone, who was rocked forward in his chair to confront her. Then Marge would stand up and move back to sitting near and like her mother.

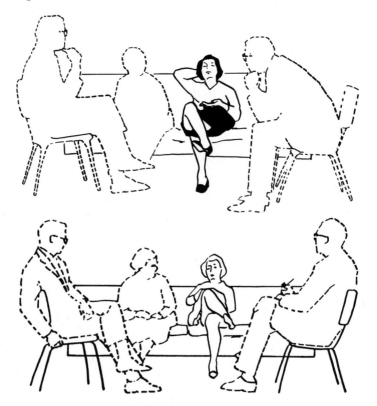

Figure 6-7: Behaviors in the Disaffiliation of Marge and
Whitaker (End of Period 2)

It is difficult to claim that participants in sequences like these are merely responding to each other. Such reciprocal escalations occur again and again in the same form. They appear to follow a format and thus be programmed.[6] They do not seem to be innovated for the occasion or arrived at by trial and error.

Many of the reciprocals of common culture are like this. In courting, for example, there may be an alternation of actions, but these escalate toward an ultimate goal and follow a traditional format.

In a game the moves follow each other, but usually they do not simply alternate in a cyclic way. Each move requires a progressive countermove and, once it has been made, the situation is no longer the same.

So I will reserve the term interaction for sequences in which it appears that each action does induce the other.[7] But I will speak of sequences as reciprocal relations if they seem to be precalibrated (Bateson 1958). If the participants are following a customary program they will respond not only to what the other person has just done, but also to what they can expect as a usual next step. For example, in the case of the disaffiliation between Marge and Whitaker, I do not think either of them were simply responding to a rejection. The pattern could be initiated by either of them. It occurred just as Malone rocked forward. Although the series was exaggerated by Marge's particular manner of performance, it is a common reciprocal in a transaction, used to terminate an inappropriate relation and get back to the usual definition of that situation.

Whenever participants are engaged in such programmed reciprocals they are likely to show synchronous and postural parallelism, just as they do when they are behaving in a complementary alliance. It is therefore likely that parallel postures and interactional synchrony indicate common involvement in some traditional format of behavior, whatever their roles and relationships.

MULTIPLE SIMULTANEOUS RELATIONS

I would like to remind the reader of something about relations which I detailed in Section B. In Session I the participants were not in complementary reciprocal relations exclusively. They were, rather, almost always in both simultaneously, side by side with one participant while facing another. Marge, for instance, would disparage her mother's behavior in complementarity while she looked at and appealed to Whitaker.

This type of multiple engagement occurred throughout Session I and unified the various relations to make a single social organization. Thus Whitaker and Malone related reciprocally to the women and in complementarity to each other and so did the women. And Whitaker would relate reciprocally to Mrs. V while in complementarity with Marge.

From the standpoint of any individual, we would say he is multiply engaged. He may sit side by side with one person, speak to another, and touch a third. Marge is shown in such relations in the upper drawing of Figure 6-8. She is in the act of shifting back to a side-by-side relation with her mother and away from Whitaker. In the process she temporarily addressed Malone.

From the standpoint of the group a configuration of multiple simultaneous relations coexists. In the lower half of Figure 6-7, Whitaker and Malone are partly side by side, each facing the women. The women are side by side, oriented to the men in their torso position, but face to face with each other.

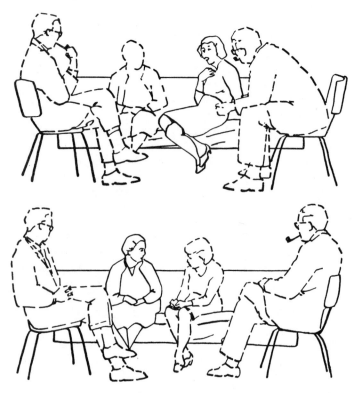

Figure 6-8: Multiple Simultaneous Relations in Session I

COMMENT: CUSTOMARY RELATIONS IN
A NARRATIVE TYPE OF TRANSACTION

In the main the relations which I have described here are characteristic of narrative and conversational transactions like Session I.

The Customary Side by Side, Complementary Relations

Some features of the mother-daughter relationship in Session I are by no means usual. We would not usually see the bizarre exaggeration of postural shifting or of courting behavior which Marge used, nor the huddling against her mother. But the basic features of side-by-side relations with intervals of turning toward each other are quite characteristic of a mother-daughter relationship in conversation with outsiders. Whenever two or more people have an established relationship in which they are not afforded an equal status, they will be expected to sit side by side.

In Figure 6-9 I have drawn the configuration of seating in another psychotherapy session. A husband and wife here are facing a therapist.

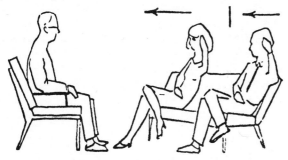

Figure 6-9: A Threesome Arrangement in Which a Husband and Wife Sit Side by Side Facing a Therapist

It is also characteristic for partners in a side-by-side relation to turn to each other whenever they disagree or need to recalibrate their shared role. They may indicate nonagreement by dissociating. If one of the partners initiates a flirtation, or even if he merely looks unrelated and searches the room with his eyes, he invites relationship from someone outside the partnership and the complementarity may break down with the formation of new alliances as it did periodically in Session I.

We assume that an established relationship is reciprocal in private. The members turn to each other and service each other. But in public the established reciprocal opens up to provide access to others. It becomes a complementarity for exchanging information with outsiders and a developing relationship with these outsiders may be allowed. Thus a dyadic mother-daughter vis-à-vis relation is periodically formed to feed, groom, and teach the child, but it will open to allow mother and daughter to relate to a husband-father and later to a suitor or a psychotherapist (see Chapter 9).

In our culture, at least, when members of an established relationship come together with relative strangers the rule for orientation and seating seems to be something like this. The members of the established relationships will sit on the same side of the room facing each other. The status figures of each subgroup will be afforded the primary vis-à-vis positions and their juniors will array at their sides.

Each partner in a side-by-side arrangement ordinarily carries out a specialized subpart in a customary role. In this case the side-by-side partners will use postural parallelism and synchronous movement. If these partners are of equal status, they will usually sit at the same height and at the same distance from the others in the vis-à-vis. Thus when Marge contested Mrs. V's occupation of the floor she sat upright exactly like Mrs. V. If one partner is subordinate he will sit lower, farther back, and tend to keep his head down. He takes a less active part, at least in speaking. His behavior is essentially supplementary, though he may be afforded a 'turn' for more active participation.

Thus I think of Mrs. V as the primary, initial narrator in Session I. In Phase I Marge was a 'supplementary' narrator. She was sometimes afforded a turn by Whitaker and she sometimes tried to usurp the position, whereupon she was confronted and rejected.

The Reciprocal Relations in a Narrative

In a conversation some narrator addresses the other persons who are in a vis-à-vis relation with him. His remarks are ordinarily addressed to all of those of roughly equal status. Thus the supplementary narrator and the other side-by-side partners are not directly addressed.

At sites where conversation is traditionally held, the furniture is usually arranged for such a configuration. Large chairs face each other, for instance. In large groups a lectern or rostrum faces rows of chairs for the audience. In a semi-circular arrangement, major chairs are often at the ends of the semi-circle.

Session I was held in a room which was arranged as a living room, with two chairs facing a sofa.

If three principal speakers are present, the seating arrangement may be triangular and each narrator traverses his head to speak to two other vis-à-vis partners, as Mrs. V did when Marge was dissociated.

If only two people are present they may sit facing each other, but they will not usually close their orientations into a complete vis-à-vis unless they are on very intimate terms. In psychotherapy, for instance, where there is one patient and one therapist, the two participants will ordinarily sit somewhat at right angles to each other, as I have depicted in Figure 6-10.

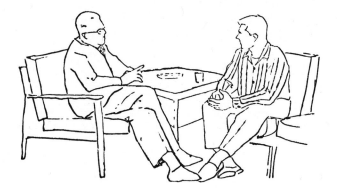

Figure 6-10: Therapist and Patient Sitting at Angles. They thus include each other and the camera with only a turn of the head. They also avoid a full vis-à-vis of total bodies which makes leg room scarce and implies an intimate relationship.

But the therapist and patient will come into a more and more complete vis-à-vis relationship as they enter a state of rapport. In a group larger than two, such complete vis-à-vis relations will exclude the others and break the group into subgroups.

The listeners in a conversation conventionally are enjoined to face the speaker, remain relatively quiet, and from time to time provide comprehension signals and affirmations.

Whitaker and Malone were co-listeners at the beginning of Session I. Accordingly they at first used the positions which are typical in this role. They suppressed their own speaking, addressed the narrator, and sat back slightly hunched down in their seats. They assumed attentive facial expressions and occasionally signaled comprehension (see Chapter 4).

Proper listeners are thus constrained to limit their speaking to questions and points of order and support the narrative with attentiveness. They are also constrained to limit nonrelevant behavior. They are to avoid attention to participants other than the speaker.

If you recall the times you have tried to complete a complicated narrative in the presence of an itchy child, you can gain some recollection of the amount of activity which could occur as noise in a transaction and you can guess at the years of training it takes to make a disciplined participant. Also recall the amount of irrelevant or partly relevant mental activity you carry out during a transaction. A tremendous amount of 'nonperformance' thus occurs in accommodating as a listener.

Such suppression is evident in a kind of active nonmobility. The body shows signs of hypertonicity or tension. The hands are often held crossed or closed, or over the genitals or the mouth, and one hand may actively restrain the other. And the legs may be crossed and one foot locked behind the other ankle. If listeners are smokers, they will commonly smoke while listening. Psychotherapists discipline themselves to an even more marked immobility in the position of listening. Sometimes they hardly move at all.

But even the most disciplined listeners are not entirely impassive. They will show perceptible microbehaviors. Their eyes narrow, their nostrils flare. The skin blanches and reddens. The lips are pursed and sucking movements may occur. Rings are touched, the fingers are steepled. The feet are pointed, shaken, waved, and so on.

It is therefore possible to make psychoanalytic inferences about the participants' cognitive and affective states, even though they are not speaking. In communicational language, some of these behaviors are metacommunicative reactions, which may refer to attitudes about the speaker's behavior and they thus may influence and alter it. And others of these behaviors represent abortive performances which indicate suppressed plans from which we may infer motives. So the listeners' nonparticipation is relative. When Mrs. V narrated, Malone was markedly controlled, Whitaker less so, and Marge continually was overtly active.

The Narrative Format

The narrator will follow some format in developing his narrative. He may make a generalization, then fill in details or substantiations. He may list details and then draw a conclusion. Or he may narrate events in a chronological order as Mrs. V did.

But the format will ordinarily include intervals for questions or comments. Mrs. V sometimes paused, I think for this purpose, but ordinarily she was interrupted. The narrative format may also provide time for the supplementary narrator to add ideas or details. Occasionally Mrs. V did invite Marge to speak more audibly. And the format ordinarily provides that a principal narrator will complete his account, and turn over the floor to some other narrator for the presentation of his views.

Thus there is an over-all format for a conversation which provides parts for all the participants. This format is generally known in common culture, followed by the participants, and enforced when it is violated. We ordinarily abstract the rules of the format as etiquette.

Chapter 7

THE TOTAL STRUCTURE OF SESSION I

In general each cycle in Session I followed the narrative programming I have described. Mrs. V would take the position of explaining and begin the narrative. Marge would use the supplementary narrator's role in the position of passive protesting. Whitaker and Malone would take the position of listening and questioning.

But five full cycles and a like number of partial cycles appeared. Then at twenty-three minutes a second phase of the session appeared. These divisions of the session were diagrammed earlier in Figure 6-1.

The successive repetitions of the cycle were similar in structure, but by no means identical. Certain dimensions of behavior showed progressive change or escalation from cycle to cycle. Thus the total transaction had phases and an agenda, so there was at least one level of behavioral integration higher than the position and the cycle.

The three following interdependent developments were especially noteworthy and will be described in this chapter:

An Accural of Information
A Progressive Development of the Marge-Whitaker
    Relationship
A shift in the parts and relations of the session.

THE ACCRUAL OF INFORMATION
IN THE SUCCESSIVE CYCLES

Although the women kept repeating the same basic positions, each recurrence brought further elucidation of the two main

162

subthemes of the narrative — the history of Marge's illness and the early history of the V family. These are, of course, typical topics in a psychotherapy session.

Thus the positional configurations kept repeating, but the content progressively changed. Consequently information accrued, which is also typical in a narrative conversation such as psychotherapy.

The Initial Topic: Marge's Psychotic Episode

The story of Marge's illness was a primary topic. Malone explicitly and repeatedly asked Mrs. V about the subject and Mrs. V spoke of the issue in three of the cycles. In the first Period 1, you will recall that Mrs. V spoke of Marge's helplessness.

In the third Period 1 Mrs. V began at a chronologically earlier place and added an account of the events that preceded the request to be helped upstairs. Mrs. V said, 'She came home for lunch and she . . . she often did. She says, 'Mother, I feel sick.' 'Oh', I says, 'take a cup of tea.' 'No, Mother, you don't understand, I'm really sick.' 'Oh' I says. I don't wanna have it on my soul, so I called the doctor and he gave her a prescription. And, then, uh, 'Gimme a glass of water. Hold me up, Mother, to drink it. Help me upstairs ta . . .' Oh, an eighteen-year-old girl. I got nervous. Is she . . . was she that sick? The next day she . . .'

In the next Period 1, Mrs. V started at the place marked by the phrase, 'the next day she,' and continued the narrative of Marge's psychotic break with a next episode: 'She . . . The next thing I thought she was gettin' better, then she starts to vomit . . . .'

Then Mrs. V told of Marge's vomiting, calling in the relatives, leaving her to go to mass, calling in a priest, sending her to her aunt's house, and eventually to the hospital. The reader can follow the account beginning at twelve minutes in the transcript in Appendix A.

The Second Topic: Earlier Episodes in the V Family History

Marge and Whitaker pushed Mrs. V to talk about other episodes in Marge's childhood. Marge would insinuate that a significant experience was being ignored, then she or Whitaker would question Mrs. V about it. In this way a number of episodes from Marge's childhood were aired.

In cycle A Marge hinted she was mad at her mother. Mrs. V dismissed this comment by saying everyone gets mad.

Marge backed down and in fact blamed men for 'watching her get angry at her mother.'

In cycle B Marge claimed that her mother had laughed when the father died. Mrs. V vigorously denied this charge and Marge backed down. Mrs. V did admit she had not missed her husband at first.

In cycle C Marge made a series of accusations, each of which Mrs. V denied. She at first denied talking about her hallucinations to Marge. She denied that Marge was psychotic. She denied neglecting her son. She denied that her husband was nervous and that there had been a problem between Marge and the father. She denied ever committing a mortal sin and insisted that her husband, not she, was the boss of the family.

In cycle D Mrs. V again denied memory of an incident that Marge considered important — a scene in which Marge recalled seeing her parents struggling on the bed.

In cycle E Marge held that Mrs. V had attacked her husband with a knife and the neighbors called the police. Mrs. V reluctantly admitted that part of the story was true.

Directly Observable Information About the Women

Since the men were able, of course, to observe the women's behavior, they obtained information beyond that which the women revealed in their language. As I will describe later such observation was one of the explicit purposes in Session I, and they told us later that they moved in at 23 minutes because they had collected sufficient ideas about the women to act on these and impinge on the pattern.

We cannot assume that nothing is happening in a transaction simply because the same basic positions and relations keep recurring. Each of the formats of Session I were used in the service of progressively developing plans. So the format for behavior in a transaction is not a rigid, stereotyped imposition, but a guideline for a type of activity. A format may be altered and used in a variety of ways.

DEVELOPMENT OF THE
MARGE-WHITAKER RELATIONSHIP

Although the Marge-Whitaker alliance dissolved and reformed in every cycle, it showed a progressive development. At each recurrence it was more overt, more stable, more quickly enjoined, and more aggressive in its confrontation of Mrs. V.

The Structure of Each Recurrence

Consider once again the pattern of address in each recurrence. At the beginning of a Period 2 (or whenever Marge
attempted to initiate one), Marge and Whitaker would briefly
face each other. Then, Marge would turn to confront her
mother. After the confrontation Marge and Whitaker would
break off their alliance and Marge would return to sitting with
her mother in passive protesting.

This sequence could be diagrammed as follows:

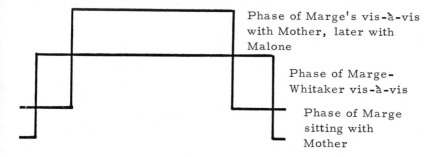

Phase of Marge's vis-à-vis
with Mother, later with
Malone

Phase of Marge-
Whitaker vis-à-vis

Phase of Marge
sitting with
Mother

It was as though Marge had to turn to Whitaker to form a
relationship, which she would then use as a supportive alliance
in contending with her mother. In later sessions she used the
alliance with Whitaker as a base for flirting with Malone and
talking about sex with him.

The Pattern of Escalation

Marge kept returning to sitting with her mother, but each
time the phase of active confrontation lasted longer. And each
time she was more aggressive in her insinuations and challenges.
She and Whitaker also came to be closer and closer in interpersonal distance as Whitaker moved in toward her. And Whitaker
took more and more an overt role in supporting Marge's challenges.

Decreasing Interpersonal Distance

In any small group there are conventional spacing arrangements. There are relatively standard distances between the
participants, depending on their relationships and dominance
and what they are doing.[1] Since the distances are standard within a culture, but vary with social class and ethnic background,

they communicate to others something of the character of the transaction and instruct the participants about the propriety and expectations of the situations. A man and a woman, for example, will use one distance in an intimate interchange, another in a personal conversation, and a third in a formal meeting (Hall 1963, 1966).

In early Period I's the interpersonal distances were as follows: Mrs. V and Marge sat together on a sofa, close enough that their bodies were touching, a distance more usual for a mother and small daughter in the presence of company. The men began the session at such a distance that their faces were about six feet from the women's faces, a usual distance for non-intimate conversation and for the initial stages of family psychotherapy.

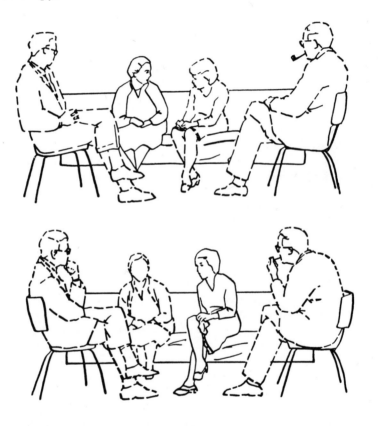

Figure 7-1A: Marge and Whitaker in Cycles B and C

At each cycle Marge moved farther from her mother and closer to Whitaker. In later Period 2s Marge was about four feet from her mother, a marked distance for a side-by-side pair. The same moving away brought her closer each time to Whitaker. In later Period 2s she was less than three feet from him. Whitaker also moved. At each six-minute interval he moved forward in his chair until he came to be closer than three feet from Marge. Thus in successive Period 1s, even though the girl went back to huddling against her mother, she was increasingly closer to Whitaker.

Thus, moving together occurred in such stages that some parameter of greater closeness was introduced periodically, adapted to, then further increased. The four stages of Whitaker's approximation are depicted in the sequence of drawings in Figure 7-1.

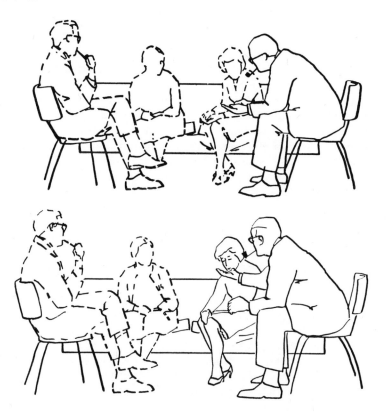

Figure 7-1B: Marge and Whitaker in Cycles D and E

The net result of these moves was the establishment of a usual rapport distance between Marge and Whitaker (see Chapter 11).

This process is ordinarily accomplished in gradual stages and the maneuvers in the series remind one of a dance. The therapist may move in, whereupon the patient may lean back and away. The therapist withdraws, but later moves forward again. In the Whitaker-Marge series Whitaker did not retract his moves. Marge would move back, but gradually come forward to meet his new distance. When she apparently had adapted to that distance, Whitaker would move again.

Although this kind of sequence is typical in psychotherapy (see Chapter 11), it is seen in other types of conversation when people are getting acquainted or when they become progressively involved in an interesting topic, a flirtation, or an argument.

Marge became more and more direct in her accusations and so did Whitaker. In cycle B, Marge accused her mother of laughing when father died. She conceded rather quickly with 'Didn't you sort of laugh?' But she also accused her mother of being mentally ill. In cycle C, Marge openingly argued with Mrs. V. She took her mother's arm, looked directly at her, and insisted that Mrs. V was afraid of Marge's father, even though Mrs. V denied this vigorously. In cycle D, Marge also directly disagreed with her mother, and she bluntly told Whitaker that it was not true that her mother had never been sick. Whitaker also made a blunt challenge to Mrs. V in cycle D, asking if she had had a psychotic breakdown and pressing her on the subject. In cycle E, Marge stated flatly that she thought her mother was crazy. Whitaker pursued this theme.

The Increasingly Overt Quasi-Courting and Tactile Reciprocals. Marge also was more and more overt in her courtship-like behavior to Whitaker. And at 12 and 24 minutes tactile contacting occurred.

THE PHASE II SHIFT

At 23 minutes Whitaker took the floor and explained the purposes and plans of the session. Then he took a relatively less active role. Malone moved in at 24 minutes and stayed forward. He started an explanation but ended in active interaction with Marge. Mrs. V sat back and began to take a more passive part.

At 29 minutes Whitaker moved back to his initial position and no longer took an active part. At 31 minutes the men stood up and ended the session.

I interpret these changes as follows: When the men had sufficiently involved Marge in rapport with Whitaker and gained
enough information about the family, they changed their tactics.
Whitaker explained the sessions and, in the process, dismissed
Mrs. V from further participation. Malone stopped intervening
and allowed Marge to keep the floor. He then shifted to relating
directly to her. Mrs. V became the supplementary narrator.
These dimensions of the structure are described in detail in
Section E.

THE CONTEXTS OF SESSION I

In the Preface I described the background in which Session
I occurred. In doing so, of course, I indicated some dimensions
of the context in which this transaction was located. Now I want
to review these, for the basic principle of context analysis is
that the larger behavioral integrations (contexts) determine the
meaning of and govern the events at lower levels.

We can visualize certain aspects of the immediate context
by direct observation. The others we must infer. Having studied
many psychotherapy sessions, I can achieve some comparative
assessments of the usual structure of this event, but we have
nothing more than educated guesses about the larger contexts of
these participant's lives.

The Immediate Contexts of Session I

The Visible Indications of the Immediate Context

There are customary sites for standard transactions which
have evolved in a culture: theatres, workshops, kitchens, living rooms, and the like. Such sites have evolved together with
the transactions which are to occur there, and with the appropriate props, tools, furniture, controlled lighting and temperature, and so forth.

Conditions conducive for conversation are ordinarily provided by a room such as a living room or consulting room.
Here walls and doors minimize noise and interruption by outsiders. Temperature control and lighting provide reasonable
comfort and visibility. And furniture is placed for appropriate
distancing and orientation. Optimal conditions exist when physical comfort allows sufficient freedom for people to attend to
each other's behavior and the arrangements allow them to see
and hear each other.

Just as the participants can observe these elements of the
physical ecology and get an idea about what is supposed to take

place, so can the research observer.

Session I was held in the living room of a house that had been specially prepared to accommodate psychiatric patients and that still had the character of a dwelling (Scheflen 1960). The room was relatively quiet. A sofa replaced the usual chairs characteristic of group and family therapy. The furniture was placed so that the participants were close enough to hear, see, and touch each other easily. The temperature was comfortable, though the lighting was brighter than usual for a conversation.

For a given kind of transaction certain types of people will convene. The participants and observers as well are instructed about what is to happen by recognizing the character and the social roles of the others present.

In psychotherapy, of course, one (or more) of the participants has a problem and the social role of patient or client. One (or more) of the participants is to do something about that problem, and has the social role of psychotherapist.

In Session I Marge was a legally committed psychiatric patient, hospitalized at a nearby mental hospital with the diagnosis of schizophrenia. Mrs. V was later hospitalized as a patient in the same hospital with the same diagnosis. Marge lived in the experimental unit where the sessions took place for the two weeks of study. Mrs. V lived at home.

Sometimes the transactional type is governed by the occasion. For example, particular transactions occur on Yom Kippur or Christmas, or on Sundays, or whenever certain crises or times of the year have arrived. Psychotherapy is held when a patient is adjudged in need of treatment or institutionalization and an appropriate group is convened for the procedure.

A participant who is experienced in common culture can usually guess what he is to do by observing these tangible contextual indications, but certain enforcing behaviors will appear if there is ambiguity. Here are a few which occurred in Session I:

1. Briefing. Before the session a member of the research staff explained the sessions in the course of obtaining a history and a permission for the filming. The sessions were also explained to Marge when she was admitted to the experimental treatment unit. The women were also told about the status and competence of the men.

2. Statements of Need and Purpose. The women often referred to their problem. We could say that they had a 'felt need'. Whitaker explained what they were there to do.

3. The Presence of the Hosts. It is often conventional to accept the host's definition of the situation. In Session I the

researchers who had briefed Mrs. V and Marge remained at the
scene. Also Marge had been admitted to the Temple treatment
unit for the experimental sessions and the attending staff had
instructed and groomed Marge for the occasion. The assistant
remained upstairs during the session.

While the treatment room was decorated to resemble a private living room, the building was located in the immediate setting of Temple University Hospital. The surroundings, then,
were clearly recognizable as a hospital compound and this ecology must have provided instructions for the procedure.

The host prerogatives were granted to Whitaker and Malone.
In general these men espoused the same system of transaction
as the psychiatrists who were host to Session I.

When Marge's behavior deviated, the head of the research
team cleared his throat and the others shifted around in their
chairs. So Whitaker and Malone were not alone in enforcing
the definition of the situation (English et al. 1966).

4. Monitors and Other Mechanisms of Enforcement. As
I have already described, kinesic monitors, interruptions, and
confrontations occurred when Mrs. V and Marge did not follow
the program.

Walls and the placement of furniture not only minimize in-
trusion but they tend to keep the people together. Usually the
site of a transaction is demarcated in visible physical ways,
but the participants may also provide barriers by their posture.
When standing, the members of a small group generally complete a circle or splay their feet to 'point' a boundary for the
group (Goffman 1963) (see also Section B). When seated, the
participants at the end of a row or semicircle tend to close the
aperture by crossing their legs in such a way that the upper
leg projects across the space or they place a leg on the furniture so that it blocks off the space and confines the group.

In later sessions when Mrs. V was not there and the men
had established more intensive rapport with the girl, they
placed their legs on a coffee table in such a way as to block off
their activities from the observers and camera, thereby boxing
in Marge.

Prohibitions may be placed on leaving. Participants may
even be held in the grouping by force. In Session I no one tried
to leave or seemed anxious to do so. Despite the fact that
Marge often seemed to be dissociated from the others she seemed keenly alert to everything that had happened. (The other
patient that Whitaker and Malone saw in Philadelphia did try to
leave. They held him physically in his chair.)

The Invisible Aspects of the Immediate Context

We could infer that there were cognitive dimensions of the immediate context that we could not see directly. Each person presumably had an image of what was to occur, a plan for managing his own behavior, and metasystem of values and beliefs about these matters.

We can gain some indications of these cognitive dimensions by observing what the people did in Session I. We can also make psychoanalytic inferences about their individual psychological makeup through three other conceptual routes.

1. Maneuvers, Tactics, and Suppressed Performances. We can observe what the participants tried to do and could not accomplish. We can note the paralinguistic and parakinesic maneuvers which they used. We can note also the abortive performances which they concealed or suppressed (see Chapter 8).

2. Paracommunicative Inference. By noting the communicative styles and the histories of the participants, we can identify their usual social roles, their institutional memberships, and their cultures of origins. If we know about the traditions of these subcultural categories we can predict the kinds of things they might do (see Chapter 10).

3. Metacommunicative Inference. If we study the metacommunicative comments of each participant and the behaviors of others which he monitors and avoids, we could develop a picture of the value systems and metaconceptions of each participant. We could cross-check these inferences against the usual value systems of the institutions, social classes, and ethnological backgrounds to which each person belongs.

Presumably these processes of inference which are characteristically carried out by psychological scientists are also carried out in everyday life by the participants in a transaction. And the inferences they achieve are one determinant in their behavioral communication (see Chapter 10).

Recognition of the Expected Formats

To an experienced member of common culture, all of these occurrences are recognizable and make clear what performance is expected. Although Mrs. V did not, we can guess, understand the details of the psychotherapy approach in general and the methods of Whitaker and Malone in particular, she did know about narrative formats and interviews. There are probably formats similar to these in any Western culture. And though Whitaker and Malone did not know the details of the women's plans, they were familiar with the general patterns of schizophrenic, mother-daughter relations, and with Sicilian culture. Also the men were briefed by the researchers about the women's history.

What happened in Session I then was roughly predictable. The general formats for narrative conversation were in main adhered to, but special variations were used according to individual plan and certain procedures were necessary to bring the variations into line. These principles governed the integrations of performance in Session I.

The Less Immediate Contexts of Session I

Session I as One Session in a Series

In the first place Session I was but the first transaction in a programmed series. Relationships and historical information were thus established in Session I for use in later sessions. Long-range planning probably affected the plans of all the participants.

Arrangements for Residence

Provisions were made to house the participants. As I have already said Marge lived in the experimental unit. Mrs. V returned home after each session. The therapists returned each evening to their families who were staying in Philadelphia in order to maintain a simulation of their usual life-space arrangements.

The Maintenance of Other Affiliations

Ordinarily it is important that a given transaction maintain rather than disrupt the ordinary social organization. Participants have families and institutional memberships to which they return after the event. Marge had an ongoing relationship with Mrs. V that would persist beyond the sessions. It was important not to disrupt this relationship without due and considered cause. Marge also had a psychotherapist at the hospital where she ordinarily stayed, and this relationship was protected as much as possible by the researchers and the therapists.

In psychotherapy, however, the sessions may be intended to change or even break up the social relationships in which the patient ordinarily participates. This was the case in Session I (see Section E). Accordingly the group composition was changed as the course of sessions proceeded — Mrs. V was dismissed and did not appear after Session II.

It is not usual, however, that a given transaction results in ideas or plans which disrupt the social organization or change the basic structure of the culture. Session I produced a view of some innovative techniques for psychotherapy, but did not produce a result which totally changed the institution. The research, too, was hopefully innovative, but many of the traditions were preserved. And some of Marge's and Mrs. V's ideas were to be affected, but the transaction did not revolutionize Catholicism or Sicilian culture.

So the principles of remote contexts, those of the society and the cultures involved, are, in the main, preserved, and these govern all of the events of the transaction level by level from its being held at all to the style of the smallest phoneme and gesture.

If we had enough data we could systematically reconstruct these larger contexts level by level as we did the shorter units which were captured on film. Then we could depict contexts as larger unit integrations, instead of describing physical objects and abstractions which represent these contexts.

COMMENT: TYPES OF COMMUNICATION. HOW THEY ARE MAINTAINED AND ADAPTED

The term communication covers social level processes of the greatest range of complexity — from simple perceptions to the most complicated systems of transaction. Any given transaction can be a simple, routine enactment of a customary program or a very variable affair which takes a great deal of negotiation, improvisation, and adaptation to keep it in progress. I would like to comment on these dimensions of communication.

Pertinent Levels in Communication

Processes at multiple levels of organization are essential to the understanding of communication. At the social level processes of group assemblage and regulation must occur so that participants can see, hear, touch, and smell each other. Processes at social levels of organization higher than the small group are essential in understanding and explaining these events. At the organismic level the participants must behave in coded or patterned ways according to some tradition of behavioral integration. They must also approach and address each other. At still lower levels of systems organization, brain, cell, and molecule, certain processes occur to sustain and mediate this information processing.

Logical Types of Communication

It is worthwhile to distinguish four logical types of communication in ascending order of complexity:

1. The Simple Perception of a Coded Enactment. If someone behaves in a meaningful patterned way and someone else of a similar background sees or hears this performance, a simple form of communication can occur. It is not essential that the behavior be intended to communication or that the process be mutual. Thus someone may brush his teech, change a tire, or talk to himself, and thereby provide information about a state, event, and context.

2. The Joint Enactment of a Routine Program for Social Maintenance. In any culture there is a repertoire of customary programs for carrying out the tasks which are necessary (or are deemed necessary) to provide for the members and maintain the social organization. Whenever these need to be carried out, appropriate participants gather and enact a replication (or else the appropriate transaction is enacted in anticipation of such need. Thus babies are washed when they need it. Or people may feed and eat when they are hungry or at regular times in anticipation of hunger. Some such transactions are very complex. Thus food is planted by one program and harvested months later by another one.

In such performances the participants recognize their own performances and those of the others. They can thus adapt and regulate the processes. Social organizations hold people together for enacting programs but the enactment and its consequences also maintain the social organization. Any transaction, then, is an event at one level in a larger schedule of transactions which collectively maintain the society. Thus Birdwhistell (1967) has defined communication as a system of integrated behaviors which mediate and permit social relationships.

3. The Use of a Program for Educating and Correcting Participants. Members of a society have to replace themselves, so there are programs for training and initiating novitiates to take necessary parts. In some cases deviant performers are taken aside and subjected to programs for discipline, rehabilitation, and punishment.

Psychotherapy seems to have evolved as one variant of such correctional procedures (G. A. P. Report 1969). The program for psychotherapy makes use of customary formats for conversation and narration and of those for developing relationships. It also makes use of medical formats for listening to symptoms and making a disposition and it uses medical metaconceptions. But in the psychoanalytic era particular specialized formats of meta-behavior have evolved for altering the patient's metaconceptions and for forming a particular kind of durable and influential relationship.

    4. <u>Programs</u> <u>for</u> <u>Producing</u> <u>Innovative</u> <u>Programs</u>. Mead (1964) has suggested that new formats have to be evolved in a culture when no one remembers what is ordinarily done or when existing programs do not meet the contingencies of the situation. Miller, Galanter, and Pribram (1960) have described 'plans for making plans.'

    Whitaker and Malone had developed innovations of the psychotherapy format and wanted to allow others to learn these. The researchers were interested in finding out how psychotherapy was done by psychotherapists who were presumably successful with schizophrenic patients. Thus Session I was a transaction in a program for evolving new programs.

The Maintenance of a Transaction

    Any transaction, however complex, may be performed efficiently and coordinatively if the participants have learned the same program and have worked out their differences in the experience of former enactments. But the matter is often not so simple. Contingencies arise from outside, participants disagree, or they hold to other investments and refuse to accommodate to this performance. I would like to describe briefly how such a situation is recognized and what mechanisms are conventionally applied to deal with such an eventuality.

The Characteristics of a Well-Coordinated Performance

    Among experienced performers a transaction may have the following characteristics. The actions of the participants are smoothly coordinated and the performances move on from one step in the format to the next. The group members are not usually awkward or hesitant, and they do not ordinarily give indication of being anxious, restless, or angry. They orient themselves to each other and do not endlessly search the room and each other's faces for cues about how to proceed.

Signs of Disconsonance in a Performance

    If, however, the participants do not perform their expected parts or coordinate them, characteristic signs of difficulty are observable. Progression in the performance comes to a stop.

The participants may repeat their behavior or begin another action, only to abandon it for still another. Often certain steps of the sequence are repeated again and again until an expected behavior is contributed. I call this repetitiveness <u>pattern looping</u>. The steps A-B-C, for instance come off as expected; then the participants may start over. Or else C is repeated again and again instead of D occurring. Or B-C, B-C, B-C keep recurring. In Session I there was much oscillation which reflected the disagreement between the women and their competition for the floor.

In a dissonant performance there is characteristic individual behavior. The participants look away from each other. They freeze and refuse to provide signals of comprehension or approbation. Then they glance at each other in a search for cues. They may show signs of boredom, restlessness, anxiety, or anger. They keep enacting monitors, like frowning, nose wiping, or lint picking. They may lexicate statements of disapproval or cirticism or question the procedure (Scheflen 1963). And they show hesitancy, uncertainty, and awkwardness in their behavior. These behaviors occurred in Session I and have already been described. Other examples will appear in the chapters to come.

In Session I the difficulties were intermediate in severity. The participants were from dissimilar backgrounds, but these fell within a broad category of traditional commonality. The session was carried on in English. The men seemed to be familiar with Italian American culture. And the women had lived in America for many years; Marge, in fact, had been raised here. The participants were similar in their understanding of psychotherapy and their expectations of the session. But, as I said, Marge had been a psychotherapy patient for six months and Mrs. V was acquainted with interviewing. Some difficulties in mutual comprehension were to be expected but there was a general basis for common understanding.

Mechanisms for Coordinating and Regulating a Conjoint Enactment

If the estrangements are gross, the group will break up or another transaction must be intercalated to change the ecology, work out the differences of opinion, service the sick or angry participants, or recruit and train others. Many transactions are of such a recalibrative type: psychotherapy, itself, is a prime example. On the other hand, if the participants have some degree of common knowledge about a progress of activity, they may be able to adjust their performances by simpler procedure of negotiation, mutual support, and mutual correction. Each of these kinds of metacommunicative activity occurred in Session I and they are characteristic of any conversational transaction.

I can mention these mechanisms briefly because they have already been described. My purpose here is to draw them together in a systematic account.

1. Negotiating a Common Program. Ordinarily the basic features of the transaction are constrained by custom and indicated by the context, but there are often details to work out: who will take a certain role, who will speak first, and so forth.

Without necessarily saying anything about his plans, a participant may run through an abbreviated performance or synopsis at the beginning of a transaction. He will preview the facial and postural patterns of the programs he will use later.

Birdwhistell (1969) believes that participants always preview. He claims that all of the major units which a person will later perform appear in token form in the first minute of a transaction. In Session I, for instance, all of the later programs of the session appeared in abbreviated form in the first minute. Mrs. V characterized Marge's illness. Marge briefly and hesitantly made facial and gestural commentary about this description and muttered inaudible comments. Whitaker invited Marge to speak up. Marge crossed her legs and made an abortive appeal which she quickly renounced. And Malone started to rock forward but did not complete his intervention. Then, all four participants settled back for a five-minute period of Mrs. V's presentation.

There are traditional provisions for doing this. The early stages of a transaction often show a prephase (McBride 1966), a stage of arrangements, trials, and previews followed by negotiation and decision. A tentative definition of the situation may result, although readjustments and realignments may occur later.

We could describe the negotiation process as follows: At any given point one or more definitions of the situation are up for consideration (Goffman 1956). Any next performance may support the existing definition or challenge it. Each participant may react to this new definition, then attack, refute, ignore, support, and so forth. At each step any performance can be held to or recalibrated until some compromise or agreement is reached.

In fact customary programs have evolved for negotiation itself. Debates and policy meetings, for instance, have a format which arranges for presenting all sides of an issue. This kind of provision was used in Session I. The oscillation was an arrangement by which Mrs. V and Marge would take turns pleading their cases.

It must not be supposed that a participant dichotomizes anoth-er definition. Rarely does he accommodate or challenge in toto. He will support at one level and alter at another.

2. Support for a Proper Performance. If one participant enacts a format which the others consider proper or suitable, they can establish a favorable definition by supporting it. They will suppress the tendency to interrupt or metacommunicate crit-ically. And they may exhibit this support by showing approval and postural parallelism. By the same token a participant can try to solicit support for his definition of the situation. He may command, flirt, promise, or whatever.

3. Cross-Monitoring the Performances. Finally, participants monitor each other's performances to keep them in line and ad-vance the enactment.

Programs for Communication and Their Apparent Function

If a progressive relation in structured by convention and there-by prescribed in advance, we can say that the behavioral relation is programmed. I have described the characteristics of a trans-actional program elsewhere (Scheflen 1968). Some of these are:

1. There are formats at all levels for the parts an individ-ual can take. These are made up of units and common variants. They are marked by junctures and a transfix. Consequently we can say they are coded.

2. These units are addressed and held in relation in custom-ary configurations of physical distance and mutual orientation.

3. 'Proper' performances are enforced by conventional meta-communicative signals (Scheflen 1963).

4. There are traditional agenda which often prescribe se-quences of relationships and steps of conjoint performance toward a common goal and point of termination.

5. A repertoire of different kinds of programs are known in any culture, each one specific to particular kinds of contexts, to given kinds of relationships, types of occasions, types of institu-tions, and so on.

One can take a functionalist view of the matter — he can presume that the behavioral programs of a culture have evolved to adapt organisms to the ecosystem and, where possible, adapt ecosystems to the organism. Whenever the organism and his en-vironment are out of dynamic equilibrium, the organism adapts itself by the use of an evolved system of changes that are struc-tured as programs of behavior.

Man's adaptation has depended on social organization. Ac-cordingly the evolution of a system of adaptive behaviors and a

system of recognizable and codified forms have occurred together. It is not that some separate system is adaptive and another communicative. The same systems of behavior that are
adaptive are recognizable and communicative.

Evolution and Cultural Transmission

In lower animals the forms of behavior presumably are transmitted genetically. The adaptive relation of behavior to context
may be learned soon after birth by imprinting (Lorenz 1935;
Klopfer 1962). In the case of man, varieties of form and patternment have evolved differentially in various cultures and have been
transmitted from generation to generation by processes of learning, such as imitation. As a consequence, all members of a giv-
en culture have had the opportunity to acquire common forms.

Individualness

On the other hand we can abstract the individuality of a participant on the basis of two successive criteria. He has learned
a particular repertoire of parts and formats at many levels. And
he plans and manages allowable variations in particular ways.

ADDENDUM TO SECTION C:
COMMUNICATIONAL STRUCTURE IN SESSION I

Consider again the operational complexities in portraying the
synthesis of behavior in a transaction. At one and the same time
the units at any level are arranged in a sequence according to a
format, and related among the participants according to traditional configurations of address and relationship. So we could
proceed along either of two pathways of synthesis, so long as we
cover both of these and show their interrelations; i.e., we could
first reconstruct the sequencing of units through time, or first
examine the structure of the relationships.

What I have done so far is to diagram the temporal sequencing in some detail. But I merely have described the relationships and abstracted their customary forms. To complete the
synthesis of Session I, I must construct, diagram, and name units of relation level by level, place them in context, and so forth.
I have not wanted to burden the reader with this much detail in
the body of the narrative. But I will produce some of this data
diagrammatically here in this Addendum for the reader with a
special interest in communicational structure of the session.

ANALOGY TO AN ORCHESTRAL PERFORMANCE

There were so many performances and structural units in Session I that presenting them is virtually impossible unless the data is organized economically and articulated in familiar and digestible terms. It is helpful to us, until our own language of communication becomes more settled and familar, to borrow from analogous, better known communicational forms. The language of music is one that serves us well.

If we assume that the form of musical composition in general is analogous to the structure of American communication, particular variants of music (e.g., a symphony, a concerto, etc.) can be seen as analogous to special communicative structures (e.g., psychotherapy). Thus, a fugue for a string quartet is a fair analogy to psychotherapy in a group of four. Both the quartet and the psychotherapy structure are performed. In each case, the performance will show a style and set of pecularities of its own, but the performance will also follow a general form and pattern. The difference between the two structures is that musical composition has an explicit score that is written down and consciously learned and practiced. The 'score' for communication has not been written down, and, to some extent, has been learned out of awareness. But certain orchestral performances, too, use a nonwritten score.

If we were to take a Bach fugue and construct a twofold table which illustrates its hierarchical structuring, the first column would contain the hierarchical integration of notes, measures, passages, and movements coded for each instrument. The succeeding columns would show the various relations of instrumental parts at each level. The total orchestral integration would appear in the right hand column. Note that we can read the table in any direction. For example, we can switch at any level from examining a part to examining a relation of parts among instruments or among sections of the orchestra. And we can examine it by analysis or synthesis (see Figure C-1).

Level	Performance of individual instruments	Performance of instruments in harmony	Performance of instruments in counterpoint	Total orchestration
Total Composition				Total orchestration
Movement				Constituent ↑ ← Unit
Passage				Constituent ↑ ← Unit
Measure				Constituent ↑ ← Unit

Figure C-1: Performance of a Fugue by a String Quartet (Blank squares are constituents)

An analogous schema can be composed for the communicational structure of Session I, as I have done in Figure C-2.

Level	Individual Performances	Complementary Performances	Reciprocal Performances	Total Units
Presentation				Structure of Session
Position				Constituent ↑ ← Unit
Point				Constituent ↑ ← Unit
Syntactic Sentence				Constituent ↑ ← Unit

Figure C-2: Communicational Structure in Tabular Form

But we can simplify the schema by combining the columns for individual performances and the column for complementary performances, because these are interchangeable or substitutable. That is, the complementary relation carries out a single performance (Figure C-3).

vis-à-vis

Level	Individual Complementary Performance	Individual or Complementary Performance	Total Unit
Presentation			Structure of Session
Position			↑ Constituent ←— Unit
Point			↑ Constituent ←— Unit
Syntactic Sentence			↑ Constituent ←— Unit

Figure C-3: Communicational Structure (Simplified)

Accordingly, in the remainder of this Addendum, I will deal with the relations of complementary performances to each other and not with individual performances. Complementary performances are related to each other reciprocally in this schema of communication.

RELATIONS AT THE LEVEL OF THE POINT

At the level of the point, five common complementary relations of point units regularly appeared. I will list these, then the reciprocal units of relation in which they occurred.

COMPLEMENTARY POINT PERFORMANCES

1. Complementary Recounting

    Recounting (Mrs. V)   Vis-à-vis
    Disparaging (Marge)   ←——→

2. Complementary Attending

    Attending (Whitaker)   Vis-à-vis
    Attending (Malone)   ←——→

COMPLEMENTARY POINT PERFORMANCES   continued

3. Attacking the Narrative

       Accusing (Marge)   Vis-à-vis
       Insinuating (Whitaker, Marge)   ⟵ ⟶
       Challenging (Whitaker, Marge)

4. Defending the Narrative

       Defending (Mrs. V)   Vis-à-vis
       Confronting Marge (Malone)   ⟵ ⟶
       Ironic Supporting (Malone)

5. Complementary Interruption

       Confronting Mrs. V (Whitaker)   Vis-à-vis
       Shocking (Marge)   ⟵ ⟶
       Restarting (Malone)

UNITS AT THE LEVEL OF THE POINT
IN RECIPROCAL RELATION

These complementary performances, together with individual performances, were integrated into isolatable units at the level of the point. Six types of lexical point units are diagrammed below. The nonlexical ones follow. Notice that the units are more highly organized than the complementary points in that each point or complementary pair of points has the vis-à-vis or reciprocal relation required for the completion of a unit.

The 'lexical' point units (those that had linguistic components) were:

1. Interviewing

    Complementary   Complementary
     Recounting   Vis-à-vis   Attending
                  ⟵ ⟶

2. Disagreeing

    Attacking the   Defending
     Narrative   Vis-à-vis
                  ⟵ ⟶

3. Making up

| Conceding (usually Marge) | Vis-à-vis ←——→ | Conciliating (usually Mrs. V) |

4. Breaking up

| Rejecting (usually Whitaker | | Repelling (Marge) |
| Confronting (Malone) | Vis-à-vis ←——→ | |

5. Allying

| Appealing and/or Lamenting | Vis-à-vis ←——→ | Attending (Whitaker) |

6. Interrupting

| Complementary Interrupting | Vis-à-vis ←——→ | Recounting |

The nonlexical (kinesic or postural) point units were:

1. Reciprocal Contacting

| Contacting (Whitaker) | Vis-à-vis ←——→ | Contacting (Marge) |

2. Inviting Rapport

| Appealing for Empathy (Marge) | Vis-à-vis ←——→ | Attending (Whitaker and Malone) |

3. Inviting Contact

| Kleenex Play (Marge) | Vis-à-vis ←——→ | Attending (Whitaker or Malone) |

or

| Hand Play (Whitaker) | Vis-à-vis ←——→ | Attending (Marge) |

RELATIONS AT THE LEVEL
OF THE POSITION

Six complementary relations of positions occurred again and again in Session I. These were related in four main reciprocal units.

1. Pleading the case. The two women, in parallel positions, addressed the men. Mrs. V gave her narrative and Marge modified it with metamessages. This complementary performance corresponded to Period 1, as described in Chapter 4.

2. Interrogating. The men, in tandemic complementarity, listened and questioned the account.

3. Complementary contending. Whitaker and Marge formed a complementary alliance and challenged Mrs. V's account. This complementarity and number 4 (following) correspond to Period 2, Chapter 4.

4. Complementary maintaining. It consisted of a complementary defense of the story by Malone and Mrs. V vis-à-vis Complementary Contending.

5. Fostered quasi-courting. It consisted of Whitaker's or Malone's (whichever reciprocated to her flirting) attending to Marge. The other man fostered it by noninterference. This activity occurred (kinesically) in periods of (lexical) contending and included the position number 7 (Hand Playing, Kleenex Displaying).

6. Fostered contacting. No monitoring or interference attended the contacting of Whitaker and Marge.

Reciprocal Relations of
the Complementary Positions

The reciprocal relations of these complementarities might be diagrammed as follows:

1. Pleading the Case   2. Interrogating

Explaining (Mrs. V)	vis-à-vis ⟷	Listening and Questioning (Whitaker)
Passive Protesting (Marge) Resigning		Listening and Questioning (Malone)
UPPER BODY PARALLEL-ISM		PARALLEL POSTURES

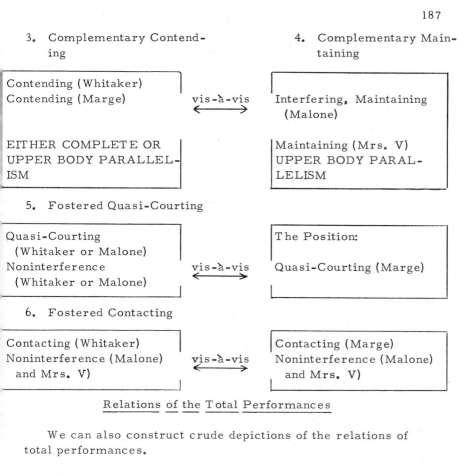

3. Complementary Contend-
ing

| Contending (Whitaker)
Contending (Marge) |
| EITHER COMPLETE OR
UPPER BODY PARALLEL-
ISM |

vis-à-vis ⟷

4. Complementary Main-
taining

| Interfering, Maintaining
(Malone) |
| Maintaining (Mrs. V)
UPPER BODY PARAL-
LELISM |

5. Fostered Quasi-Courting

| Quasi-Courting
(Whitaker or Malone)
Noninterference
(Whitaker or Malone) |

vis-à-vis ⟷

| The Position:
Quasi-Courting (Marge) |

6. Fostered Contacting

| Contacting (Whitaker)
Noninterference (Malone)
and Mrs. V) |

vis-à-vis ⟷

| Contacting (Marge)
Noninterference (Malone)
and Mrs. V) |

Relations of the Total Performances

We can also construct crude depictions of the relations of total performances.

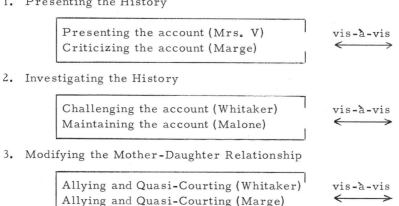

1. Presenting the History

| Presenting the account (Mrs. V)
Criticizing the account (Marge) |

vis-à-vis ⟷

2. Investigating the History

| Challenging the account (Whitaker)
Maintaining the account (Malone) |

vis-à-vis ⟷

3. Modifying the Mother-Daughter Relationship

| Allying and Quasi-Courting (Whitaker)
Allying and Quasi-Courting (Marge) |

vis-à-vis ⟷

4. Continuing the Mother-Daughter Relationship

        Presenting her account (Mrs. V)   vis-à-vis
        Maintaining the account (Malone)

The complementaries were related something as follows:

Developing the History (lexical)

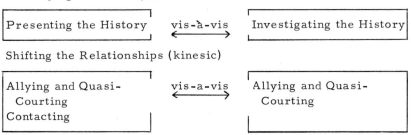

Shifting the Relationships (kinesic)

But we have now produced greatly oversimplified diagrams.
I will try to clarify these complex relations in the following chapters.

PART II

Special Aspects of Behavioral Communication
in Session I

Emphasizing specific styles and particular
management and adaption which the participants
made in accordance with their own plans and in
reaction to the special situation of Session I.
Section D treats the behavior of the women and
Section E described strategy and tactics used by
the men.

SECTION D

Some Features of the Women's Performances

Introduction:

INDIVIDUALITY IN COMMUNICATION

While the women conformed generally to the structure of a psychotherapy session, they did so in their own ways. In common culture, we would say they acted individually. They carried their parts in ways that were in some measure particular for them and in some measure typical of people of their class, background, and diagnostic category. Three kinds of such format variation in the performances of Mrs. V and Marge will be discussed in this section:

1. One kind of variation was particular to their backgrounds and social role. Both were southern Italian-American, Catholic, female, and unmarried. Marge was a late adolescent, Mrs. V a middle-aged widow. They showed behavioral features character- istic for these determinants and we can presume that they could not have changed these features at will. I will call these kinds of features style. These features are of special communicational significance. They provide information about the backgrounds of a participant.
2. Other features of the women's performances were change- able, and, in fact, did change throughout the session. They appear- ed to be in the service of particular plans or purposes which were regulated by larger contexts of their lives. I will call these varia- tions tactical.
3. Still other features of their performances were not typical for women, for Catholics, or for southern Italian-Americans. These features were deviant — not merely foreign or alien. The deviant styles are not, however, rare or unknown. They are also

191

customary and, to some extent, predictable in people classified as schizophrenics.

I cannot, of course, make rigid distinctions on the basis of the data of one transaction. We would have to have comparable filmed transactions involving many southern Italian-Americans, for instance, to attribute certain variations to ethnic background with any degree of certainty. And it is also hard to say definitely that a given behavior is schizophrenic or tactical. In fact it can be argued that schizophrenic behavior is tactical. However, some approximate distinctions can be made from general cultural and psychiatric experience. I will devote one chapter in this section to each of these variations.

The data of this section provide us with an opportunity to speak about the psychodynamics and neuropsychology of communication. So in each chapter I will comment on these matters. After describing styles (Chapter 8), I will discuss how these gave indication of the tactical variations. In Chapter 9, I will discuss theories of cognitive processes and the neuropsychology of information processing. Then in Chapter 10, when deviant behavior is described, I will discuss theories of the nature and development of schizophrenia.

Chapter 8

THE PERFORMANCE STYLES OF THE WOMEN

A participant's style tends to be persistent and pervasive, characterizing everything he does in a transaction. And it is not likely to be managed consciously. This chapter describes some of the stylistic features in the women's performance. Later I will deal with the exceptions — those transient features of style which were manipulated at phases of the transaction.

These persistent styles, I believe, were reliable indicators of a participant's life situation and his lifelong states and backgrounds. So I will end the chapter by describing how styles provide information about the mediate and remote contexts of a participant's life. These contexts are determinants in a person's performance at a given transaction, and therefore of some predictive value. Hence, they are of communicational importance.

PHYSICAL APPEARANCE

Each of the women presented a behavioral set at Session I which did not change with movement. We usually designate such features as physical appearance.

Attributes Usually Considered Phenotypical

Both women were slightly swarthy, and appeared to be of Mediterranean origin. Mrs. V was pyknic or mesomorphic-endomorphic. Marge was mesomorphic, but not obese. These types have been associated with cyclothymic personalities and with southern Italian culture. Both women appeared to be in good

194

health. They were reasonably good-looking and without any evident physical defects. In a Period 2 demeanor Marge impressed
us as being sexually attractive.

We tend to attribute the stable features of physical appearance to heredity. I think this is an oversimplification, since
posture, facial demeanor, styles of bodily movement and dress,
cosmetics, and hairdo are also highly stable and make up part
of the Gestalten of physical appearance. In fact, patterns of bodily movement learned early in life may affect the development of
the muscloskeletal system (Birdwhistell 1962).

Dress

Marge dressed in the manner of American working-class
girls, while Mrs. V dressed like any postmenopausal, peasant
woman from a central or southern European culture. Her hair
was combed back in a knot, and she wore a large, long polka
dot dress, cotton hose, and flat shoes. Thus Mrs. V's dress
indicated European, peasant background, though not specifically
Italian. Her leg posture indicated that she was postmenopausal
and somewhat obese — she allowed her knees to drift apart but
covered herself by pulling down her dress. Both women showed
working-class dress, cosmetic usage, and hairstyles.

In later sessions Marge fingered a Catholic medallion. In
some transactions participants wear uniforms, emblems, or
other indicators of categorical membership[1] (Ekman 1969).

The gender of Mrs. V and of Marge was obvious from their
appearance and dress. There was no evidence of gender con-
fusion in the behavior of the women, as is often the case with
mental patients. In many cultures postmenopausal women may
be afforded male roles. There was no evidence that Mrs. V had
taken such roles, a point of possible significance in the problem
the two women were having (see Chapter 10).

Presence

Mrs. V was persistently stolid in Session I. She did not
show the presence that some people show — the command of
gaze and space and the certainty of behavior that goes with longstanding dominance. Nor did she show signs of habitual submissive behavior — a tendency to avoid the gaze of others or
the hunched-down posture which goes with behaving apologetically
and hesitantly.

Marge showed a variable presence. In a Period 1 she would
look away, mumble, avoid eye engagement, and huddle against
her mother. But in Period 2 she sat upright, becoming very

assertive and commanding. We could generalize that Marge oscillated in presence as she did in behavioral form in the cycles
of Session I.

PERSISTENT BEHAVIORAL STYLES

Vocal Qualifiers of Paralanguage

Collectively the nonlanguage sounds and the vocal qualifiers
have been termed paralanguage (Trager 1958). In linguistics
these dimensions of speech behavior are distinguished from the
structural features and content. Characteristic vocal qualifiers
are: rasp, nasality, overloud or oversoft volume, overfast or
overslow pace, clipped or drawling intonation.

Mrs. V tended to speak oversoftly and flatly, using few variations of vocal qualifiers. Psychiatrists abstracted expressive
and schizophrenic qualities from Mrs. V's speech (see below).

Marge, on the other hand, showed a wide range of paralinguistic qualities. She would mumble inaudibly one minute and be
overloud the next. She changed her rate of speech from overslow
to overfast. She sometimes spoke in a sing-song rhythm. Psychiatrists judged Marge's speech to be highly affective or emotional and used these qualities as one basis for diagnosing her
'schizoaffective-schizophrenia' (see Chapter 10).

Vocal qualifiers have been of special interest to psychological scientists since they provide indicators of mood and personality (Gottschalk 1961; Eldred and Price 1958; Pittenger,
Hockett and Denehy 1960).

We should bear in mind, however, that certain patterns of
vocal qualifiers are also indicative of dialect, class, and ethnic
background. For example, drawl occurs throughout the southern
United States, and oversoft is highly valued by middle-class Americans (Trager and Smith 1956). I do not know what the usual paralinguistic patterns are for Sicilian-Americans.

Word choice also varies with regions of the country, social
class, and other categorical memberships. The women spoke of
'mind-pictures,' for example. Word choice and pronunciations,
together with favored paralinguistic qualities, occur together as
typical dialectical patterns.

Marge and Mrs. V used a clearly recognizable dialectical
pattern which is typical of the large southern Italian-American
enclave in South Philadelphia.

Parakinesic Qualities and Regional Uses of Kinesic Styles

As with language, posture and movement can have a variety
of qualities. One can move languidly or jerkily, in small or

grand excursion, and so forth. Accordingly, we may speak of kinesic and postural styles or of parakinesic qualities (Birdwhistell 1969). As in paralanguage, these features may characterize a dialectic area or institution and are not necessarily an idiosyncratic feature of one individual's behavior.[2]

A parakinesic quality may pervade all of a participant's behavior. The parakinesic qualities of Mrs. V and Marge paralleled their paralinguistic traits. Mrs. V was underactive to the point of moving depressively. Her lack of movement was especially noteworthy in view of her Italian background, for members of this culture ordinarily move often and in a wide range of arm and hand excursion.

Marge was overactive. She sat up, sprawled, stood, crossed and uncrossed her legs, and so forth. She also moved rapidly and broadly, throwing her arms and body around in a wide excursion. Although so much movement is abnormal for an adult, it did show the mobility of Italian-American kinesics more typically than did Mrs. V's behavior.

In southern Italian culture, gesticulation is characteristically carried out from the shoulder. This use of bodily organization contrasts markedly with the mode in old American cultures of British extraction and with the mode in Eastern European Jewish culture. In the latter, for instance, the elbows are held close to the body and the arms are moved from a fulcrum at the elbow. These differences are quite indicative of cultural origin (Efron 1941; Birdwhistell 1963).

Marge varied her demeanor and parakinesic styles with the positions she used. When she was sitting with her mother in a Period 1, she was slow, dissociative, and noncourting in style. During a Period 2, when she was contending, her face and body were animated. She showed a range of styles. Her body came into the hypertonus of the courtship state. She was alert, overfast, and widely excursive in her range of movement. Her demeanor changed kaleidoscopically with facial expressions of anger, depression, dominance, humor, and so forth. Also, Marge used characteristically Italian gestures during periods of sitting with her mother.

I would make the following guess: Marge had learned two paralinguistic and parakinesic styles: one which she used in her family, at least when relating to her mother, and the other which she used in relationships with people outside the family, perhaps with men. Possibly she had learned the second from her father, from some other relatives, or from peers in her neighborhood.

After this I will use the term paracommunicative to refer to the performance styles of any unit of behavior, condensing the current uses of the terms paralanguage and parakinesics.

The Use of Culturally Specific Unit Forms

Many transactions occur in wide distribution across ethnic and class lines. So the same basic activity is carried out by many peoples, but the people of a given cultural category use specific unit forms for the activity. Thus all peoples eat, but each culture has its own dishes and manners. And certain word choices are characteristic for particular dialectic areas. Smiles and quasi-courting routines are typical ways of attracting a relationship in certain classes and traditions. So the use of a particular and typical pattern of alternative unit forms can be indicative of a participant's background. Similar generalizations could be made about some personality types within a cultural category. Therefore, the characteristic alternatives which a person habitually uses characterize his repertoire, that is, the repertoire of his background.

We cannot judge the limits of a person's repertoire by watching him in one transaction, but we can note that he uses certain alternatives over and over. Such repetition becomes especially significant if it is stereotyped — if, for instance, a participant keeps using forms that are not acceptable to the others or which do not accord with his other purposes. Thus, if a participant does not make use of the full repertoire which, given his background, he should have learned, we can suspect either that he is operating under some special constraint or that he is a deviant.

I do not know enough about the tactical variants of Mrs. V's and Marge's backgrounds to comment about their cultural specificity. But in many cases, as I will describe in Chapters 9 and 10, their behavior did appear to be stereotyped. They did not use the full range of behavioral alternatives allowable in psychotherapy or, I think, in Sicilian-American culture. In Chapter 10 I attribute this to deviance, more specifically, to schizophrenia.

OTHER BEHAVIORS THAT INDICATED THE LIFE CONTEXTS OF THE WOMEN

Stated References to Larger Contexts

We interviewed Mrs. V and Marge before the session. They gave information which identified them as South Philadelphian, Catholic Sicilians of the working class. Mrs. V also told us she was a widow, who had lived alone since Marge had been hospitalized. We also knew Marge was a hospitalized mental patient with a diagnosis of schizophrenia who had been in psychotherapy for six months.

Most of this information could have been inferred from the behavior of the women in Session I. Some of it was stated in their utterance to the men. Mrs. V told the men she was widowed, for instance. Both women used words like <u>mass</u>, <u>confession</u>, and <u>mortal sin</u>, and Marge made the sign of the cross. Mrs. V spoke of being given wine by her father. She mentioned <u>ice</u> (Italian water ice) and <u>street carnival</u> (an enclave custom in Italian South Philadelphia). Marge showed an apprentices' knowledge of psychiatric terms and concepts (see Chapter 9).

Consistent Metabehavior
That Indicated Values and Beliefs

There are a number of ways by which the women indicated their metaconceptions. Sometimes they stated them by metacommunicative intercalations about their own or their partner's behavior. Through these intercalations they also indicated their conceptions about proper behavior by their kinesic monitoring behaviors and facial gestures when others took a position. And by psychoanalytic inference we can derive certain of their values by the innuendoes, denials, rationalizations and concealments they used.

Operationally we can inventory all of the metacommunicative behavior of each woman, abstract some consistent themes, and interpret these within any of a number of psychological frames of reference. I do not want to get involved in controversial and debatable frames of reference, but a few clear themes did emerge.

Mrs. V's Ideas About Marge's Behavior and About Family

As we might expect of a mother, Mrs. V consistently monitored Marge's sexy and provocative behavior. But Mrs. V also wiped her nose and prepared to stand whenever Marge started to reveal a secret of the V family history, and whenever she allied with Whitaker. Sometimes Mrs. V also verbalized her disapproval of these actions by Marge. She expressed disagreement, however, about other kinds of behavior which she did not monitor. She denied that Marge was crazy. She denied discord between Marge and the father and also tended to minimize the violence, separations, and disagreements which beset her marriage. She also minimized Marge's anger at her. And she did not like the fact that Marge did not level with her.

It was my impression that Mrs. V's main concern was to cover up disagreements among family members and hold together what was left of her family. A high value on family cohesiveness has been reported by many observers as a characteristic of southern Italian culture, as well as a characteristic of families which have a schizophrenic member (Wynne et al, 1958).

Mrs. V's General Values

We could also infer that Mrs. V set store upon Marge's and her husband's intelligence. She disapproved of being nervous, crazy, sexy, violent, and suicidal, and apparently thought it improper to laugh about her husband's death. On the whole she seemed to espouse Catholic values.

Marge's Attitudes

Marge repeatedly referred to going to hell, being dead, being operated on for sin, and so on. In Session III we found that Marge had become pregnant and had had an abortion. But Marge poked fun at other of her mother's values. She burlesqued her mother's classical health advice and the idea of seeing into the future. She teased her mother about being unable to commit 'mortal sin,' and she especially mocked her mother's injunctions against being sexy. Marge was serious about being angry at her mother and she insisted that the older woman was mentally ill. She did not concur in the idea of family closeness and harmony.

The reader can make his own inferences from the transcript in Appendix A. We can generalize that the women's metacommunicative behavior was consistent with the other indications of their background.

Indicators of Health and Persistent Affect

Illness may be indicated by flushed cheeks or pallor, by weakness and poor tonus, by corneal dullness, inattentiveness, coughing, wheezing, and wincing in pain, and so on. None of the participants in Session I gave any indication of poor health.

As I described above, Marge showed styles of behavior which we ordinarily associate with anger. She protruded her jaw, she made direct face-to-face confrontations to Mrs. V, and she raised her voice. But these qualities were transient and related to immediate contexts in Session I. We would not say she was essentially an angry person. The same thing can be said about her tendency to fall into slow movement and the facies of depression. These indicators did not persist in her facial demeanor. We would say she was intermittently depressed in Session I, rather than saying she had a depression.

But Mrs. V did show persistent signs of depressive affect. She consistently spoke and moved slowly; her face sagged and her lids appeared heavy. In cases like hers the affective indicators did not appear to vary with the vicissitudes of the transaction, so they suggested a continuing state related to the larger contexts of her life situation.

COMMENT: THE PERSONAL CONTEXTS
OF A PERFORMANCE

The Contexts of Cultural Experience

Emic Systems of Behavior

The cultural heritage of a people prescribes what Pike calls an 'emic system' of behavior.[3] It provides a repertoire of formats for all occasions, a communicative system of language, gestures, postures, and spacing patterns, and a metacommunicative system of beliefs and values. Each child who grows up in a culture learns these systems of form and style and replicates them at subsequent transactions. As a consequence a knowledgeable observer can identify a participant's culture of origin by watching his behavioral style and the repertoire of forms that he uses. So we have no difficulty recognizing that Mrs. V is of southern Italian extraction. And at least traces of such ethnic background are evident in Marge's behavior.

There are usually a number of subtraditions in any ethnic tradition. There are several social classes, each of which has distinctive behavioral qualities, and there may be a number of religious, occupational, and regional subcultures. Features of these subcultural traditions are also recognizable in the performances of their members.

If an individual has learned a single emic system of culture, we can assume that this system determines his behavioral repertoire. The occurrence, then, of any culturally recognizable sample of behavior in his performance will predict the remainder of that emic system. If he speaks Sicilian like a native, for example, we can expect that he eats Sicilian food, uses Sicilian gestures and postures, and shares Sicilian values. But there are a number of exceptions and difficulties to keep in mind.

For example, all members of a tradition do not use the full repertoire of possible forms and styles. They probably recognize the full range, but they use only some subset prescribed for their gender, age grouping, marital status, institutional affiliation, and so forth — a constellation we can abstract as a role.

Furthermore, people may change their ethnic, class, and institutional memberships. They may be upwardly mobile in the class system, for instance, or they may migrate to another

place and begin to acculturate. Mrs. V and Marge had thus in
some degree acculturated, and Marge showed traces of middle-
class style. [4]

Temperament and Personality

Even if we should categorize the expected forms of behavior
for a participant by taking into account all the known divisions of
his ethnic background, class, religion, age grouping, and so
forth, we would still find variations, some of which we attribute to
temperment or personality. Thus there are sad and happy and
open and paranoid Catholic, Sicilian-American working class
members. Maybe there are genetic differences in temperament,
but certainly there are idiosyncratic experiences in an individual's path to maturation through the various emic systems of his
background.

Some of these seem to cut across culture. Thus psychiatrists find basically similar schizophrenic reactions in many
Western cultures. Maybe specific cognitive disorders and overly close mother-daughter dyads develop in all Western cultures
and lead to certain consequences regardless of the emic systems
in which they occur (see Chapter 10). In any event we could see
deviant behaviors in Mrs. V and Marge that seemed to override
their cultural experiences. Mrs. V's immobile body and face,
as we have noted, seemed to be quite atypical for a southern
Italian background but common in schizophrenia.

Consequently we ordinarily postulate some interaction between culture and personality. At this point in history it is
difficult to visualize the role of genetic transmission. Within
the limits of cultural experience each individual develops modes
of behavior which further determine his niche in the society.
Thus some interrelations of cultural experience, social niche,
potential, and idiosyncratic experience sustain each other and
form a persistent and consistent pattern of behavioral determina-
tion. Borrowing an idea from Langer (1953) I will call this system of determinants the remote content of an individual's present
performance. [5]

We can hold only that the total cultural experience of an individual determines the limits of his repertoire — determines
the forms of behavior that he is able to learn. More immediate
contexts shape the actual behavior he will use.

The Mediate Contexts of
the Women's Performance

Some of the stylistic features of the women's behaviors were
not indicative of permanent cultural constraints. Rather, they

had reference to phases and eras in their life situations or life spaces.[6] Such arrangements certainly persisted beyond Session I but were not in all probability lifelong. The following indicators seemed to belong to such mediate contexts: Mrs. V was in an era of middle-aged, noncourting widowhood; she had once been single and once been married. Marge was unmarried and sexually active. The history indicated that she sometimes used these behaviors in prostitution.

Marital status, sexual activity, parenthood, and age grouping define the mediate context in a woman's life. Ordinarily there are culturally prescribed roles and established constraints for her at each of the stages from childhood to old age.

During a person's lifetime he may belong to several ethnic, regional and class subcultures, and a number of institutions. At any era of his life, he may be affiliated actively in some and inactively in others. Thus he may remain an active, practicing Catholic or become unaffilliated and therefore retain only residual behaviors and values of this institutional membership. Similarly a daughter may remain actively affiliated with her family and its values or she may move away into other relationships and hold other metaconceptions. The stress upon certain indicators, their frequency and overtness, for instance, may indicate the current life-space memberships of a participant; with this information we can make a rough estimate of his more influential mediate contexts.

In Session I both the mother and daughter gave every evidence that they were actively involved, even preoccupied with each other (see Chapter 10). Marge and Mrs. V also showed an active investment in Roman Catholicism. They used Catholic signs and Catholic phrases. They spoke of mortal sin and told stories of visits by the priest. Marge also gave indications of current membership in the role of mental patient. She spoke the words and ideas of psychotherapy. She showed brief evidence of the bizarre qualities and autism of the institutional, schizophrenic patient (Scheflen 1965).

People who have learned more than one ethnic and social class pattern can behave in more than one cultural mode. Marge at times used Sicilian styles, although she did not have to. She sometimes used forms which, I would guess, she learned in school. Marge's use of these modes seemed to be related to her relationships in the Periods of Session I. In Phase I she used Sicilian-American styles more frequently. When relating to Whitaker, she used more American class styles.

We might guess, therefore, that Marge had played roles in three mediate contexts; one as a daughter in the V family (evident in a Period 1); another as psychotherapy patient in a mental

hospital (evident in a Period 2); and still another outside of these
institutions (evident in relating to Whitaker in transition to a Period 2).

Context and the Choice of Performance

So we say that contexts determine a performance. But since
we do not, in a systems concept, picture relations with linear
arrows, we must also comment on the other side of the arc.
Whenever Mrs. V behaved as a widowed mother of an adolescent
daughter in an extended family of an Italian Catholic enclave,
she contributed to the maintenance of these contextual systems.
In a more adequate formulation, then, we say that contexts and
performances are interdependent.

The quality of being Sicilian tends to dictate that of being
Catholic, just as these qualities together tend to dictate mother-
daughter dependency and the resulting behavior of this relationship tends to dictate efforts which prevent separation. At the
same time, the act of blaming, the appeals to loyalty, authori-
tarianism, and other behaviors of cohesiveness in the mother-
daughter relationship tend to maintain the family, which in turn
maintains and transmits Catholicism and Sicilian culture.

We could predict that Mrs. V's performance would be ded-
icated to maintaining the existing contexts of her life. She did
not seem to have any ties outside her family. She had no immediate relatives other than Marge, and Marge's behavior was
threatening even this relationship. Thus Mrs. V was tied essentially to a single immediate context. When this was threatened she must have been prompted to a strong and sustained effort
to re-establish its conditions. Hence, her performance in Session I was likely to be stereotyped.

A participant thus joins a transaction under certain constraints. The immediate context requires of him a certain performance. He must behave communicatively and appropriately
for the immediate situation. But he maintains cognitive images
of mediate contexts which he must maintain by his performance
and he can only perform formats which lie within his life experience. In some measure he has to accommodate these various
considerations and he may have to make choices or compromises.

In the simplest instances this might not be an issue. If a
person stays within his culture he will not necessarily encounter
alien behavior or be asked to perform an unfamiliar part. If he
stays in a stable institution his role is established and he shares
with others the same occasions, transactions, and performance
expectancies. Thus a religious man stays with others of the
same persuasion. When he behaves in a 'proper' program within

that group he simultaneously maintains his affiliations, abides by his beliefs, forwards a plan to spread 'good,' and increases his institutional status. Thus, most of the potential incongruities of a transaction are avoided by established order in larger social systems.

But the matter was not so simple in Session I. The men and women were, as noted, strangers to each other and members of different institutions, social classes, and ethnic groupings. Also the women had strong disagreements between them. Even though the structure of the psychotherapy session provided some latitude for these differences, certain discrepancies had to be faced. We might guess, for instance, that Mrs. V had to decide whether or not she should sanction Marge's relationship to the men, since it threatened to change the mother-daughter relationship.

Faced with such choices a number of solutions are possible. A participant might refuse to enact the formats expected by the others. Or he might accommodate himself to the immediate situation and thereby risk a disequilibrium in higher contexts. Or he might partly accommodate. In Chapter 9 I will describe some ways in which the women managed these possibilities. We can surmise that they had plans for the session which they modified with the contingencies of its progression.

Thus we can order determinants in a performance by levels of context. The remote contexts of a person's life — which we abstract as genetic, cultural, and psychic determinants — would limit the possible repertoire of a performer.

The mediate contexts of his life — which we represent by factors such as goals, social position, and affiliations — would constrain his performance inasmuch as it would supposedly maintain these contexts. And the immediate context of the transaction would further limit his performance.

At each level of context a participant has some latitude of choices. He may attend or avoid certain transactions. Once there, he may or may not have a choice of roles. If he is versed in several cultural traditions he may have a choice of formats. The performance expected of him may or may not allow him to support existing affiliations, beliefs, and goals. So we do not maintain dichotomously either an idea of free will or an idea of predestination. Choices are possible at each level, but the choices at any level are constrained by conditions at higher levels of context.

Paracommunicative Inference
and Paracommunication

These issues of deduction are of contral concern in a psy-
chodynamic approach. Personality assessments are made by
processes of inference something like those I have just made.
We observe a participant's behavior and make inferences about
his activities in other circumstances and about his cognitive patterns. And we use these deductions to locate him in a classific-
atory system of personality or cultural types. From these operations we try to make predictions about what he may do in a
specific circumstance.

In communication theory our central interest is not in personality or enthnographic assessment, but the processes of inference about a participant's life contexts are not academic.
These same deductive processes are carried out regularly by
participants in any transaction — styles are recognized, attributed a significance, reacted to with biases, or used as a source
of information for gauging a performance.

Whitaker and Malone, for example, had been quite familiar
with Italian culture since their childhoods. Malone was experienced with Catholicism. They told us that they planned some of
their tactics on the basis of predictions about Mrs. V and Marge
when they realized the ethnic background and religion of the women.

Furthermore, we need to know about the backgrounds of participants for research purposes — to explain and understand the
significance of different communicative systems and to study issues of miscommunication. So we make paracommunicative inferences as a means to an end in communication theory.

Judgments about a participant's life contexts and the deter-
mination of his behavior are most reliably made, I believe, on
the basis of his style, i. e. , from his paracommunicative qualities.
So I call these mentalistic processes paracommunicative inference. That such inferences are an activity in communication justifies, as well, a concept of paracommunication.

But paracommunication does not depend alone on inferences
about style and variation. Participants use symbolic behaviors
to signify the traditions — ethnic, class, regional, institutional,
and role — to which their performances belong. Also they indicate their values, states, and so forth. Thus participants behave
paracommunicatively. [7]

Chapter 9

<u>TECHNIQUES</u> <u>THE</u> <u>WOMEN</u> <u>USED</u> <u>IN</u> SESSION I

In Chapter 8 I sketched possible limits of the behavioral repertoires of the women, limits imposed by the totality of their experience. And we have agreed that the women's behavior was constrained by the definition of Session I as a type of narrative conversation. But within these limits the women had a latitude for tactical management. They could pick certain topics, for instance, and avoid others.

In this chapter I will describe how they shaped and managed their behavior within the range of these limitations. I will stick to the hierarchical scheme we have been using, mentioning first their over-all performances, which I will consider as their strategy. Then I will describe how they managed positions to form tactics in the over-all strategy.

I assume that these tactical variations were determined and constrained by the mediate contexts of the women's lives. I will make some comments about the neuropsychology of planning and carrying out a plan.

THE APPARENT STRATEGY OF THE WOMEN

Review of the Women's Performances

We should go back to Chapter 6 and review briefly the over-all performances of the women.

The format of Mrs. V's performance can be summarized as follows:

A. An alternation of: Explaining (to the men) ;
                          and
                      Maintaining (against Marge
                      and Whitaker but supported
                      by Malone) ; consisted of two
                      points:

                          Defending (point 7) ;
                          and at times:
                          Conceding (to Marge)
                          (point 12)

B. Then late in the session: Passive Protesting
                      (moving into a nonlexical
                      alliance with Whitaker,
                      who had dissociated from
                      Marge)

Marge's performance was not as simple as her mother's.
She played with a Kleenex, quasi-courted, and in general maintained an active kinesic relation with the men. In addition she
used various combinations of points in her format from position
to position. We could summarize these alternative constitutents
as follows:

Passive Protesting (in relation to her mother but directed
toward the men) ; consisted of three points:

Conceding	(point 12)
Lamenting	(point 8)
Disparaging	(point 13)

then:

Contending (in alliance with Whitaker) ; consisted of five
points:

Appealing for Empathy	(point 14)
Insinuating	(point 16)
Challenging	(point 10)
Accusing	(point 11)
Repelling	(point 4)

Marge meanwhile engaged in:

Quasi-courting (with Whitaker, then Malone)	
Contacting	(point 19)
Kleenex play (with Whitaker)	(point 20)

The General Compliance with the Definition

In general these positional performances were in keeping
with the formal definition of the transaction as a psychotherapy
session. Mrs. V kept trying to narrate episodes in the history.
Marge began by sitting back and commenting on the narrative.
Even the repetitiveness of these positions is not unusual since we
would expect that a number of topics would be breached and the
speakership would oscillate if the participants disagreed.

Consistent Slanting of the Performances

But each time the women performed these positions they
slanted them in a particular direction. Three consistent tactics
can be abstracted by observing these directions.

Discrediting and Defending

In each position the women intercalated disparaging metacommunicative points about the other. And each woman added point
comments to support her own position when it was disparaged.

Seeking Alliance

Although Marge was most overt about it, both women sought
support from the men. Marge used laments and sexual appeals,
for example. When Marge achieved such support from Whitaker
she used it to contend with her mother. She did not stay in face-
to-face relation with Whitaker or converse with him unless he
questioned her.

Reconciliation

But the women did not maintain their contention. One of them
quickly conceded and offered a conciliatory statement. Then
Marge would break off her relation with Whitaker and return to
sitting with her mother. Even in Phase II when Marge had become
engaged with the men Mrs. V appealed to her to return home and
Marge said she wanted to do so.

The occurrence of these reconciliations indicates that the women were constrained not to escalate their argument to the point
of a schizmogenesis (Bateson 1958). So their argument was nego-
tiatory. Each one seemed determined to alter the other's behavior
and change the other's conceptions in order to make easier a life
together. Even their relationships with the men were used in the

service of influencing each other. My guess is that they saw no choice but to stay together (see Chapter 10).

THE TACTICAL MANAGEMENT OF A POSITION

We cannot observe directly what plans the women had and thereby substantiate this idea of their strategy, but we can note more carefully what they did to slant and tailor the usual positions of the narrative conversation.

The Selective Use of Language Points

The narrative position is performed by taking a posture of vis-a-vis orientation to the listeners and recounting a series of descriptive language points. But the narrator can choose particular points and omit others.

Mrs. V's Selective Narrative

In the simplest instance a narrator strings together a number of point units until he completes a picture of some remote context and specifies his meaning. He may then add additional point units if he is questioned or if the listeners indicate noncomprehension.

Mrs. V, however, tended to be vague. She would utter a few point units and stop speaking. At six minutes and two seconds, for instance, she said: 'I think they (hallucinations) just come into my mind, and sometimes when I think to verify what I see.' Then she stopped speaking and folded her hands. The men remained immobile, staring at her without comprehension signals. She continued with another vague comment: 'Something like that. I didn't read it. It just came in my mind.'

As she made these comments, Mrs. V gave every indication of embarrassment. She had brought up the subject only at Marge's insistence. We can assume she did not want to talk about her hallucinations.

This incident typifies Mrs. V's account. She was often vague. She did not supply much information until she was pressed to do so by Marge and Whitaker. Ethnographers and demographers generally agree that the Italian-American family member is especially closed-mouthed about family affairs when he is interviewed by outsiders. From her omissions and Marge's insinuations we can guess that Mrs. V selected her narrative points to conceal the discord in her family history.

Marge's Points of Disclosure

But Marge kept adding points of insinuation and accusation which brought to light certain incidents in the history. In fact Marge aired a series of allegations in a systematic way as if she had a list of charges. All in all, Marge managed to establish a rather unflattering picture of her mother's past behavior.

She depicted her mother as mentally ill. With reluctance the older woman admitted nervousness, hallucinations, ideas of being persecuted by some 'French people,' and an episode where she had apparently wandered the streets in a panic. And Marge depicted dissention in the family. She alleged that she was afraid of her father, that her father beat her. She brought up a struggle between her parents and an incident in which the police were called because Mrs. V was allegedly attacking him with a knife. And Marge managed to portray her mother as uncaring. She implied that Mrs. V was glad when her husband died, that she had neglected the baby brother, that she talked crazy to Marge and did not understand her.

Marge's insinuations brought to light incidents of her mother's behavior which fitted psychiatric theories of the mother's causative role in the development of schizophrenia, e. g., maternal indifference, maternal psychosis, marital discord, and so on. Her choice of these topics and the ways she seemed knowingly to catch Whitaker's ear with these insinuations gave me the impression that Marge was familiar with these psychiatric ideas. She had been in psychotherapy for six months with another psychiatrist.

In the theoretical language sketched in Chapter 8, we would say that Marge introduced tactics from the mediate context of her previous psychotherapy relationship. By labeling Marge's statements tactics I do not mean to imply that her accusations were false or unfounded. But her systematic selection of these charges indicated that she had discussed them at some length in her previous psychotherapy.

Loading the Narrative with Metacommunicative Points

Recall once more Mrs. V's opening remarks. She quoted Marge as saying, 'Help me upstairs.' Then Mrs. V added a discrediting metacommunicative point: 'A young girl like her.' Mrs. V could have said, 'Poor girl, she was so sick,' or she could have omitted any metacommunicative addition. Marge soon turned the tables. She mocked Mrs. V's advice to get more sleep

and eat. And then said, 'Gonna go to hell,' which one can guess
was also a caricature of a parental religious warning.

So it went throughout Session I. Mrs. V added such a deroga-
tion each time she told about Marge's illness and Marge used
points of disparagement whenever Mrs. V spoke. So the narrative and supplementary narrative positions were loaded with metacommunicative points that were not necessary to tell the story.
They were used to slant the narrative to another purpose — that
of discrediting the other woman's position (her metaconceptions,
as I previously called them).

If one is not the principle speaker, he may remain verbally
silent, yet be kinesically 'noisy,' thus conveying metacommunicative information and distracting attention from the primary speaker.
Marge did this continuously in any Period 1 with facial expressions
and exhibitionistic gestures. She also muttered comments. So in
one kind of tactical manipulation body language is substituted for
speech.

The Addition of Direct Accusations and Denials

As you know by now, the women periodically would turn to
each other and openly disagree, with Marge making direct accusations and Mrs. V denying them and rationalizing.

At first Mrs. V would ignore what Marge said. It seemed
that certain Gestalten had to be accumulated before Mrs. V's response was elicited. In other words, Marge had to reach a certain
plateau of insistence. Then the mother turned to her, and
Whitaker picked up her daughter's insinuations (Schflen 1966).

Modification of the Address

The position may be manipulated by modifying the behavior
of address, a tactic used repeatedly by Marge.

Loading the Address with Representational Behavior

Marge loaded her orientation to Whitaker with the behaviors
of Kleenex display and quasi-courting. And sometimes she added
facial expressions and shrugs of helplessness. Thus the representational behavior of appealing and promising can be used to
supplement the address in hopes of making it more compelling
or more attractive to a potential addressee. In other cases
forceful, amiable, or preening behaviors were added to an address.

Promoting a Point Unit to a Position

Marge used another manipulation of the usual unit forms.
She performed what are ordinarily point units in a gross, exaggerated manner by altering her basic posture. She would stand
up, for example, to make a single language point and a facial
gesture of mock incredulity and 'shock.' She would sprawl and
make an expressive point of despair or disparagement. By such
manipulation of posture she made a point unit into a full position
and thus interrupted (or tried to interrupt) the narrative.

Tactics of Introducing a Position

Holding Off

A participant may hold off the introduction of a tactic until
some propitious time — until someone else has completed a position, for instance, or met disapproval. Whitaker did this repeatedly and Mrs. V seemed to, but it was difficult to assert that
Marge did. She seemed to try to manipulate the situation continuously.

The Substitution of Alternative Point Units

In the repetition of a position one or more of the constituent
subunits may be replaced by an allomorph (Z. Harris 1951), i.e.,
by a form recognizable as being of the same class of behavior
but having a different implication or connotation. Synonyms of
speech are an example. Sometimes the allomorph may be used
to specify a meaning more exactly, but it also can be used tactically. It can be used, for instance, to make a position more
persuasive or more acceptable.

Mrs. V did not use many alternative points in her narrative.
She tended to narrate sequentially. But she did use allomorphs
in her defense, repeating a repertoire of denials, rationalizations, and avowals of not remembering. But Marge tried a number of alternatives both in appealing to Whitaker and in confronting her mother. In initiating a Period 2, for example, she might
use alternatively any or several of the following point units: appealing, lamenting, insinuating, or challenging.

In challenging her mother Marge also used alternatives. To
picture such usage one must have a knowledge of the usual sequence of forms. Recall once more the pattern Marge used in
the beginning of a Period 2 to elicit an admission from her mother.

She would turn to her mother accusingly (step A), place her
hand on her mother (step B), cock her head and use supplicant

tones, as she asked her mother if the accusation were not, in reality, true (step C). If mother ignored her, as she usually did, or
flatly denied the charge, Marge would sprawl on the sofa and dis-
associate herself from the others.

But Marge had a series of alternative tactics for steps B
and C. She would raise her voice and repeat the challenge loudly. She would turn to Whitaker and by her facial expression disparage the mother's denial or she would look appealingly to the
men or to the camera.

It was almost as though Marge tried out a series of possibilities to see which one would work and she escalated a series until
one actually did. Imagine a child trying to be heard in an adult
conversation. He may try to speak and be shushed. He may tug
on his mother's sleeve but be ignored. Finally he becomes insist-
ent enough that the conversation is broken off to attend to him.
Thus Marge mounted an increasing number of disparaging and appealing points in a Period 1, then she directly and insistently confronted her mother in a Period 2, but she varied the order and
emphasis of the point units which she employed.

Multiple, Simultaneous Tactics

These steps were executed in succession. Often, however,
they are carried out simultaneously. Speech, while it may be
used in narration and postural kinesics, also may be used to load
the address and initiate the supportive relationship.[1] So the complex business of a transaction is managed by using multiple modalities differentially but simultaneously.

Suppression and Concealment as Tactics

For completion of the discussion of tactics I should mention
a subject I have already covered (Chapter 6). For tactical reasons certain performances must be suppressed accordingly. A
participant may show as active immobility and constrain his hands
or mouth. But I think it is virtually impossible to restrain totally
a customary or highly valued enactment. The participant may in
this case perform some other unit of behavior which serves to
conceal or direct attention away from the performance he wants
to conceal. Maybe this is one reason women wear cosmetics and
perfume (Birdwhistell 1963).

In such cases it is often possible to note abortive behavior
from which one can make a psychoanalytic inference about motivations which were concealed by defenses (A. Freud 1946).

Maneuvers in Managing a Point Performance

By the same token point units can be altered as a maneuver in the tactics of modifying the position. Special syntactic sentences can be chosen, for example. But I do not want to discuss such variations in detail. I will, instead, merely illustrate two matters which I mentioned in Chapter 8. A feature of paracommunication can be stressed or manipulated to alter an implication or convey an impression.

For example, Mrs. V said (2 minutes) 'He [her husband] died. It'll be a year this December 3rd. December 3rd it will be a year.'

The initial morpheme 'died' was said oversoftly, slowly, and tremulously. Probably this is a common paralinguistic quality for such a statement, indicating solemnity, proper sadness, and appropriate hesitancy about widowhood. But the second syntactic sentence was stated in a matter of fact way without any paralanguage beyond the usual range of qualities — as though this statement were a factual answer to Malone's preceding question: 'Where is your husband?'

But Mrs. V then repeated the affirmation about his death. And this time she loaded it with paralanguage. Haltingly, slowly, oversoftly, she said, 'December 3rd it will be a year.' We might surmise that having answered the question with data, Mrs. V then put in indicators of sadness, lonliness, dependency, and the like.

Marge did this sort of thing continuously. She imitated her mother's vocal qualities and facial expressions to mock her. She switched from middle class to Italian-American styles. She stressed qualities of lamentation and depression, used qualities of coyness and cuteness and so on.

The form of the point unit is also maneuvered in the use of innuendo. This will be described in Chapter 11.

COMMENT: PLANS AND THEIR EXECUTION

The Idea of Plans

From the tactical variations which we see a participant use, we classically infer his goals, drives, or motivations. We usually arrive at these abstractions by assigning behavioral variations to Aristotelian classes of theories about instincts, needs, and so on. But it is problematical to define such hypothetico-deductive categories. The participants in a transaction are acculturated, socialized people. Since they are not embryos, we cannot realistically speak of instincts as a determinant. And concepts of need and drive have yet to be defined in the terms necessary for systematic usage. These terms refer to organized systems of suborganismic, organismic, and contextual events. They are only represented intrapsychically. They do not occur there. So we had best stick to behavioral terms and to contexts and their cognitive representation. A schema for doing this has already been advanced by Miller, Galanter, and Pribram (1960). They speak of 'Plans,' which they describe as follows:

> 'Any complete description of behavior should be adequate to serve as a set of instructions, that is, it should have the characteristics of a plan that could guide the action described. When we speak of a Plan in these pages, however, the term will refer to a hierarchy of instructions, and the capitalization will indicate that this special interpretation is intended. A Plan is any hierarchical process in the organism that can control the order in which a sequence of operations is to be formed.
>
> A Plan is, for an organism, essentially the same as a program for a computer, especially if the program has the sort of hierarchical character described above. Newell, Shaw, and Simon (1958) have explicitly and systematically used the hierarchical structure of lists in their development of 'information-processing languages' that are used to program high-speed digital computers to simulate human thought processes. Their success in this direction — which the present authors find most impressive and encouraging — argues strongly for the hypothesis that a hierarchical structure is the basic form of organization in human problem solving. Thus, we are reasonably confident that 'program' could be substituted everywhere for 'Plan' in the following pages. However, the reduction of Plans to nothing but programs is still a scientific hypothesis and is still in need of further validation. For the present, therefore, it should be less confusing if we regard a computer program that stimulates certain features of an organism's behavior as a theory about the organismic Plan that generated the behavior.'

The plan, then, is cognitive representation of a traditional way to behave — a way appropriate for a given context. The

plan[2] makes use of preferred alternatives. Thus a choice of
pathways is made. Theoretically, at least, a plan can be altered at any time and at any level to adapt it to the contingencies
of particular communicational process (see below).

Planning and Executing

In situations like Session I the participants know in advance
that they will participate in a given transaction. They have some
idea or phantasy about what they will be expected to do. Presumably they scan their memories of past experience to find some
similar transaction and tentatively they select a format and a set
of preferred alternatives.

I know that Whitaker and Malone planned their parts in Session
I at length because I sat with them as they did so. I had the impression that Mrs. V and Marge enacted a more stereotyped plan
from a customary repertoire. Bateson (1962) speaks of such an
automatic plan as calibrated behavior.

So the process of planning can vary from the most detailed
thinking out of subvariants to a spur-of-the-moment production of
a usual or traditional part. In either event we must suppose that
the participant matches a percept of the immediate context with
the formats in his cognitive repertoire and selects a plan congruent to multiple contexts in his view of the hierarchy.

Miller, Galanter, and Pribram (1960) postulate a 'Tote'
mechanism, by which a plan can be tested first in imagination
and then in operation.

The participant presumably practices his plan in imagination — he imagines he is performing it. He receives retroactive
or feedback information as he calls on his past experience to imagine the responses of the others. He also perceives his own
affective and autonomic response. He can, then, alter the plan
or some subplan and rehearse his approach.

At some point the participant enacts his plan. He produces
motor actions that replicate the form of his imagery. Miller,
Galanter, and Pribram (1960) speak of execution as follows:

> We shall say that a creature is executing a
> particular Plan when in fact that Plan is control-
> ling the sequence of operations he is carrying out.
> When an organism executes a Plan he proceeds
> through it step by step, completing one part and
> then moving to the next. The execution of a Plan
> need not result in overt action — expecially in
> man, it seems to be true that there are Plans
> for guiding actions. An organism may — probably

does — store many Plans other than the ones
it happens to be executing at the moment.

At any point in its performance the plan can be recalibrated.
The participant may accommodate the plan at any level, substi-
tuting a syntactic sentence or gesture, a point, or a position,
adding certain units and so forth. Or he may withhold or conceal a motor activation of some portion and 'think it' instead of
enacting it overtly. Or he may substitute a metacommunicative
commentary (facial, gestural, or lexical). Thus the participant
has various logical types of options in enactment.[3]   He matches
and adapts these to his percepts of the immediate context and to
his images of personal contexts.

A series of feedback loops are necessary to such recalibration. These are sometimes described as 'external' — (the ex-
teroceptive observation of the responses and monitors of others)
and 'internal' (self observational and proprioceptive systems).
Some of this retroactive information is experienced consciously
as metacommunicative thought about the performance and some
is experienced emotionally.

Mechanisms for Recalibrating a Performance

Pribram also marshalls evidence of continuous inputs from
suborganismic levels. Biased homeostats in the walls of the
third and fourth ventricle apparently provide information about
any parameter in metabolic or physiological state that is not
compensated for with reflexes (Pribram 1963, 1966). These
inputs constitute parameters which can lead to a modification
of the plan.

Possibly these continuous sources of information are integrated in the temporal lobe. We can visualize a continuous
cerebral process in which all inputs are continuously scanned
and all percepts and images are matched (Pribram 1963).

Such concepts of neuropsychological functioning remain
hypothetical but they do include the ideas of systems operation
which have proved useful in other sciences. And they take us
away from the reductive reflex arc and S-R conceptions of neuro-
systems which forced earlier psychological theorists like
Wertheimer (1925), Koehler (1925), and Freud (1913) to depart
from neurological considerations. Any theory of neurophysiological functioning must be complex enough to account for that
which we can see the human organism do (Pribram 1967).
Ideas like those of Miller, Galanter, and Pribram (1960) and
subsequently of Pribram (1954, 1963, 1966) are based on
neurophysiological research and on complex models which could

be so. This was not the case with the simplistic S-R or expression conceptions which Osgood calls 'kiddie-car models' (Osgood 1963).

If an adequate theory of the nervous system can be developed, one obviates the need for a separate psychological theory. To put the point another way, the old dichotomy between brain and psyche can be eliminated by an adequate theory of either one. The behavioral science movement has contributed to the demise of simplistic theories of instinctual expression and simple stimulus reaction by showing the complexity of behavioral integration. At the same time the new neuropsychologies (Pribram 1954, 1965) have contributed to communication by developing an adequate idea about the mechanisms of communicative behavior.

Chapter 10

SCHIZOPHRENIC CHARACTERISTICS
IN THE BEHAVIOR OF THE WOMEN

Although Marge's illness was specifically diagnosed as schizophrenic reaction and she was hospitalized for this condition,
Mrs. V also showed typical features of this state. She was later
hospitalized and her illness was diagnosed as schizophrenic reaction, paranoid type. Although the psychiatric observers con-
curred that this diagnosis applied to each of the women, it was
difficult to identify accurately the behavioral features which are
pathonomic for this condition, and so I will have to use my own
judgment. I will therefore abstract in this chapter certain features of the women's behavior which I think were deviant, but not
necessarily schizophrenic, and I will point to certain features
which I think are characteristically schizophrenic.

SCHIZOPHRENIC QUALITIES IN THE
INDIVIDUAL BEHAVIOR OF EACH WOMAN

Schizophrenic Qualities
in the Behavior of Mrs. V

Mrs. V's behavior showed three qualities which are ordinarily considered schizophrenic.

Flattened affect. Mrs. V showed a definite diminution of
facial mobility and paralinguistic variance. She spoke in a mono-
tone and was kinesically immobile most of the time. She did not
react by changing her vocal qualifiers, her facial expression,
and her other kinesic qualities. This diminution of paracommunicative quality is called flattened affect in psychiatry and is considered a classical indication of schizophrenia (Blueler 1950).

219

Cognitive defect. Mrs. V explained her behavior with rationalizations and denials that seemed almost absurd at times.
It was hard to believe that she believed them or expected others
to do so. And in presenting these she often skipped steps and
left unsaid elements of her argument that were important in making it hold water. Finally she showed little apparent awareness
either of the incredibility of her statements or of the dubiety of
the other participants.

Indications of schizophrenic misconceptions. There are sug-
gestions that Mrs. V held conceptions that have typically been
reported in schizophrenic patients, and she reported experiences
that sounded typically psychotic. Here are the two most obvious
examples:

1. Mrs. V seemed to have little appreciation of the
   gravity of Marge's difficulties. She wrote off
   Marge's psychosis as a minor illness and she
   seemed to think Marge could return to her home
   without any particular problems. It seemed as
   though she had no understanding of the matura-
   ational process of the young woman or of the
   changes in classical Sicilian family structure
   which were occurring with acculturation. It
   might be inferred that her own devotion to the
   mother-daughter symbiosis overrode any other
   perceptions she could have achieved. And maybe Marge's difficulties seemed trivial to her because she had known them all her life.
2. Mrs. V described two personal experiences that
   seem typically psychotic. She apparently felt
   influenced by certain 'French people' and had
   hallucinations (mind-pictures). Apparently she
   once left her marital home and wandered in the
   streets in a panic, which clinicians identify as
   paranoid and depersonalized in character.

Marge's Deviant Behavior

Marge, of course, produced the most obvious deviant and inappropriate forms in Session I. She stood up a number of times
in a sudden, dramatic way. She sprawled on the sofa. She exhibited her thighs. She made shocking comments like, 'I want
to be raped.'

Some of these behaviors are deviant — they would not appear in common culture; not even, for the most part, in schizophrenic behavior.

Marge's standing shocked was an example. My guess was that she contrived these behaviors to disturb her mother and used it tongue-in-cheek. Her bizarre sexy behavior gave the same impression. She seemed to be satirizing sexiness.

Other of Marge's behavior was unfamiliar in this context, but we might expect to see it regularly in another situation. Her sprawling behavior is typically seen among children — possibly up until about the eighth year. Her mugging at the camera is also characteristic of the children and so were some of her paralinguistic patterns. Her sexual behavior in appealing was inappropriate for a formal transaction but it is seen in modeling, courtship, and possibly in prostitution.

Notice, however, that none of Marge's behavior was unrecognizable. It was borrowed from other contexts or loaded with qualities which would not be seen in usual conversation, but it was not wholly unique, unrecognizable, or disordered. This point is worth emphasizing because there is a myth that schizophrenic behavior is somehow original, random, or unlawful. The behavior of schizophrenic patients may be much more bizarre than Marge's was, but it is so patterned that it is awarded a standard diagnosis and it is usually rather stereotyped and nonvariegated.

Marge showed some subtler deviant behaviors that did not appear contrived. She was almost never quiet. She changed her facial expression often, showing a gamut of configurations from anger to anguish. And her hands were usually in action, stroking her legs, waving a Kleenex, or gesticulating. Her gross movements were often overfast, jerky, arrhythmic, but at times slow and writhing. Her changes in pace and style were more noteworthy than any given pace or style.

Certainly Marge did not show a flattened affect. In fact, Birdwhistell (1963) suggested it be called a fattened affect. Unlike her mother Marge's behavior was replete with paracommunicative changes, well above the usual range.

This sort of variation has been a puzzling problem in schizophrenia. A generation ago most psychiatrists agreed that flattened affect was a necessary symptom of schizophrenia, but so many exceptions appeared that a diagnostic class of schizoaffective types was developed, types for people like Marge with a very labile paracommunicative style. Thus schizophrenic patients may have either a flattened or a fattened affect. In either event they show paracommunicative deviance. As a matter of fact all kinds of measures of physiological and behavioral variables have shown a hypernormal variance in schizophrenic patients.

The contrast in the affective indicators between mother and daughter is striking. It appears that Marge had the job of affective indication for both of them, just as she had the role of metacommunicatively qualifying the historical data of Mrs. V's account. Maybe Mrs. V was affectively flat because Marge has taken over all of this behavior and vise versa. Maybe the wide paracommunicative variance in schizophrenia is often the result of such specialization of communicative function, a specific instance of the general symbiotic complementarity which has been described in the family relationships in schizophrenia (see below).

Marge's Dissociative, Autistic Behavior

The particularly schizophrenic quality of Marge's behavior was most evident in her manner of relating. The grossest example was her oscillation from huddling with her mother one minute to eliciting an alliance from Whitaker and attacking Mrs. V the next. And she would work hard to solicit Whitaker's support, then quickly abandon it. Thus her rapid positional shifts reflected a tendency to flit from relationship to relationship.

Marge used a wide variety of address and transfix behavior in making these shifts. She placed a tactile hold on her mother when confronting her. She occasionally addressed the cameraman. Sometimes she turned to her mother or to Whitaker, but overprojected her voice as if speaking to a large audience. Most often she looked down, muttered inaudibly, and did not project to the others. When her eyes were visible on a few occasions, they did not seem to be appropriately converged. Half of the time Marge did not directly address the others. Yet her remarks were obviously related to the others and were intended to evoke their attention.

At other times Marge dissociated herself from all the others. She seemed for a few seconds to be out of contact. But a closer examination of this behavior showed that she remained in contact in at least one modality. Sometimes she would turn away from the others or sit back and cover her face. Her body would fall into a marked hypotonus. She was not in postural parallelism with the others and she did not move synchronously with anyone. Yet she spoke appropriately and showed that she had been listening to the others. In short Marge was in contact in one modality — a kind of partial, unimodal association which I already described and pictured in Chapter 6.

At other times Marge reversed this unimodal dissociation. She would speak irrelevantly and address her remarks to the camera or to herself but hold her body in parallelism and active hypertonicity.

And her intervals of dissociation were dramatized or exhibited. She would throw herself back on the couch, for example, or stand up and speak to an empty portion of the room. In my experience this kind of gross but partial dissociation is characteristic of schizophrenia. In chronic severe schizophrenia the patient appears totally autistic for months or years but may later give evidence of a keen awareness of what is going on. Or conversely he talks actively to you, but you sense his detachedness or remoteness. This mixed picture is reflected in his own subjective experience. He feels at once detached and overly dependent or enslaved. I believe that one who is schizophrenic is inordinately attached to and dependent upon a parental figure, but he denies, hides, and conceals such attachment with an exhibited detachment. And analysis of his behavior shows these incongruent types of relation: one evident in some modality, usually postural-kinesic, and the other shown in some other modality, often speech and subjectivist conception.

I suspect that this ambivalence in Marge's behavior was related to her tendency to quickly form and break relationships. There was yet another manifestation of interpersonal difficulty in Marge's behavior. She seemed constrained to relate either to her mother or to Whitaker in a mutually exclusive way, as if she had to choose between them and could not sustain relatedness to both. When she broke with her mother in a Period 2 she did so dramatically and then confronted her mother. When she broke with Whitaker she did this completely and dramatically. I think this sort of difficulty is also typical of people with schizophrenia. These patients seem to be able to relate only in a one-to-one relationship, with this becoming so hazardous for them that they tend to dissociate into aloneness and autism.

I think these difficulties may explain a finding which Davis (1968) reported in the Laban or effort-shape analysis of schizophrenic behavior. She found that these patients do not coordinate their body movements in what I have been calling multiple simultaneous address. It is also reported that schizophrenic patients show unusual patterns of interpersonal distance Horowitz 1966; Hampe 1967). These findings are suggestive and deserve more systematic behavioral description.

It is interesting to note that despite the obvious deviances in Marge's behavior, we would clinically consider her mildly schizophrenic or a patient in partial remission, but Mrs. V's behavior, which was not grossly deviant, was undoubtedly schizophrenic and her prognosis was poorer than Marge's. As it turned out, Marge was later discharged from the hospital, but

Mrs. V was admitted and has remained hospitalized for years.
This is often the case. The dramatically deviant behaviors are
not what is typically schizophrenic; rather, the subtle difficulties in relating are.

A SCHIZOPHRENIC CHARACTERISTIC
IN THE RELATIONSHIP OF THE WOMEN

We would expect to find concomitant difficulties in the
mother-daughter relationship when we observe it at the social
level. This proved to be the case.

It would seem likely that a mother and daughter in such a
situation would devote most of their attention to the men, rather
than form only transient relations with the men and huddle together, continuously confronting each other. I have already
described the tendency for the women to huddly together, then
disaffiliate and have a confrontation. And we have also seen
Marge's tendency to court Whitaker, then disaffiliate with him
in a bizarre caricature of sexiness.

There were other features of this mother-daughter attachment that I have not yet sufficiently brought out.

Cross-Monitoring in the
Mother-Daughter Relationship

Each time either woman formed a relationship with one of
the men the other woman interrupted it. Birdwhistell (1963)
has called such an arrangement cross-monitoring.

Marge's Interruptions of Her Mother

Marge was almost continuously trying to gain the attention
of the men by one device or another. She would escalate her
interruptive behavior until it succeeded or until Malone intervened. One of her dramatic tactics was the position I have called
standing shocked.

Marge also used the position which I called resigning in
such a dramatic way as to make it potentially interruptive.

Mrs. V's Monitoring of Marge's Relations to the Men

Altogether Marge crossed her legs ten times in Session I.
These occurred as five pairs of leg crosses. Each pair began
with a proper quasi-courting action, followed within a moment
by the bizarre type described above. The first appealing leg
cross always initiated an alliance with Whitaker, and the bizarre
formation always terminated it.

We would expect a mother to monitor this kind of sexy, exhibitionistic behavior and sometimes Mrs. V did. But the mother's monitoring was usually directed at Marge's appealing behavior. What Mrs. V monitored, then, was a relatively normal coquettish behavior of appeal to a man.

In addition Mrs. V monitored Whitaker's response to the girl.

Whitaker used to light his pipe just before he moved in toward Marge and after the pattern was repeated three times, Mrs. V began to monitor Whitaker's pipe lighting. My belief is that she monitored pipe lighting because she had learned it preceded Whitaker's alliance behavior with Marge. Thus, I think, she evidenced disapproval of the alliance behavior between Whitaker and Marge, with far more regularity than she did Marge's grossly deviant sexy behavior.

Oscillation as a Locked Relationship

This cross-monitoring seemed to lock the women into relationship. Neither one could relate to a man without the other's interference. Marge would try to relate with sexy behaviors, then disaffiliate with a bizarre behavior we could regard as 'de-courting' (Figure 10-1).

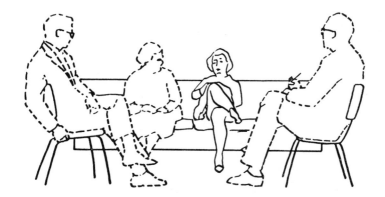

Figure 10-1: Marge in Bizarre 'De-courting' Behavior

THE HISTORY OF A LOCKED RELATIONSHIP

The women's history gave the impression that such locked-in, regressive stasis had been going on for years. They did not seem to be able to break it. If we pool the manifest content of their statements, as Jaffe (1958) does in 'dyadic analysis,' we can make clinical inferences that seem analogous to what we have observed in their communicative behavior.

The statements of the women can be classified into one of
four categories of psychoanalytic inference:

1. Statements of symbiotic relatedness in which one of the
women cared for (or did not care for) the other who was helpless, overdependent, or having symptoms often considered to
reflect such states.
2. Statements of rivalry or anger between them that seemed to be related to the need to pull apart.
3. Statements of sexuality or of one woman relating to a
male.
4. Statements suggesting that the deserted woman was alone
or unconscious while the other was guilty or about to face punishment.

The first seven repetitions of these ideas are summarized in
Figure 10-2. By referring to the transcript reproduced in the
Appendix of this volume the reader can check these interpreta-
tions and see that the themes continue throughout the session.

It seemed that these two women were in the position of not
being able to live together or to live apart. When alone together,
one of them seriously regressed while rejecting regressive or
any other satisfactions — the typical schizophrenic dynamic,
in my view. When apart, great guilt and anxiety developed, presumably because they shared a fantasy that separation and hetero-
sexuality meant death. It seems the women believed that only
one of them could relate to a man, but in doing so she deserted
the other and caused her death. Therefore, they seemed to be
forever escaping from and then re-establishing their mutual dependency.

Type Theme	Approx. Frame Numbers	Content
1	0- 200	Mother helping daughter upstairs
3	200- 300	Daughter having a doctor's prescription
4	300- 360	Daughter ought to sleep
1 & 2	450-2190	Anger and denial of hatred between moth- er and Marge
3	2300-3040	Daughter's sexual and animal behavior Information about father's death
4	4100	Daughter says she is dead
1 & 2	4100-5340	Mother didn't miss father: mother and daughter argument

3	5400	Daughter 'hallucinates' father
4	5500-5830	Daughter says she died and is the 'only one'
1	5920-6650	Daughter's sick stomach; mother feeding her
3	6650-6820	Calling the doctor
4	6820-6900	Daughter's dying
1	7200-7550	Mother's illness: The world makes her nervous
3	7550-7810	Mother's hallucinations: French people
4	7810-7850	Mother's unconsciousness
3	9600	Mother's hallucination about God and daughter's hallucinations with a sexual implication
4	10900-11350	Death, lack of control, and inability to sin
1	12320-12500	Mother denies collapsing
3	12500-14260	Husband as a family man: father hits daughter and prevents her from going out (dating)
4		Mother denies father's slapping was dangerous or that she had to stop it

Figure 10-2: Lexical Themes in Mother-Daughter Relationship
(First Ten Minutes of Session I)

Mrs. V and Marge appeared to have no way to break their attachment. They were able to oscillate from attempting to separate and form other relationships, to returning to their symbiotic attachment. Their relationship lacked a progressive program. It seemed to me that this was evident both in their history and in what was observable in their behavior during the session.

COMMENT: ON THE NATURE AND
ORIGINS OF SCHIZOPHRENIA

Varied Theories About the
Origins of Schizophrenia

There are widely divergent opinions on the nature of schizophrenia. Disorders at all levels of organization, from the molecule to society, have been postulated. Whatever the origins, the clearest evidences of disturbances are manifest at the organismic level (in disordered thought and behavior) and at the social

level (in deviant relationships). Some theorists see the disturbances of thought as a consequence of abnormal genetic development and as the cause of the overdependence and autism. Others see the disordered parent-child relationship as a consequence
of difficulties in the family and consider the social or communicational problems as the cause of the deviant thought and behavior.

It would be widely agreed that a difficulty in the mother-child
relationship is characteristic in schizophrenia, whatever the
cause and significance of this difficulty. The problem I have described in the relationship of Mrs. V and Marge is typical. There
is a degree of symbiotic, hyperdependent attachment admixed
with a degree of discord, rejection, and withdrawal (Mahler
1958). In some cases the autism is apparent while the ties are
denied. But in either case the ambivalent combination of interdependence and distance feature the disorder (Hill 1955;
Limentani 1956).

We cannot say how this symbiotic attachment developed.
Some theorists claim that it begins when a mother notices her infant is defective (Bender 1945). Others hold that the mother re-
jects the child at an early age (Rosen 1953) and the child then
tries to cling to the relationship. Still others hold that the mother
was possessive and the child has developed autistic behavior in an
unsuccessful attempt to fight free from the symbiosis (Levy 1943;
Mahler 1963). Recent theorists attribute the mother-child symbiosis to disturbances in the total family (Spiegel and Bell 1959;
Ackerman 1966; Bowen 1966; Jackson 1962) and even in the relations of that family to the larger society (Speck 1967)

Thus we do not know how the schizophrenic relationship develops. But, however it begins, a symbiosis is maintained by
vicious cycles at each level of social organization. Suppose I
first describe this phenomenon of stasis and then come back to
the other, controversial issues.

The Phenomenology: A Deep Belief
in the Need for Interdependency

The Symbiotic Myth

In cases of symbiotic relatedness, the partners seem to
share a myth about their need for each other and this phenomenon is regularly described by schizophrenic patients (Searles
1955; Wynne et al. 1958). The partners seem to believe that
one of them will die if they become separated. The dependent
partner, usually the patient, feels he is helpless without the
support of the other, but he nevertheless feels guilty about

deserting the partner (Galvin 1956; Rosen 1953). The anxiety and guilt on this score is so great that it amounts to a demoralizing panic at any threat to the cohesiveness of the relationship. This fantasy accompanies a tendency to distrust all other relationships. In short we can claim a subjectivist triad consisting of a sense of personal incompetence, a deep, guilty loyalty to the partner, and a suspiciousness about other, potential relationships.

The Behavioral Coding of Constraints

These fantasies seem to be maintained by metacommunication among the partners and by events in their lives which seem to confirm the myth (see below). The cross-monitoring behaviors I described earlier are but one type of such systems-maintaining activity. There are also likely to be kinesic signs which represent impending illnesses, imaginary sexual disaster, and the like (Sherman et al. 1968). Such kinesic signals remind the partners of their social incompetence, their debts to each other, and so on, but they are not ordinarily in awareness.

Enacting the Necessary Roles

The maintenance of such a symbiosis when a child grows up into adulthood requires that he remain infantilized, helpless, sick, incompetent, or the like. Accordingly the patient-to-be has to enact such a role. And the relationship must develop a rationale because its deviance becomes increasingly apparent. Consequently a myth is held about the sacrificing parent, the helplessness of the child, and so forth. To debate whether this situation leads to the cognitive defects of schizophrenia or is a consequence of them takes us back to the chicken-egg argument which characterized presystems theories (Singer and Wynne 1965). In any event, belief is shared about the incompetence of the schizophrenic partner. This is reinforced by metacommunicative suggestion and re-enacted in everyday life.

The mother-daughter relationship ordinarily consists of a set of reciprocals for the feeding, discipline, and training of the child. These are applied according to a maturational scale which progressively reduces the mother-infant relationship and leads to a growing competence for work, sexuality, marriage, and so forth. This did not happen in the case of Marge and Mrs. V, nor does it generally in cases of schizophrenia. The history indicated that Marge was unable to live outside a hospital. She

had engaged in sex, but had not managed a sexual relationship.
In the session she showed childish or regressive behavior.

The parent enacts the reciprocal part to the incompetent
patient. Although she may critize, and reject as Mrs. V did,
she fosters the dependency. She complains about her responsibility, but continues to nurture and encourage the child to remain
with her (Levy 1943; Mahler 1958).

Maintenance by Double-Binding

A double-bind theory of schizophrenia was developed in the
1950s to conceptualize these relations (Bateson et al. 1956);
Haley 1959; Watzlawick, Beavin and Jackson 1967).

In double-binding a covert series of instructions conflicts
with the open and acknowledged definition of the situation. The
conflicting messages cannot be visualized comparatively because
they are not of the same logical type. Thus the paradox cannot
be resolved. For example, one set of instructions, usually verbalized, criticizes the child's dependency, but another set, im-
plicit in the relationship and signalled kinesically, may censure
and interdict the learning and experience which make maturation
possible.

In the case of Marge and Mrs. V, the mother alleged her
competence and depreciated Marge's dependency. Yet there was
every indication that Mrs. V had not been able to handle the problems of her life. And Marge kept questioning this competence,
but she would sprawl and exhibit childishness just at the point of
making her accusation stick.

So the myth of the competent mother and helpless child was
partly maintained despite Marge's ambivalent assault upon it
(Abrahams and Vacron 1953).

The signals of monitoring which tended to maintain the relationship were coded kinesically. They did not appear as conscious
or lexicated interdictions. I would imagine that Mrs. V did not
know she performed them.

Layers of cognitive and metacommunicative myth may be
built upon this conflicting system of behaviors. Marge was criticized for enacting her dependent role. Then her psychosis was
written off as insignificant. And the women affirmed the value
of living together and spoke of going back to the days of Marge's
childhood.

Maintenance by the Failure of Other Relationships

The symbiotic relatedness is maintained by the failure of the
partners to develop other relationships. The partners unwittingly

exclude others, they unconsciously cause other relationships
to fail, and they simply lack the experience and communicative
skills to maintain courtship, marriage, and friendship.

The Exclusion of Others

Whatever their origin, the cognitive and metacommunicative
difficulties in schizophrenia and cross-monitoring behavior make
it difficult for anyone else to join in or intervene in the relationship. In such cases the history often indicates a vicious cycle
with the father-husband. The more he is excluded the more remote a figure he becomes, and the lesser his importance, the
greater the interdependence between mother and child. Sometimes a father-child symbiosis similarly excludes a mother
(Lidz et al. 1957).

Unsuccessful Attempts to Break Out

Marge seemed to be trying to break out of the dilemma.
From her standpoint the situation may have seemed something
like this. If she continued to relate to her mother as a dependent child she lacked the status or power to alter the relationship.
She could not take over, solve problems, or persuade her mother to grasp what was going on. If, on the other hand, she left
her mother she was apparently regarded as a distrusted outsider,
who had to be brought back to the fold.

In this setting Marge's behavior makes sense. She was trying, I think, to solve the metacommunicative problem — pre-
serve the mother-daughter relationship by changing the ground
rules, by attacking the cognitive distortions. Thus she tried to
expose Mrs. V's psychosis and incompetence. In a Period 1,
however, she seemed unable to gain her mother's attention and
so made ineffectual insinuations. In a Period 2, allied with
Whitaker, she was an antagonist.

I would guess, from my knowledge of psychotherapy, that
Marge's tactics were learned in her previous psychotherapy.
She used ineptly but unmistakably a first approach in the psychotherapy of schizophrenia — a tactic for discrediting the mother's hold, a tactic of confrontation and interpretation.

Another of Marge's behaviors could be construed as an
attempt to compromise the dilemma. One of these we heard
about in subsequent sessions. Marge was allegedly a prostitute.
We could interpret this as a way of relating temporarily to a
man. And we could argue that this kind of hit-and-run behavior
was reflected in her relationship to Whitaker.

Social Incompetence and the Self-Fulfilling Prophecy

In any event, when Marge did relate outside the home, her relationships were unsuccessful. Her pregnancy and abortion precipitated her regression and psychosis. We can guess that her difficulties with men stemmed partly from her inexperience. She seemed to be afraid of her father (Lidz and Lidz 1949; Frazee 1953). Her Sicilian background did not suit her for courting without a father or brother to monitor the process. Her way of relating to men in Session I probably reflected her general approaches which were, we can guess, either remote or purely sexual contacts which she probably terminated as she did with Whitaker early in the session.

Mrs. V's behavior seemed to cycle similarly. Her story of leaving her husband when Marge was a child apparently ended in a psychotic panic reaction.

Thus the myth of helplessness is a self-fulfilling prophecy and the interdependency is maintained in the immediate life situation.

Inadequate and Idiosyncratic Communicative Behavior

The development of secret and special communicative behaviors further maintains the attachment. Unsuccessful in communications, the partners keep falling back on each other where their unusual tactile, kinesic, spacing, and metabehavior is understood. I suspect this was the case with Marge. Her crazy pattern of appealing and rejecting with the use of sexual behaviors could not have enabled her to maintain a courtship. Since her attention-getting behaviors, for example, could easily be seen as seductive, she may have ended up having sexual intercourse in whatever kind of relationship she attempted.

Maintenance by Institutionalization

Whatever the genetic or childhood origins of the dependency, once it is manifest it can be stabilized by becoming institutionalized in the social system.

Family as a Total Institution

A total institution restricts the behavior of its members (Goffman 1961). If a person belongs to one total institution without other social relationships his behavior is constrained almost entirely to the stereotyped roles he serves in that institution. In

the case of Marge and Mrs. V, the family constituted a total institution.

This stereotyped performance, which is deviant and overdependent in schizophrenia, justifies the institutionalization.
Thus the mother or father feels it necessary to protect the developing schizophrenic child, keeping him home and away from
other people. If the schizophrenic child does leave he is likely
to marry a counterdependent partner[1] or form a homosexual
symbiotic relation which perpetuates the behavior; after all,
'it is only natural' to take care of someone who is 'sick.' So the
parents may take the patient away from a psychotherapist or
spouse or college or whatever other relationships the patient is
involved in. They take him home to bed, chicken broth, or whatever family means are used for unconscious reindoctrination.

Mrs. V exemplified such activity. Even though Whitaker
had explained the sessions, and promised to try to help Marge,
Mrs. V's last appeal was for Marge to come home to her. She
even promised to move back to the house where Marge had lived
as a child.

Sanctions in the Larger Social System

Such systems of deviance also seem to be supported in the
larger social order. Counterdeviant roles are officially recognized, e.g., those of policeman, custodian, and mental-health
professional. There is also evidence that deviances have more
general sanction. It seems to be universal for a community to
have a town drunk, a known prostitute, a religious fanatic, a
comic, a hatchet man. Such official deviants can be counted on
to show up at public functions and perform their characteristic
deviation.[2] Despite many complaints about them, such people
never seem to be effectively silenced or disposed of. If the
holder of these roles should leave town or die, another seems to
take his place.

If a deviant is unable to sustain himself in private institutions such as the family or gang, a public institution may take
over the role of supporter and custodian. Marge was being indoctrinated into such institutionalization at the time Session I
occurred.

The public institution must of course maintain itself and so
it unwittingly recruits counterdependents and patients. It may
thus maintain the symbiotic relationship and further 'protect'
the patient from other relationships. In addition the patient is
labeled with a diagnosis which announces his incompetence and
confirms it officially.

234

The Cultural Context of the Problem

In some measure the old country pattern of the cohesive extended family is a background for this sort of difficulty. In many old country traditions the family is to remain cohesive and all offspring are to remain living in the extended family clan for the duration of their lives — sometimes in the same household. In these social arrangements they do not assume leadership until all senior members of the group have died. The Sicilian culture from which Marge and Mrs. V were derived is such a culture. Marge was raised in an Italian enclave where such arrangements were maintained unacculturated.

The Culturally Derived Expectations of the Women

With such a background we could expect that Mrs. V and Marge both would think they must remain together for life. At the end of the session Mrs. V said, 'My grandfather's house was my house.' In fact, we would anticipate that the attempt to leave would produce intense guilt in those indoctrinated in such values.

Usual Provisions in an Extended Family

But an extended family social organization ordinarily would provide for the sexual maturation of the children and provide them with regulated courtship and marital partners. This does not happen, however, if nuclear families become separated in migration or if for some reason they do not effectively intervene in closed mother and daughter relationships. If the father and brother are detached or dead, as well, there would be no chance for such intervention. In southern Italian cultures also there would be no protection for the courtship of the daughter. In such closed families the members are not likely to allow outsiders to fulfill these roles. Consequently the extended family tradition may result in difficulty for its members if it is destroyed without the survivors knowing alternative ways for child rearing.

The Dilemma of Partial Acculturation

Other cultures, such as middleclass American, demand that children leave home in their early twenties or late teens, establish separate households, and assume leadership there. In fact the failure to do so is deeply criticized as an evidence of immaturity. But there are no provisions for learning these abilities in an old country model of development. On the contrary, the child has been taught to remain within the parental domain.

A considerable conflict of values can develop in the children of extended families who are partly acculturated and accept middle-class American values. Marge was, of course, in such a position. We cannot expect that Mrs. V would understand. Thus in acculturation a discrepancy in child-rearing behavior may increase between the metacommunicative values and the actualities of existence.

So we could speculate that the women were caught in a progressive narrowing of opportunities by migration, marital discord, the loss of an effective larger family, and finally by the death of the husband. We can also postulate that a confusing clash of value systems led to distorted metacommunicative conceptions. Mandel and Fischer (1956) have developed a three-generation theory of cumulative neurotic difficulties.

Causation in Schizophrenia and Psychosis

The genetically oriented scientist and the classical psychologist, in fact, might advocate a different view of deviance. They might hold that is a consequence of defective inheritance or destructive early experience. But this view in no way contradicts the idea that traditional dependency and deviation are maintained in the social system. It seems that dependents are selected at an early age, even within the family, and induced into traditional roles which shape their behavior. Whether this training and reinforcement cause or merely maintain the deviance must remain an open question.

We can hold to the general idea that traditional roles and social sanctions have evolved which provide for the care of dependents and deviants and that these provisions maintain deviant behavior. Obviously those who are recruited and who accept a given role have personality traits and motivations suited for its performance.

But we do not have to understand the earliest origin of schizophrenic condition in order to understand it. Once a closed cycle occurs it can maintain itself. With a systems model we recognize that retroaction can maintain a system of effects, even though the original triggering or kicking-off mechansim has ceased to operate (Marayuma 1963). Perhaps, then, a congenital defect, a family crisis, a childhood illness, or any circumstance delays the process of individuation, and the vicious cycle, once in progress, is maintained by forces like those I have described.

Whatever the chains of circumstances, a persistent symbiotic dyad has inevitable vulnerabilities which will lead its members into trouble. The partners will disavow it and others will disapprove, unless it is attractively rationalized. So the partners try to withdraw from each other; hide and deny their affiliation, blame and hate each other. The schizophrenic syndrome emerges as the child approaches maturity. And the lack of experience and social competence make both partners vulnerable to the panic of separation when sexuality, education, induction into military service, and progressive intolerance force the symbionts to separate. Then, I believe, one or both of them may develop a psychotic reaction. Once the psychosis becomes public, a second chain of circumstances may be instituted and the patient assumes a socially sanctioned role. When these continue, the schizophrenic patient may develop the advanced picture of institutionalization with autism, loss of interest, and so forth (Scheflen 1965). Thus symbiotic attachment closed by double binding may lead to schizophrenia which leads to psychosis. These conditions may thus be probable consequences of each other, rather than the same states.

SECTION E

Some Behaviors of Psychotherapy

Introduction:

THE EVOLUTION OF PSYCHOTHERAPY

Metacommunicative units can be applied for the correction of deviant behavior at any level of integration. A point can be intercalated in a transaction or whole transactions in an institutional procedure can be directed toward educating novitiates or changing the behavior of deviants.

In the last century there has been a progressive evolution of special transactions for changing the behavior of neurotic and schizophrenic subjects. Freud (1933) developed a strategy for extensive review of the patient's conceptions and a specialized transaction evolved which is called insight, expressive or psychoanalytic psychotherapy. This transaction usually has the following features: fifty-minute sessions are held one to five times a week. The therapist and patient form a special relationship which is descriptively called rapport. Over time the patient tends to re-enact his childhood patterns of behavior in the relationship with the therapist, whereupon his relationship is called a transference. This behavior is then observed for critical examination, interpretation, and discussion. Through insight the patient thus can unlearn his existing concepts, values, and patterns of action and perhaps (Alexander and French 1946; Mowrer 1950) learn new ones (Bibring 1954; Devereux 1956; Rogers 1958; Shands 1960; Ford and Urban 1963).

In the 1940s these approaches were applied to schizophrenic patients (Fromm-Reichmann 1950; Bychowski 1952; Rosen 1953). In the social science era, the 1950s, the methods of psychotherapy were increasingly applied to groups, including the family. It became common practice for co-therapists to manage

237

238

the therapy group, and the relationships of the group members came to be scrutinized as well as the behavior of a particular patient-member (Jackson 1962; Ackerman 1966).

Whitaker, Malone, and the Atlanta group played a prominent part in these developments. They developed special applications of psychotherapy for the schizophrenic patient (Whitaker
and Malone 1953). They pioneered in family therapy (Whitaker
1958) and co-therapy techniques (Whitaker, Malone, and
Warkentin 1956). Session I was an example of their technique.
It shows features of classical psychotherapy, as described in
Chapter 11, and features of the family and co-therapy approaches, as described in Chapter 12.

Chapter 11

THE TACTICS OF THE PSYCHOTHERAPISTS
IN SESSION I

As is characteristic of psychotherapy, the men sat back at first and permitted the women to lead off, but they progressively imposed on the relations and subject matter a structure to which the women more or less accommodated. In this chapter, I will describe four tactics which the men used. Then I will compare these to the customary tactics of insight psychotherapy in general.

THE TACTIC OF OBTAINING INFORMATION

The first step in classical psychotherapy is to obtain information about the patient. To do this the therapist gets the patient to talk about his problem, then sits back and restrains himself from commenting, except to ask questions and encourage the patient to go on.

A typical demeanor is used in this stage of psychotherapy. In strict applications the body is held immobile, and the face is set in an impassive, deadpan expression. This kind of expressive control is believed to minimize cues which may influence the patient's selection of topics and viewpoints.

In addition a psychotherapist keeps his distance at the beginning of a course of sessions. He can converge his eyes at a point beyond the speaker and overproject his voice so as to speak to the room at large. He can avoid tête-à-tête relations and keep physically beyond the usual distance for rapport. And he may maintain formal paralinguistic tones. Whitaker and Malone began Session I with these classical behaviors.

239

Influence from the Position, Listening

A therapist can exercise a great deal of influence from this position. He can reinforce or discourage certain topics by the use of minimal kinesic cues. He can interdict certain violations and thus maintain the definition of the situation. He can maintain the distance or else decrease it and foster rapport. When there are family members or multiple patients he can subtly foster a relationship with one of them and discourage rapport with the other. Such maneuvers in the tactic of listening direct the subsequent behavior of the patients and set up the more specific definition of the transaction. And the appearance of such weighting in the early behavior of the therapist previews his later technique.

Whitaker and Malone seemed to influence the topics and behaviors of the women by the use of such maneuvers from the first minute of Session I. Thus I called their position selective attending. The maneuvers they used were (1) influencing the topic, and (2) monitoring certain behavior:

1. Influencing the topic. On three occasions Malone asked Mrs. V to talk about the day Marge became psychotic. But Whitaker questioned her, at Marge's instigation, about her own illnesses and about earlier events in the V family history. Thus the two themes of Session I were in part chosen by the men.

In a similar way, Whitaker screened what Marge had to say. He selectively attended her when she spoke about problems in the family and ignored her other comments. And Malone made it clear that the did not want Marge to talk about her sexual behavior and 'her sin' at this point in the session.

2. Monitoring Certain Behavior. Since the therapist is generally impassive, the few cues he does furnish may be doubly influential. Certain kinesic monitors, not recognized in common culture, have escaped the censorship of psychiatric self-discipline. Three examples are nose-wiping, looking away, and lint-picking (see Chapter 5). It is usual in psychotherapy to see psychotherapists pick lint from their clothing or wipe their noses, despite their dead pan expression, when the patient acts in ways or speaks about behaviors which are not socially approved. When we see which behavior of the patient elicits these monitors we can sometimes predict the areas which the therapist will later choose for confrontation and correction.

Thus in Session I Malone wiped his nose at Marge's sexy behavior and Whitaker picked lint and looked away. The men also picked lint and frowned when Mrs. V denied and rationalized.

Selective Attention to Marge

As the reader knows Whitaker overtly supported Marge and encouraged an alliance with her. He did not do this with Mrs. V, and Malone, who overtly supported Mrs. V and scolded Marge, contributed to the rapport formation with Marge by his covert behavior. Thus rapport with Marge was selectively escalated, while the initial distancing was maintained with Mrs. V. This was appropriate since the men were going to dismiss the mother from further participation. Here are some of the maneuvers by which this was done.

1. Whitaker's selective support. Whitaker picked up Marge's comments and sharply questioned Mrs. V about them. He also moved in toward Marge. And he developed an informal style with Marge which he did not extend to Mrs. V.

2. Malone's ironic support of Mrs. V. Malone said the words which would support Mrs. V's arguments, but remained formal with her and tended to load his comments with innuendo which suggested a failure to accept the woman's allegations. At times these loaded comments amounted to subtle confrontations of Mrs. V's position, so I will describe them more fully below.

3. Malone's kinesic attentions to Marge. Finally, Malone scolded Marge but he moved in synchrony with her for the first five minutes of the session and again from 23 minutes on.

Numerous instances of this behavior are depicted in the multi-modality transcript in Section B. Malone moved his leg exactly as Marge had done at 28 seconds. From 1 minute: 30 seconds on, Malone and Marge both made stroking movements with their hands — Marge on her leg, Malone on his chair. These were carried out in perfect synchrony and lasted nearly a minute. At 4 minutes and 52 seconds Marge took out a Kleenex and blew her nose. Immediately afterward Malone took out a handkerchief and did the same thing in the same rate and rhythm of movement.

As I stated in Chapter 7, such synchronous behavior is an indication of a developing relationship which later will become manifest.

In summary we can say that the men began the session in the classical manner. They listened and questioned, maintained psychotherapist impassivity, and at first avoided any instructions. But their later tactics were presaged by their initial kinesic behavior as invariably it is in a transaction.

THE TACTIC OF FOSTERING RAPPORT

As Session I proceeded Whitaker escalated his selective attention to Marge into a developing relationship of the type which psychotherapists call rapport.

Characteristics of the Rapport Relationship

In Phase I rapport existed temporarily. It was formed late in a Period 1 and dissolved at the end of each Period 2. In Phase II it became lasting and persisted throughout subsequent sessions.

At each formation of rapport the following sequence would occur: Marge and Whitaker would address each other in a tête-à-tête and converse briefly. Then Marge would shift to sitting like Whitaker and would confront her mother.

Thus the rapport relationship was a temporary vis-a-vis which was used as a transitional step to a side-by-side alliance. It was thus open to interaction with other people. It was not closed by cross-monitoring, for instance, as was the mother-daughter relationship. Marge used the relationship to argue with her mother. In Phase II and subsequent sessions she used it to relate to Malone, perhaps to learn flirting, tactile contact, and other nonsexual behaviors under Whitaker's protective aegis.

Thus the rapport relationship is not a sexual relationship per se. It is also not a closed dyad in the sense that a marriage or a parent-child relationship may be in traditional cultures. If rapport does become a closed dyad it ceases to serve its tactical and strategic purposes and becomes an end in itself. Like other dyads it is supposed to be temporary.[1]

The Progressive Moving-In Series

I have already described the pacing by which Whitaker moved forward every six minutes, and I have described how he stepped up his proximity and support of Marge at each step (see Chapters 1, 6 and 7).

Maneuvers in the Fostering of Rapport

Schizophrenic patients are notoriously fearful of new relationships and premature, tactless attempts to induce such relationships may result in an increased autism and distrust from the patient. It may also result in intervention by family members. In Session I Mrs. V monitored Whitaker's and Marge's approaches to each other and Marge did pull back and repel Whitaker. So

part of the psychotherapist's communicative skills involve his
judicious use of the tactic of rapport inducement.

We already know that Whitaker moved forward in steps. Here
are some other maneuvers and tactical modifications that he used
in Session I.

1. Whitaker moved in when he received an invitation from
Marge and not at other times. Participants may indicate their
readiness for an address and thus invite a relationship by using
kinesic behaviors. Marge used them all. She would trail off
in her contention with her mother and drift away from the older
woman. Correspondingly she would lean toward Whitaker, uncross her arms, and turn toward him. She would search his face
with her gaze and show hesitance or uncertainty in her behavior.
At 6 minutes she lamented and quasi-courted. At 10 minutes she
dropped her handkerchief near him.

Whitaker moved in when Marge made this appeal. [2] She did
make appeals at other times which Whitaker passed up. The
safest interpretation is to say that Whitaker selected Marge's
appeals at six minute intervals to conform with the pacing of the
session.

2. Whitaker did not court Marge. Whitaker engaged in tete-
a-tete and contacting behaviors with Marge but he did not act se-
ductively toward her. I have elsewhere described such behavior
as quasi-courting (Scheflen 1965). It is used by psychotherapists
in general. This pattern is not seductive in middle-class America. [3]

3. Whitaker avoided the persistent exclusion of Mrs. V
from his relation to Marge. A full body vis-à-vis excludes
third parties from participation. Whitaker and Marge avoided
a full vis-à-vis. In the first tactile contact, for instance,
Whitaker looked and talked to Mrs. V. He did not even look at
Marge when he handed her the Kleenex. In the second, Whitaker
turned only his face to Marge.

Thus by relating to Mrs. V lexically and to Marge kinesically, Whitaker maintained the multiple simultaneous relations I
described in Chapter 7. We can hold that such a procedure is
necessary in any transaction which involves more than two people.
But in Session I special tactical considerations were involved.
We can guess that a persistent Whitaker-Marge twosome would
have brought intervention from Mrs. V and Malone, and Marge
might have returned to huddling against mother. Insofar as
Whitaker and Malone encouraged multiple simultaneous relations,
then, they were acting tactically to encourage rapport.

4. Whitaker did not try to hang on to rapport with Marge
when she broke off to return to her mother. When Marge would
break off with Whitaker and return to sitting with her mother,

Whitaker would also turn away from her.

It seemed that Marge exhibited dissociation from Whitaker to conform to the plans for maintaining the mother-daughter interlock. Maybe Whitaker shared in this behavior for tactical reasons.

The Tactic of Metacommunicative Discrediting

A basic technique of the expressive or insight psychotherapies consists of the use of metacommunicative behavior to discredit certain metaconceptions of the patient which are adjudged unrealistic.

In Session I such tactics were employed gingerly toward Mrs. V's story. In later sessions they were directed to some of Marge's ideas.

In Session I Whitaker more overtly used the metacommunicative tactic, but Malone participated subtly.

Subtle Metacommunicative Qualities in Whitaker's Attending

Whitaker used subtle kinesic behavior in attending and questioning. He would 'suggest' through facial expression that Mrs. V question her own story.

One kinesic technique for doing this is in general usage. When someone makes a dubious statement, it can be questioned by assuming a dead pan expression, staring at him, and withholding any signals of approbation or comprehension. Whitaker did this whenever Mrs. V used denial or rationalization.

There are other kinesic metabehaviors or gestures which make a discrediting or questioning comment more directly. A shrugging of the shoulders is one of these. Raising eyebrows and holding these while slightly cocking the head is another. Whitaker used these subtler indications of dubiety, rather than the gross discrediting kinesics which Marge employed.

Selective listening steers the direction of a speaker's topic. One can act bored when he takes certain directions and interested when he takes others. Thus a therapist can make notes when a patient discusses certain topics or nod his head and attend closely. Then, with other subjects he looks away, doodles on his note pad, yawns, and so forth. Thus the patient can be conditioned to operate along certain lines of behavior. Whitaker used a variant of these maneuvers of selective attention. He would glance at Marge when Mrs. V related certain incidents and get more involved in kinesic representational behavior with the girl.

The systematic use of all of these maneuvers can alter a definition of the situation. Searching glances to others, signaled inattention to the speaker, the withholding of comprehension and approval, and indications of boredom can turn off a speaker and invite someone else to interrupt him.

Whitaker and Marge allied to interrupt Mrs. V. They did so by escalating such subtle indicators. Ultimately there would be a gross interruption of Mrs. V by one of them. It is usually this way in an interaction. Covert kinesic behaviors develop progressively until one party finally performs an obvious act. The practice of assigning an originator can thus be misleading. We erroneously blame the person who took the first obvious step in the reciprocal sequence. We may realize the difficulty when we try to decide who initiated a fight among siblings or who started a lovers' quarrel.[4]

Malone's Use of Metacommunicative Innuendo

The innuedo is an instance of metacommunicative manipulation. A participant qualifies his behavior in such a way as to suggest another possibility. Malone often did this in Session I.

At one point when Mrs. V was under fire because of an insinuation that she had neglected her baby, Malone supported her ironically. What Malone said was, 'You would do anything for her,' allegedly affirming that Mrs. V would not have been guilty of neglect. But his paralanguage and stress pattern conveyed a different implication. He placed so strong a primary stress on 'anything' and so retracted a drawl on the word that a sharp incongruity was evident. This configuration usually serves to exaggerate a comment of praise to render it plausible.

Malone also used innuendo as a confrontation early in the session (see page 3 of the transcript at 2 minutes and 1 second). He asked Mrs. V, 'Where is your husband?' The husband had not been previously mentioned during the session, so the usual structure would call for the primary stress to be placed on the 'where' or on 'hus-(band).' Malone put the primary on 'is' — a structure used when the person in question is then under discussion. He thus acted as though they had been talking about the husband all along.

This usage makes no sense except in a very special context. Marge had been talking about getting sexy. Malone thought she was unwittingly referring to her father and subtly made a connection. This is a technique sometimes used in psychotherapy to suggest an interpretation to a patient by innuendo, such that the patient can pick up the connection if it is not too disturbing.

Malone is generally aware of such behavior, using it as a covert, but purposive, technique of psychotherapy. I think he used innuendo to make subtle confrontations and qualify his overt role of supporting Mrs. V. This behavior, coupled with his kinesic relation with Marge, presaged and fostered both the withdrawal of Mrs. V and the rapport between Marge and Whitaker.

Metaconceptual Connecting:
The Special Use of Confrontation
by Whitaker and Malone

Whitaker and Malone do not believe that it is necessary that the patient have a systematic and fully conscious picture of his discrepant conceptions. They believe that the necessary ideational connections can be made out of awareness. In fact they believe that the schizophrenic patient's misconceptions are preverbal and are not even coded in the conceptual systems which are derived from language.

Accordingly their techniques for changing metaconceptions are not aimed at conscious linguistic expression. They do not require that the patient be able to talk about his insights. In fact they prefer that he not do so and they do not interpret in the classical psychoanalytical sense. In a sense they see their efforts directed at helping the patient make connections of some sort between experience in the immediate relationships and his symbolic representations of experience.[5] They use at least the following maneuvers to this end.

1. They call attention to a connection between ideas they believe are related by restatements which link the ideas together in a single syntax. For example, late in the session Mrs. V was talking about her family home in childhood, her present home, and her expectation that Marge would return there. Marge was talking about going to hell. In this context Malone said 'You mean hell?' And Whitaker detailed this reference by saying: 'You mean hell is her home? Kinda like it was yours, huh?'

2. If the therapists have a thought which seems to refer to the patient's problem, they will state this thought even though they cannot formulate its connection explicitly. Thus they may tell the patient a fantasy or affective response they have had, much as a patient is expected to do in a classical insight therapy. They may then discuss this idea with the patient, but they believe a connection may be made whether or not the matter is discussed. For example, in Session IX Whitaker told Marge that he visualized her with a hole in her head. It was not clear what this imagery referred to.

3. They may simply respond to representational behaviors of the patient with other representational behaviors without explaining or being able to explain the significance. For example, Whitaker made tactile contact with Marge.

The smelling incident is interesting in this regard. 'Why,' the researchers asked, 'did Whitaker have Marge smell the object in his hand?' As he did so, he said the object was Parmesan cheese. Whitaker intercalated this behavior in the middle of an explanation of the sessions which would end with Mrs. V's dismissal from future sessions. My own guess is this: Whitaker used a representational behavior whose reference was Mrs. V. Mrs. V was the Parmesan cheese, and Whitaker was attempting to convey his metacommunicative attitude about the quality of her mothering.

Whitaker thinks this may be so but is not sure why he did it. He said it intuitively seemed the correct maneuver to follow. Such refusal to explain each action characterizes the men's metabehavior about their method. When they teach it, they often comment that they have no explanation. In part this lack of explicit rationale is a result of their application of a maneuver even when they cannot explain it. In part, I think it is a purposive opposition to the classical insight therapist who insists upon a conscious rationale before acting. Whitaker and Malone feel this is poor practice because therapists who act on this injunction may fabricate complicated rationalizations for their behavior in therapy and eventually set an example for the patient who gets lost in 'intellectual' rumination.

THE TACTIC OF EXPLAINING

During the first twenty-three minutes of the session Whitaker had progressively moved forward into the position of principal narrator. At this point he took the floor and explained the purposes and plans for the sessions. In doing so he carried out two actions. First, at 24 minutes, in the middle of the explanation, he placed his palm under Marge's nose and asked her to smell the object he held there. The second or 24 minute physical contact was made.

I have described this action before, but a drawing is reproduced as Figure 11-1 to refresh the reader's memory.

Then, Whitaker went on with the explanation. As he described the plans for future sessions he made it clear that Mrs. V was not to attend them.

Whitaker's explanation and his dismissal of Mrs. V completed the progressive engagement of Marge in the session. She was brought into the prominent role that Mrs. V had occupied.

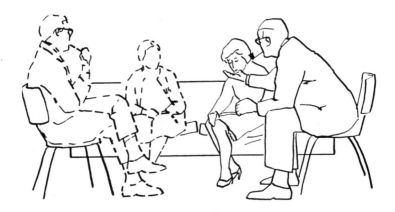

Figure 11-1: Whitaker's Position at 24 Minutes for Explaining
and Tactile Contacting

Malone then engaged her actively in vis-à-vis and Whitaker became relatively quiet. This Phase II structure was maintained
throughout the other eight sessions of the series; Malone became
the active therapist with Marge, while Whitaker assumed the less
active position of intermittent intervention that Malone held before 24 minutes. So the 23-24 minute intervention was a critical
turning point in the course of this session and of the series of psychotherapy sessions.[6]

COMMENT: CUSTOMARY AND UNCUSTOMARY
FEATURES OF THE WHITAKER
AND MALONE TECHNIQUE

The Whitaker and Malone approach is to be classified with
the expressive or insight therapies. In classical psychiatric
terms, feelings and thoughts (misconceptions in metasystems)
result in behavior that is inappropriate to reality (to the actual
life contexts). Accordingly, the strategy of an insight therapy
calls for the patient to become aware of his behavior and his
conceptions in order for these to be altered.

The Usualness of Their Tactics

The following interdependent tactics are used in any expressive or insight therapy:

1. Tactics for learning about the patient's behavior
   and conceptions, followed by: Tactics for encouraging the patient to learn about his behavior
   and metabehavior, and

2. Tactics for fostering and regulating the rapport relationship.

2. Tactics for fostering and regulating the rapport
   relationship.

Whitaker employed these techniques in Session I and Malone
did in subsequent sessions. It is also characteristic in initial
interviews to explain the purpose and plans of psychotherapy.
So the four tactics which Whitaker used are customary in psychotherapy.

The men also used the basic demeanors of psychotherapy —
the restraints of facial expression and movement which tend
to minimize metacommunicative instruction to the patient.

Figure 11-2 shows some features of tactical progression in
another psychiatric interview. In this particular session the following phases occurred.

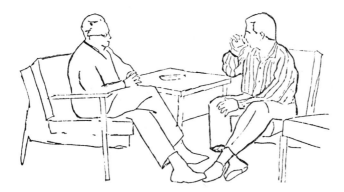

Figure 11-2: Regularities in Another Psychotherapy Session.
          Above, In this psychotherapy session the patient
          would drink from a glass of water and make a
          reference to his father. The psychotherapist
          would then make an interpretation about his de-
          pendency. Below, This complex occurred every
          fifteen minutes in two sessions. The structure
          is analogous to that of the tactile contacting in
          Session I. The therapists would 'use his tech-
          nique' at 15 and at 30 minutes in response to a
          characteristic representational behavior of the
          patient.

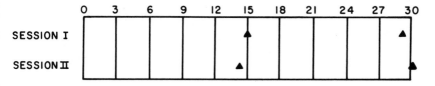

The therapist listened as the family members recounted experiences. He did not move in very much, but he did escalate his participation after the seventh minute. At fifteen minutes the patient took a drink of water and mentioned his father. Then the therapists interpreted the patient's dependency on his mother. Immediately afterwards the patient and therapist shifted posture and returned to their original positions. In the next fifteen minutes this sequence was repeated. And in the second session the same format was used.

A format like this appeared in all but two of the psychotherapy sessions I have studied. Some of its features are illustrated in Figure 11-2.

Progressive uncrossing of extremities

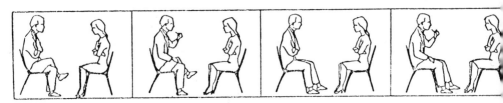

Progressive movement toward the patient

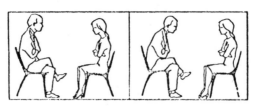

Less conventional progression, leading to physical contact

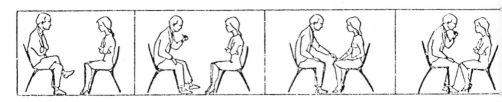

Figure 11-3: Types of Progressions in Therapists' Positions.
[Reprinted from Psychiatry]

The diagram in Figure 11-3 represents the timing of steps in customary program of progression.

The implication of this finding is clear. Though this progression is not explicitly taught in psychotherapy, it must be learned in the preceptor system of teaching psychotherapy by identication, or else it has a prototype in many such transactions in the culture. In any event the procedure is institutionalized and Session I is a replicate of a basic transactional form that is in widespread use. In other words, though the participants may have modified the procedure and given it their own style, they did not invent it for the occasion. They must have held some similar cognitive image and plan for the units of behavior (Miller, Galanter, and Pribram 1960), brought it to the session, and enacted it.

Other features of Session I might not usually appear in the psychotherapy of the neurotic patient, but they are often employed with schizophrenic patients. The moving-in series is not usually pronounced in the therapy of neurotic patients. The therapist will move only slightly toward the patient. And the use of tactile contact was unusual in the 1950s except in the treatment of the psychotic patient. By and large, psychotherapists feel that more intense and heroic measures are necessary to gain rapport with the schizophrenic patients.

Comparison with Other Sessions of Family Therapy

The Whitaker-Malone series was in one way usual for family therapy. Family therapists and group therapists tend to alternately support one group member after the other in presenting his case — a technique Whitaker and Malone did by taking sides complementarily. In family therapy it would not be usual to dismiss the mother after two sessions. Some therapists use this approach, but it is more characteristic of the previous tradition of family interviewing in child psychiatry. In some measure Whitaker and Malone's dismissal of Mrs. V was influenced by the research team who had invited them to Philadelphia to demonstrate individual therapy.

In making these comparisons it is important to bear in mind that Whitaker and Malone have been pioneers in developing these methods of therapy for schizophrenic patients and for the family. Many of the strategies that were relatively unique in 1959 have now been widely adopted.

So the program of psychotherapy has come to be institutionalized. Particular arrangements are made for it, therapists and patients both have come to know the rules, and the timing has been

pre-established. Thus an interview takes thirty to fifty minutes,
a series of sessions are planned for, and certain strategies are
phased in and out in a course of multiple sessions.

As I have described, Whitaker and Malone used special variants of confrontation. They also tend to speed up the rapport-
making procedures and add tactility and representational exchanges.

The Structure of Session I as Compared
to That of Other Psychotherapy Sessions

The tactics of psychotherapy are programmed. They are applied in steps in an over-all strategy.

The psychotherapy session ordinarily consists of a series
of phases. There is an introductory period for taking seats and
arranging the initial positions and orientations. In this phase
the participants usually preview the patterns of behavior they
will employ — as they did in Session I. Then they settle back
for a first phase of narration and presentation. The patient re-
counts his difficulties or history, and the therapist attends the
account. After ten to fifteen minutes, most therapists move forward to initiate rapport and step up their questions and comments.
Then, when rapport has been established, the therapist makes
the more active intervention which characterizes the technique
of his approach reassuring, confronting, interpreting, making
physical contact, etc. Then these three phases are repeated and
the session is then terminated.

The second cycle tends to vary in several ways. The patient
is encouraged to associate his current life behavior (which he
described in the first sequence) to past experiences. The ther-
apist-patient closeness and rapport are likely to be deepened or
intensified, and the second intervention will be more comprehensive than the first.

Chapter 12

<u>THE WHITAKER-MALONE STRATEGY</u>

In a psychotherapy session like Session I, where there are
two patients and two therapists, the program not only provides
for phases of technical employment, but also for a complementary relationship between the co-therapists. And techniques are
tailored to the patients and their relationships. Also, since a
given session is but one encounter in a programmed series of
sessions, the strategy of psychotherapy is more complicated than
the mere phasing of techniques described in Chapter 11.

These matters are the subject of Chapter 12. I will describe
first the complementary relationship between the men, then
sketch an overview of their strategy for the ten sessions they
held with Marge. In concluding I will comment on behavioral
change in psychotherapy.

THE WHITAKER-MALONE
COMPLEMENTARITY

Consider once again the format each man used for the session. Whitaker changed his behavior according to the following
phases:

1. He began the session by sitting back with his arms and legs
crossed, listening and questioning. He moved forward in three
shifts at six-minute intervals, stepping up the pace of his attention to Marge, his support of her, and his challenges to Mrs. V's
story.

2. At 23 minutes he explained the sessions, at the same time making his second physical contact with Marge and dismissing Mrs. V from further attendance.

3. In Phase II Whitaker became relatively inactive. He held his position near Marge and continued to talk to both women, but Malone moved forward, too, and afterward participated lexically and kinesically with Marge.

Malone behaved as follows:

1. Malone started the session in a position almost identical to Whitaker's: sitting back in his chair with his legs and arms crossed. From this position he intermittently rocked forward and intervened, censoring Marge and inviting Mrs. V to continue.

2. At 24 minutes Malone rocked forward and confronted Marge as usual, but this time he did not sit back again. He stayed in the forward position until the end of the session, adding to Whitaker's explanation and contending actively with Marge.

At 29 minutes both men ended the session. Malone glanced at his watch, whereupon Whitaker made a customary gesture of completion. He brushed his palms off on each other. Then he sat back in his initial position, leaning back in his chair, crossing his legs and arms. He remained silent until 31 minutes when he and Malone both stood up and terminated the session.

The Complementary Program
of Postural Progression

Notice that both men moved in toward Marge but they did so differentially — Whitaker moved in step by step, while Malone held back until 24 minutes and then moved all the way forward in one jump. Nevertheless, these moves were interrelated. They were parts in a larger, complementary program of progression which the men shared. In review, the following sequences show this complementarity:

1. During the first six minutes both men sat back with their legs and arms crossed. Thus they were in parallel or congruent postures. (Since Malone had his left leg over his right and Whitaker had his right leg over his left, this isomorphism was 'mirror-imaged'.)

2. At 6 minutes Whitaker took one step forward in his format of moving in, but Malone did not shift his basic posture. As a consequence the parallelism of positioning which had obtained for the first six minutes no longer was in effect.

At 12, 18, and again at 23 minutes, Whitaker made a further shift toward Marge which Malone did not duplicate.

3. At 24 minutes Malone did move in. He moved all the way forward to the position that Whitaker had attained by his step-by-step progression. Thus the two men again came into parallelism or isomorphism of positioning. They remained in this complementarity until minute 29.

Thus the men remained in parallelism for the first 6 minutes and again from 24 to 29 minutes. Even though each of their moves was not complementary, their progression of positions was. Technically, we would say that the complementarity was evident at the level of their total parts of performances — in their program of positions.

Note also that the rate of progression was a function of their role in a given session. In Sessions III and IX, when taking the active role, Malone moved in at six-minute intervals while Whitaker retained the initial, baseline position during these four moves. The more mobile man in any session related most actively and explicitly to Marge. The other encouraged or inhibited that vis-à-vis. These roles were exchangeable in the system. The relation of these two progressions are diagrammed in Figure 12-1.

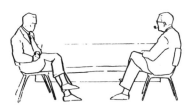

Leaning back in chair, arms and legs crossed

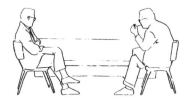

Leaning forward in chair, arms uncrossed, legs crossed

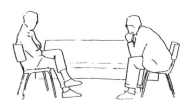

Leaning forward, legs uncrossed, arms together on chin

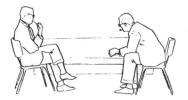

Leaning far forward, forearms extended toward Marge

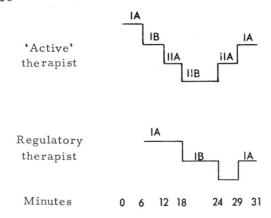

'Active'
therapist

Regulatory
therapist

Minutes   0   6   12 18   24 29 31

Figure 12-1: The Complementary Program of Moving In.
1. The Basic Postures.   2. Diagram of the
Temporal Relations.

The two men did not, at any point, speak to each other or
even fully look at each other. The progression was regulated
by a set of signals we called pipe signalling. About one minute
before each shift in the postural progression, the man who was
going to shift would make a pipe signal.[1] The other man would,
within a minute, respond with a pipe signal. Then, and only
then, would the active physician shift his posture.

In systems, each move in represented (or is a signal of)
the occurrence of a parameter, the state of relationship differ-
ing after the parameter has been introduced. Presumably, the
time of such introduction follows some assessment of the readiness of the group members. In this case, the order and nature
of the shift is dictated by the tradition of these men's approaches
or the tradition of psychotherapy in general; i.e., it is programmed. This may be analogous to the process of education,
in which the order of subjects is dictated by tradition, with the
time of their introduction representing some assessment of the
student's readiness.

The General Nature of the
Whitaker-Malone Complementarity

The Whitaker-Malone relationship can thus be described in
behavioral terms as a complementarity of performances. The
relation of their postural shifts was but one indicator of a conjoint performance which had the following general characteristics:

1. Open. Although their relationship was continuous and progressive in the postural and kinesic modalities, the two men appeared dissociated in the lexical modality. They never spoke to each other and only once exchanged glances. Covertly, then, they appeared unrelated. Their relationship was not closed, impenetrable, or excluding, but rather receptive and open.

Thus, the Whitaker-Malone twosome contrasted with the oscillating, closed, cross-monitored, mother-daughter dyad. We could conjecture that this openness offered a paradigm to the women, who seemed to have no model of being allied while also being open to other relationships. At any rate, the openness seemed to be a factor in the relationship that formed. It tended to break down subgroups or exclude twosomes and establish a larger group.

2. Multilayered in Communicative Modalities. The complementary relation sustained simultaneously two layers of communicative activity. Lexically, there was a relation of positions that corresponded to the narrating of the women's history. Kinesically, by splitting, the girl was brought into relationship to the men by quasi-courting and contacting. Rapport was initiated and the mother was eased out of the active group.

3. Programmed. That the men did not speak to each other, used little search behavior, and moved forward in highly regular steps indicates that these patterns could not have been created de novo in the session. They must belong to an institutionalized procedure evolved earlier in the relationship of the men. Often the men moved together like practiced dancers or musicians following a well-known score.

THE OVER-ALL STRATEGY

The men told us that they employed two strategies in Session I: (1) they obtained a history of the women's problem, and (2) they established rapport with Marge. I would like to reformulate this second strategy more comprehensively. I would say that the men gradually supplanted Mrs. V with Whitaker in the parental role and then began re-educating Marge in the context of this more favorable social structure. They accomplished the first of these steps in Session I; I will try to conceptualize this process first and then I will tell briefly about their usage of the new situation in subsequent sessions.

Step 1. The Replacement of Mrs. V

As I have already theorized, a premature attempt to break the mother-daughter symbiosis would have failed (Chapter 10).

Psychotherapists, having discovered this, have developed techniques for tactical maintenance of patient dependencies until they can replace them with more workable relationships such as the alliance with the therapist. Whitaker and Malone, I think, tried to kill two birds with one stone in Session I: they replaced Mrs. V with Whitaker and they obtained Mrs. V's blessing on the exchange. Theoretically this move may have made Marge more tractible or cooperative by relieving her guilty loyalty to her mother.

But Whitaker and Malone added another aspect to the pursuit of this strategy. They split the usual function of juggling which the individual therapist may find so difficult: i.e., maintaining the existing social relationships of the patient while changing them. They separated their roles in the session and assigned each of these tasks to a role. Whitaker took on the job of inducing rapport with Marge while Malone supported the mother, regulated the pacing of the Whitaker-Marge rapport, and took the villain's part in preventing a premature coalition so that Whitaker did not appear rejecting.

Let me try to explain these ideas in social systems terms.

Maintaining a Cohesive Group for Enacting the Transaction

Simmel (1902) pointed out that in a group of three, there was a striking tendency for two to pair off against the third. More recent experiments by Mills (1953) seem to confirm Simmel's work. Looking at Session I, one could argue that in this group there were tendencies to form excluding or opposing twosomes. It may be that the tendency in any group is to break down into subgroups which are at variance with each other or which at least tend to go off in divergent directions. However, if a group is to carry out certain purposes for which it is assembled, it must maintain itself for a time in integration or stability. Some mechanisms, then, are required to offset any tendency toward disintegration or schizmogenesis (Bateson 1958; Parsons 1961). This may well be one of the functions of oscillation.

There seemed to have been an unwritten rule in Session I that no participant be 'left out' by the formation of a new relationship. When Marge and Whitaker formed a relationship, Malone turned to Mrs. V; after Malone criticized Marge and Whitaker abandoned Marge, Mrs. V turned to her. Whenever any change occurred in the configuration of relations, some other change immediately or simultaneously occurred which for a time maintained the basic organization: two complementary relations vis-à-vis each other.

The mother-daughter relationship, it seems, was unstable in both phases, elaboration or opposition. The stability of the group, however, was made possible by oscillation. I conjecture that tendencies for clique formation or subgroup cohesion (Talmon-Garber 1959) can be offset in any group by oscillation because oscillation fosters the continuation of the larger group structure. Its function can be termed morphostatic (Maruyama 1963).

In other words, the function of the monitoring seemed to be to maintain some order of dynamic equilibrium — to prevent the continuance or dominance of either of two 'extremes': the mother-daughter symbiosis on the one hand, or the split into opposing alliances on the other.

It would be a mistake in such a system to settle for the simple inference that the monitoring person is acting solely from some personal motivation like jealousy or the fear of being left out. First of all, monitoring was an interchangeable role. If Malone did not engage in monitoring, Mrs. V did; when it was Malone who engaged in alliances with the girl, Whitaker performed the monitoring. At this writing, such monitoring seems to be a general characteristic of any group so composed. Malone, as the monitoring performer, did not simply force his actions upon unwilling others. Whenever interrupting occurred, it occurred in the face of progressive 'openness,' dissociation, and search behavior. In other words, the participants in an alliance 'invited' interruption. All four participants in Session I contributed to maintaining the oscillation between elaboration and opposition.

The Use of Covert, Kinesic Behaviors to Initiate Change

While the lexical units were oscillating back and forth from elaboration to opposition, another set of relations was occurring that was progressive and of a very different nature and significance. These were mediated by quasi-courting along with hand-playing, Kleenex-displaying, and contacting. Each step in the kinesic series brought the therapists closer to their stated goals for this session.

The alliance-forming behaviors of Whitaker and Marge, when they had lexical components (e.g., challenging), were interfered with and monitored actively by both Mrs. V and Malone. This interference terminated the Whitaker-Marge alliance and precipitated the flip-back from opposition to elaboration. The kinesic behaviors, on the other hand, were monitored neither by Malone nor (after twelve minutes) by Mrs. V. Not only did Malone fail to interrupt these kinesic units, but he encouraged them actively.

It was as if the developing relationship of Marge, first to Whitaker then to Malone, was permitted so long as it did not have overt lexical elements or maybe so long as it did not turn to challenging and opposing the mother. In any event, the kinesic units developed between Marge and the men without visible interference at a time when opposing and elaborating were continuously being monitored, interruped and terminated.

In contrast with oscillation, which seemed to maintain a steady state, the kinesic unit seemed to modify the quality of the relationship or to bring about a shift in who participated in a given subgroup. Each step in Whitaker's moving in seemed to be a parameter in the Ashby sense (1956), and the system reestablished a steady state at a new, greater intensity of Marge-Whitaker closeness and mother-daughter distance. The moving in was presumably intended to disrupt the mother-daughter interdependency, exclude Mrs. V from active participation, and bring Marge into rapport with both men.

Communicationally, we surmise that covert but progressive kinesic-postural activities can escape monitoring and lead to shifts and relationship formation when lexically manifested relations are in steady states.

Use of the Complementary Relationship in this Balancing

Thus the men seemed to encourage oscillation while introducing kinesic behaviors to change the oscillation.

At lower levels the behavior of the men seemed oppositional. For example, one man supported Mrs. V, the other challenged her. At the higher level, however, these pieces can be understood as a complementary unit for maintaining the equilibrium of the mother-daughter relationship until such time as they could alter it. The clinician experienced in psychotherapy of schizophrenia will see in these approaches a familiar idea. In individual therapy of children or schizophrenic patients, the therapist treads a line between encouraging rebellion against constricting parental introjects and preventing the patient from showing hostile or unsocial displays that engender too much guilt.

Just as a therapist sometimes backs down from pressure that frightens his patient in order to reassure or allow recalibration, Malone would interrupt to reaffirm Mrs. V's rationalizations or quiet the challengers. A moment later Whitaker would reapply the pressure and make overtures of rapport to the girl. These actions, divergent at the lower level, can be complementary in terms of holding Mrs. V out of panic, obtaining her blessing upon their relationship to Marge, and giving Marge support without stampeding her into too early a break from her symbiotic attachment.

It seems to me that this is fundamental strategy in any rapport formation, i.e., to fit in with the patient's expectations or his internalized lifelong rhythms and patterns, in order to form a common ground, a familiar and tolerable equilibrium. The therapist may have to promise to change the status quo or the patient will see no hope or use in therapy, but he had better not try to do so too soon.

The two therapists, by personifying these influences and by bringing the mother to the initial sessions, where she and Marge could play out their usual patterns, seemed to cast the scene in the interpersonal field, where it could be more readily apprehended. Maybe this is what they mean when they speak of working with current interaction rather than memory and past fantasy (Whitaker and Malone 1953, 1959; Whitaker, Malone, and Warkentin 1956).

Excusing Mrs. V from the Group

I presume the following: When the men considered the developing rapport between Whitaker and Marge to be stable, Mrs. V's dismissal was announced. In the process Whitaker explained the purposes of the session and promised an ultimate reunion between mother and daughter — thus providing a rationale for Mrs. V's absence and a hope upon which she could justify leaving the girl in the men's hands. In the process Whitaker seemed to test or affirm his relationship with Marge by making the second tactile contact.

Step 2. The Subsequent Use of the New Whitaker-Marge Relationship

In Phase II Malone actively addressed the girl and moved synchronously with her. He continued his tones of disapproval and scolding in Session I. But in subsequent sessions he flirted with Marge, combed her hair, rubbed her feet, talked about sex with her and was in general friendly and noncensoring.

In these subsequent sessions it was Whitaker who sat back and took the relatively inactive role. He did not move in toward Marge until late in a session. He also took over the regulatory role. He encouraged Marge to relate to Malone when she tried to dissociate from him and he sometimes intervened if the relationship between Malone and the girl seemed threatening or oversexualized. Thus Whitaker became the regulating therapist.

But an important difference had occurred. Whitaker maintained his rapport with Marge. He supported her and maintained a brotherly kind of attitude. He became her ally in her new venture of relating to Malone. And Malone acted the part of quasi-courting partner. He encouraged Marge to talk about sex and to make physical contact with him and care about him without sexuality. This plan was developed because the men felt that Marge needed to learn about friendship with a man without having avoidance or sexual intercourse as her only alternatives (English et al. 1966).[2]

COMMENT: BEHAVIORAL CHANGE

There was no question that Marge's behavior changed during the sessions with Whitaker and Malone. Even in Session I she became obviously less autistic and more alert by Phase II, and in subsequent sessions her behaviors of sprawling, shocking, and repelling ceased. But there was a sharp difference of opinion about the significance of these changes among the psychotherapists who observed the series. Some observers said that the changes would be transient because they merely reflected the absence of the mother. In this point of view one can argue that Marge's improved behavior was a consequence of her relationship with the men and was merely an extension of her improved behavior in any Period 2. On the other hand, some observers argued that Marge's awareness of the situation and her ability to behave realistically with men was improved by the sessions and they believed these changes would be lasting. They believed that Marge had learned some new and more realistic patterns of behaving.

A difference of opinion reflects a difference in criteria of change among clinicians. Classically it has been recognized that two orders of improvement can occur in psychotherapy.

1. A 'transference improvement' often occurs as soon as the patient forms rapport — as soon as he agrees to enter treatment and forms a trustful relationship to the therapist. But such improvements are considered to be temporary. Psychoanalytic clinicians believe that no change has occurred in the patient's conceptions, so they feel that the patient's improvement will not be carried over to relationships beyond that with the psychotherapist.

2. A lasting improvement with insight is believed to occur when the patient knowingly can change the contexts of his life and adapt his behavior and his affective state to situations and relationships other than those of the therapy.

The expressive or insight psychotherapist believes, then, that only insight and change in conceptions lead to lasting change. But other clinicians argue that behavior can be changed by altering visible behavior with techniques such as reinforcement (Wolpe 1958; Krasner and Ullman 1965).

Theoretically this argument may be doctrinal. Behavior, metabehavior, and context are but aspects of a single system, and in principle one cannot change any aspect of this system without changing the others. But practically and strategically it may make a difference which of these aspects is influenced first in the processes of psychotherapy and it remains probelmatic whether change without insight is lasting or necessary. But we can, I think, spell out more carefully what we mean by behavioral change from the study of transactions like Session I.

Consider first that an individual's range of behavior will be constrained by the immediate context, by the ongoing transaction. Given a describable phase of a known transaction, a person has a number of options for allowable behavior — maybe one or two parts, several positions and relations, maybe a dozen usual points and gestures, and a few hundred syntactic sentences. By observations we can roughly catalogue a repertoire in any immediate stable context for a given participant as I have done in this volume. Marge, for instance, had a characteristic and repetitive set of behaviors in any Period 1 and a somewhat different set in any Period 2.

As various alternative behaviors appear in the progress of a transaction, we do not necessarily have to postulate that a significant change has occurred in the participant's life situation or in his conceptions at higher levels of context. Thus Marge showed a progressively greater employment of alert, sexually active, agressive, and related behavior as Session I went on — a change a psychiatrist would regard as healthy or indicative of improvement. But this change was obviously associated with a greater and greater persistence of the Period 2 constellation and Marge had behaved in this more normal fashion in any Period 2 from the beginning of the season. We have no grounds to postulate that she had learned any new behavior or experienced a durable change in her life-space. To do so we would have to show, at least, that her Period 2 behavior persisted during a Period 1 type of context or that even with her mother present she did not fall again into Period 1 types of relationship.

In subsequent sessions Marge's improved behavior continued, but her mother did not attend subsequent sessions and there was no repetition of the Session I context for us to observe. Many of us had the impression that Marge's behavior did demonstrate new learning but the proposition is not demonstrated.

On the basis of long-term observation, however, we could probably establish that three basic types of change could occur from a participant's experience in a transaction. These, of course, coincide with the three types of context I have been differentiating throughout Part II of this study.

1. A repertoire of allowable behaviors might be extended by any change in the immediate context of the transaction.

2. A transaction (or series of them) could alter the life-space arrangements of a participant's life and permit him access to portions of his behavioral repertoire which he had been unable to use.

3. A participant could learn parts, positions, and other units of behavior which he had not previously acquired.

Presumably these changes could occur either by alterations in the actual immediate situation, life-space arrangements, or life experience, or else because of changes in the subject's conception of these immediate, mediate, or remote contexts. In psychotherapy both of these eventualities probably occur. For example a patient's concept of his relationships might lead him to change his institutional memberships and circle of friends, whereupon he might be able to have new experiences and learn new patterns appropriate for these new life contexts.

In an ongoing series of psychotherapy sessions, the various loops in complicated interacting systems changes are the subject of discussion, suggestion support, and so on. As any change occurs these are techniques for dealing with it. For example, if Marge left her mother, she would need to learn new ways of dealing with men. Whitaker and Malone anticipated this situation and they spent most of the subsequent sessions in teaching her such behaviors. If she failed to learn programs of behavior suitable to new life context, she might well have to return to the interlocked relationship with her mother and this return might have precluded further chances for her to learn. So we could conceive of psychotherapy as an applied communicative effort to impinge on strategic loops in the vicious cycles of a schizophrenic patient's life. So far as I know, courses of psychotherapy have yet to be studied by systematic and direct observation and the success of the efforts remains a debatable subject.

Appendix A

COMPLETE LEXICAL TRANSCRIPT
OF SESSION I

Mrs. V. Help me up stairs, a young girl like her, help me upstairs, and,
M.
Wh.
Mal.
Time: (in minutes and seconds)　(0:12)

Mrs. V. uh--the next day I thought she'd get better by, ah, ah, she
M.
Wh.
Mal.
Time:

Mrs. V. has the doctor's prescription---Did I say the wrong thing, dear?
M.
Wh.
Mal.
Time:

Mrs. V.
M.　You said I oughtta have a good sleep, and eat.
Wh.　　　　　　　　　　　　　　　　　　　　　　　　　Well why
Mal.
Time:

Mrs. V.　　　　　　　　　　　　　　　　　　　　　　　　/5sec. pause/
M.
Wh.　don't you say what it is you wanted to say now, Marge?
Mal.
Time:

Mrs. V. Well the next day she---　　　　　　　　ha-ha. The next day she---
M.　　　　　　　　　　　Gonna go to hell.
Wh.　　　　　　　　　　　　　　　　　　　　　Was that what you
Mal.
Time:

Mrs. V.
M.
Wh.　started to say before when mother---sorta stopped you or you
Mal.
Time:　　　　　　　　　　　　　　　(:30)

Mrs. V.　　　　　　　　　　　　Yeah, I don't care what you said, it's what
M.　　　　　　　　　　　　　　Yes, I did.　　　　　　(I did)
Wh.　stopped yourself?
Mal.
Time:

Mrs. V. sh---　　　　　　　You stopped what?　　　　　　You
M.　　I did stop it, I did.　　　　　　　Gettin' angry.
Wh.
Mal.
Time:

267

```
Mrs. V. stopped getting angry.                                              At me, at
M.                                                                          You know,
Wh.
Mal.                           Getting angry at whom, Marge?
Time:
_____
Mrs. V. me-- I remember I usta get angry, everybody gets angry
M.          you know, mother, you know who..      (              ) or
Wh.
Mal.
Time:
_____
Mrs.V.
M.          somethin'
Wh.         When did---When did you stop getting angry at mother, Marge?
Mal.
Time:
_____
Mrs. V.                                                      /3sec. pause/Well
M.          When did I sta--, start, or stop--gettin' angry?
Wh.
Mal.
Time:                      (1:00)
_____
Mrs. V. everybody gets angry, I usta get angry at my mother.
M.
Wh.                                                              When dja
Mal.
Time:
_____
Mrs. V.                             What?                      Yes, I want to
M.                        Mother----tell me somethin' (
Wh.         stop getting angry?
Mal.
Time:
_____
Mrs. V. tell you anything I can tell ya.                       No.  I, I
M.                          ) these people.  Do you hate me?
Wh.
Mal.
Time:
_____
Mrs. V. wouldn't do da tings I do do if I hated you---I'd just stay home
M.
Wh.
Mal.
Time:
_____
Mrs. V. and--wouldn't care whether---I heard from you. (ha-ha)
M.                          (                          )
Wh.                                                         What d'ja
Mal.
Time:
_____
Mrs. V.
M.                                   Me? You're watching me get angry with my
Wh.         say, I didn't hear ya?
Mal.
Time:                                                               (1:30)
```

268

Mrs. V.   No, you're, uh, not getting angry, everybody gets angry--
M.   mother.
Wh.
Mal.   It would be sa-fer for
Time:
_____
Mrs. V.   I'm nervous too.   I have reason ta---(don't cha think)
M.   What do ya think I
Wh.
Mal.   someone to watch you.
Time:
_____
Mrs. V.   Marge, don-don't talk like that.
M.   am, an animal or somethin'?
Wh.
Mal.
Time:
_____
Mrs. V. You'll be gettin' home..
M.
Wh.   Sometimes I feel like an animal, don't you feel like
Mal.
Time:
_____
Mrs. V.   You're just goofy now -- If you'll just - - -
M.   I
Wh.   an animal sometimes?
Mal.
Time:
_____
Mrs. V.
M.   don't know what you're talking about---waddya mean, feel like an
Wh.   Really?
Mal.
Time:
_____
Mrs. V.   Oh, Marge
M.   animal? Sexy, ya mean? Oh boy.   Don't say that word,
Wh.   Or mad.
Mal.
Time:
_____
Mrs. V.
M.   ya know, don't say that word, sexy.   He's
Wh.
Mal.   Where is your husband?
Time: (2:00)
_____
Mrs. V.   He died. It'll be a year this
M.   dead with myself, I get sexy with myself, you know what I
Wh.
Mal.
Time:
_____
Mrs. V. December 3rd.   December 3rd, it'll be a year.
M.   mean?   I was
Wh.
Mal.   He died when?
Time:
_____

Mrs. V.	3rd.
M.	dead. Real dead.
Wh.	Just before
Mal.	December 30th. Tur(d) /3sec. pause/
Time:	

Mrs. V.	Yeah, just before Christmas.
M.	
Wh.	Christmas time, then, huh? What
Mal.	
Time:	

Mrs. V.	He uh.. it started June 9th. He
M.	(justa) cheese.
Wh.	happened?
Mal.	
Time:	

Mrs. V.	went to that hos-pit-al doctor, he got an x-ray and, uh, his 'a
M.	
Wh.	
Mal.	
Time:	(2:30)

Mrs. V.	lung wasn't good---So they operated on him---and he come home to
M.	
Wh.	
Mal.	
Time:	

Mrs. V.	recuperate. He seemed to be doin' good, and then he had to go
M.	
Wh.	
Mal.	
Time:	

Mrs. V.	back to the **hospital**---**un** he died.
M.	/2sec. pause/ I died.
Wh.	You died
Mal.	
Time:	

Mrs. V.	But nobody could stop his death.
M.	Yup---I died.
Wh.	when he died?
Mal.	
Time:	

Mrs. V.	H-how could stop the ( ) I
M.	Did you. I cried, you laughed.
Wh.	
Mal.	
Time:	

Mrs. V.	laughed and I ( )?
M.	Did you die when he died too, mama?
Wh.	
Mal.	
Time:	(3:00)

Mrs. V. Well-a-a-I-I miss him more as time goes on as (ah) I see myself
M.
Th.
Val.
Time:

Mrs. V. alone.   I mean right away you
M.
Th.
Val.   You didn't miss him when he died.
Time:

Mrs. V. don't feel it very much.   Yeah.
M.   I didn't miss him (when he died)   No.
Th.   What
Val.   S-sort of a shock.
Time:

Mrs. V.   She
M.
Th.   did Marge mean when she says you laughed when he died?
Val.
Time:

Mrs. V.   When he died, I
M.   laughed at him when (   ) as I (though it was) after all, it
Th.
Val.
Time:

Mrs. V. laughed, Marge? I laughed? Marge, did I laugh when he died?
M.   was (   )
Th.
Val.
Time:

Mrs. V.
M.   Didn't you s-just sorta laugh at him a little--I mean, didn't you
Th.
Val.
Time: (3:30)

Mrs. V.   When he was sick you mean?   Oh, I,
M.   laugh at him, remember?
Th.
Val.   (cough)
Time:

Mrs. V. I get angry sometimes all ri(ght). I've been--ever since I'm
M.
Th.
Val.
Time:

Mrs. V. livin' in that house I've always--been so--I've never liked it
M.   Yeah, I know about it.
Th.
Val.
Time:

Mrs. V. too much and I've always been nervous.
M.   Aw skip it, I seen him standin' there...It scares me.
Wh.   I'd b
Mal.
Time:

Mrs. V.
M.   Let me tell you something
Wh.   scared if I saw him standing here too.
Mal.
Time:

Mrs. V.
M.   I'm dead mister---I am dead---dead.
Wh.
Mal.   You're the most alive dead
Time:

Mrs. V.
M.   Yeah--am I the only one who goes throug
Wh.
Mal.   person I've ever met.
Time:

Mrs. V.
M.   this?---What (I was going through) I guess I am.
Wh.
Mal.   How do you feel,
Time   (4:00)

Mrs. V..   Well I--I don't like it at all (huh)
M.
Wh.
Mal.   about, uh, Marge's upset?
Time:

Mrs.V.   I'd love to see her that sh--
M.   Remember when
Wh.
Mal.   You don't like it?
Time:

Mrs. V.   Oh, that's nothing
M.   usta get sick to my stomach, remember that?
Wh.
Mal.
Time:

Mrs. V. Anybody gets sick. Sometime
M.
Wh.   What do you think she meant when she
Mal.
Time:

Mrs. V.
M.
Wh.   said she was dead?---Did she tell you that she felt dead that
Mal.
Time:

272

Mrs. V.   Wait a minute. She come home for lu-uh, and she, uh,
M.
Wh.   first day?
Mal.
Time:
_____
Mrs. V. she often did, she says no mother I feel so, oh I says take a
M.
Wh.
Mal.
Time: (4:30)
_____
Mrs. V. cup o' tea, tomorrow if ya still feel sick. No mother you don't
M.
Wh.
Mal.
Time:
_____
Mrs. V. understand, I'm really sick. Oh, I says, I don't wanna have it
M.
Wh.
Mal.
Time:
_____
Mrs. V. on my soul, so I called the doctor---and---he gave her the
M.
Wh.
Mal.
Time:
_____
Mrs. V. perscripts-s---and them, uh, gimme a glass of water. Hold me up
M.
Wh.
Mal.
Time:
_____
Mrs. V. mother ta drink it. Help me upstairs ta--oh, an eighteen year
M.
Wh.
Mal.
Time:
_____
Mrs. V. old girl. I, I--   I got nervous, I
M.
Wh.
Mal.   Sorta like a baby, wasn't it?
Time:
_____
Mrs. V. says is sh-- was she that sick?   The next day she--
M.
Wh   (T.C.)   You ever
Mal.
Time:
_____
Mrs. V.   Have I ever been nervous?
M.   I've been
Wh.   been nervous before?
Mal.
Time:
_____

Mrs. V.   Well, I don't know, I often--I guess I, I am the
M.   nervous.
Wh.   Before?
Mal.
Time: (5:00)
_____
Mrs. V. nervous type I tink, I'm not the real calm type.
M.   She is mentall
Wh.
Mal.
Time:
_____
Mrs. V.   Well, I am, I call myself mental, uh. These things make me,
M.   ill.
Wh.
Mal.
Time:
_____
Mrs. V. the whole world makes me nervous.
M.   Mind picture, remember ya usta
Wh.   Uh huh. Had you
Mal.
Time:
_____
Mrs.V.   Wadda ya mean, your picture
M.   see them mind picture, plenty of 'em.
Wh.   ever collapsed?
Mal.
Time:
_____
Mrs. V.   Mind, oh, I, I say that I get, I think I always
M.   Mind picture, my picture, mind picture, my picture   (
Wh.
Mal.
Time:
_____
Mrs. V. got them only I never, I never---I was unconscious, I think (ha)
M.   ) for real.   But how?
Wh.
Mal.
Time:
_____
Mrs. V.   I don't know, sor
M.   But how?
Wh.   What kind of mind pictures are they, mother?
Mal.
Time: (5:30)
_____
Mrs. V. of, things that come in my mind and--
M.
Wh.
Mal.   Could you give us an
Time:
_____
Mrs. V.   Like I never studied in school but---on account of
M.
Wh.
Mal.   example?
Time:
_____

274

Mrs. V. those French people, and that comes in my mind and, (ha) I see
M.
Wh.
Mal.
Time:

Mrs. V. to verify it. When I (   ) have a call of **heresy,** when I
M.
Wh.
Mal.
Time:

Mrs. V. hear (ha)   Somehow or other
M.
Wh.
Mal.   You can see sort of into the future.
Time:

Mrs. V. I, I get a mind picture, I call it up.
M.
Wh.
Mal.   Have you any mind
Time:

Mrs. V.   No.
M.
Wh.
Mal.   pictures about Marge?   Did you have any about your husband?
Time: (6:00)

Mrs. V. Oh, I don't know, I, different, I think they just come into my
M.
Wh.
Mal.
Time:

Mrs. V. mind an' sometimes (when) I think ta see ta verify what I,
M.
Wh.
Mal.
Time:

Mrs. V. what I, see. Something like that, I didn't re-- I didn't read it,
M.
Wh.
Mal.
Time:

Mrs.V. it came in my mind.
M.   I **can't** get better---I can't.
Wh.   Do you get mind
Mal.
Time:

Mrs. V.
M.   'Bout the future?   Yes-s-s-s, um hum
Wh.   pictures too?   Yea.   (cough)
Mal.
Time:

Mrs. V.   Um,
M.   yea.
Wh.   Do you ever--tell Marge any of your mind pictures?
Mal.
Time:
_____
Mrs. V. guess maybe (hum, hum) I talk about---I never said I get mind
M.
Wh.
Mal.
Time: (6:30)
_____
Mrs. V. pictures now did I?   Yeah,
M.   You said yes you did, I remember now.
Wh.
Mal.
Time:
_____
Mrs. V. I might of--said it.
M.   I got mad at her so many time--we don't
Wh.
Mal.
Time:
_____
Mrs. V.   Oh its not bad, I mean, still at differen
M.   understand each other.
Wh.
Mal.
Time:
_____
Mrs. V. times...
M.
Wh.   Do you think you understand her any better than ya did
Mal.
Time:
_____
Mrs. V.
M.   (   )Whew---What? Oh.
Wh.   before you collapsed?
Mal.   We don
Time: (7:00)
_____
Mrs. V.
M.   I don't understan
Wh.
Mal.   understand each other either. /5sec. pause/You feel that---
Time:
_____
Mrs. V.
M.   the way she talks crazy to me, I don't understand that kind of
Wh.
Mal.
Time:
_____
Mrs. V.
M.   talk.
Wh.   Can you tell us about some of that how--how she talks crazy
Mal.
Time:
_____

```
Mrs. V.
M.                      I'm dead.
Wh.     to ya?                        I didn't hear that.  Could you say it
Hal.
Time:                    (7:30)
```

```
Mrs. V.
M.                  I'm dead              I'm dead somewhere, I'm dead--
Wh.     out loud?             You're dead.
Hal.
Time:
```

```
Mrs. V.                                                      (laugh)
M.      dead am I.  I, I can't control myself anymore.        I cannot
Wh.
Hal.            You both hold your hands the same way.
Time:
```

```
Mrs. V. (                ) myself because I can't see on account of the
M.               control myself.  I cannot control myself.
Wh.
Hal.
Time:
```

```
Mrs. V. lights out there.
M.                  I am---I can't even mortal sin.
Wh.                  Your mother control ya?  Do you think
Hal.
Time:
```

```
Mrs. V.                      That's what she says, she committed a
M.                      Ya know--
Wh.     mother can control you?
Hal.
Time:
```

```
Mrs. V. mortal sin.  I wouldn't know what she committed.
M.              yes-s.
Wh.                                          Has she always
Hal.
Time:                    (8:00)
```

```
Mrs. V.
M.                      Yes, you know what I did to my(          ), she
Wh.     controlled ya?
Hal.
Time:
```

```
Mrs. V.                      You say you committed a mortal sin an', and
M.      knows, she knows.
Wh.
Hal.
Time:
```

```
Mrs. V. I'm sorta-- wondering what a mortal sin could be.
M.              Yea                        I don't think about it.
Wh.
Hal.
Time:
```

Mrs. V.	No, I
M.	
Wh.	Do you think you've ever committed a mortal sin, mother?
Mal.	
Time:	

Mrs. V.	doubt, I couldn't say I've ever committed a mortal sin--I jus', I
M.	
Wh.	
Mal.	Ever?
Time:	

Mrs. V.	always live my life--the way it came every day--so I never
M.	
Wh.	
Mal.	
Time:	

Mrs. V.	committed a mortal sin. No. I al--
M.	Never committed a mortal sin?
Wh.	
Mal.	
Time:	(8:30)

Mrs. V.	from what I imagined a mortal sin is---
M.	
Wh.	Have--have you ever
Mal.	
Time:	

Mrs. V.	
M.	No I never collapsed.
Wh.	collapsed like Marge collapsed, ma(ma) How
Mal.	
Time:	

Mrs. V.	Well he had some
M.	
Wh.	about your husband. Was he a nervous type, too?
Mal.	
Time:	

Mrs. V.	I would say his hands used to tremble, but---but, uh, he wasn't
M.	Yea-a-ah
Wh.	
Mal.	
Time:	

Mrs. V.	nervous though, I mean he was--he was pretty intelligent to me.
M.	
Wh.	
Mal.	
Time:	

Mrs. V.	He was an intelligent guy, that's
M.	
Wh.	What kind of a guy was he?
Mal.	
Time:	

278

Mrs. V. what I would s-, I would say.
M.
Wh.
Mal.   What was he like apart from, was he--
Time: (9:00)

Mrs. V. Well, I mean he was--he was pretty good.   Yeah, he was a
M.
Wh.
Mal.   Good man?
Time:

Mrs. V. good man, I would say. He was, he was, yeah, he was a lot for
M.
Wh.
Mal.   Loyal to the family?
Time:

Mrs. V. the fam---he was a family man (you know), yeah, and---did a lot
M.
Wh.
Mal.   Stand up for himself?
Time:

Mrs. V. to take care of his family and to--- wasn't he that way, Marge?
M.
Wh.
Mal.
Time:

Mrs. V. You could say that.   He was
M.   Ye-eh (sob, sob)   (sigh)
Wh.
Mal.   Who was the boss in the family?
Time:

Mrs. V. the boss.
M.   o-o-o, o-o-o
Wh.
Mal.   Is that right, Marge? Did your father wear the pants?
Time: (9:30)

Mrs. V. Wasn't he the boss, Marge? Was I the boss?
M.   He was, yes, he
Wh.
Mal.
Time:

Mrs. V.   Oh no, he didn't scare you, he
M.   scared me, he scared me yes he--yes he did.
Wh.
Mal.
Time:

Mrs. V. never hit you even.   Wha-, he
M.   Yes he did. Mother, listen to me.
Wh.
Mal.
Time:

```
Mrs. V. hit you, daddy?                                          Aw, he would
M.                    Don't you remember when he hit me?
Wh.
Mal.
Time:
_____
Mrs. V. take her like any father would.              No, he, he tried like any
M.                        (                          )
Wh.
Mal.
Time:
_____
Mrs. V. father would when she'd wanna go out, I'll slap ya or somethin',
M.                                                 Tried to hold it in, tried
Wh.
Mal.
Time:
_____
Mrs. V.
M.        to hold it in.                                She didn't.
Wh.
Mal.                                                              How many
Time:                                                    (10:00)
_____
Mrs. V.                                  There's ten, ten of 'em.
M.                                                          She can't
Wh.
Mal.     children in your family?
Time:
_____
Mrs. V.
M.        commit one, she's crazy.  She can't commit a mortal sin, she's
Wh.
Mal.
Time:
_____
Mrs. V.                                  Nobody's saying that.
M.        crazy.  I--I'm not crazy, I'm not crazy,  I'm not crazy--I wasn't
Wh.
Mal.
Time:
_____
Mrs. V.          You're not, you've never been, and you won't be.
M.        crazy.
Wh.                                                         Have any of
Mal.                      (TC)
Time:
_____
Mrs. V.                              That's all I got.
M.                                                      (                  )
Wh.      your other children collapsed?
Mal.
Time:
_____
Mrs. V.                              My fa--
M.
Wh.      You meant you have ten children---   your brothers and sisters.
Mal.
Time:
_____
```

```
Mrs. V.  Yeah, that's right.                                              My only
M.
Wh.                        Yah.   And Marge is your only daughter.
Mal.
Time:                                                              (10:30)
_____
Mrs. V.  daughter.                                          I had a, a son
M.
Wh.                   You don't---had any other pregnancies?
Mal.
Time:
_____
Mrs. V.  that died.                              He was two weeks---- he
M.                                                                  Oh
Wh.                 How old was he when he died?                  Hum?
Mal.
Time:
_____
Mrs. V.  was ten days when he died.                              Younger,
M.
Wh.                          Ten days.
Mal.                                     Is that older than Marge?
Time:
_____
Mrs. V.  a year younger.
M.
Wh.                      A year younger?
Mal.     Younger.                        And you haven't had any children
Time:
_____
Mrs. V.                        Why he must be, he was---born in a catholic
M.             Is he in heaven?
Wh.
Mal.     since?
Time:
_____
Mrs. V.  hospit(al).                        Yes, you were baptized.
M.               Was I baptized?---after that, I gue(ss)   I was bapti--was
Wh.
Mal.
Time:
_____
Mrs. V.                Yes.                  Why I   really don't--a--at baptism?
M.       I baptized?      Did I cry?           Did I get scared.
Wh.
Mal.
Time:                            (11:00)
_____
Mrs. V.        A-a-you're too young for--to get scared at that age--3 months.
M.       Yeah.
Wh.
Mal.
Time:
_____
Mrs. V.                            Yes.               At three months---
M.       you don't know.   Didn'cha see me?   Oh my gosh.
Wh.                           You know.                  you know what the
Mal.
Time:
_____
```

Mrs. V.   They say pneumonia.
M.   Yeah.
Wh.   boy died from?   Pneumonia.   Did you feel he
Mal.
Time:
_____
Mrs. V.   Well, I, I would say so, he sorta had a
M.
Wh.   was well taken care of?
Mal.
Time:
_____
Mrs. V. cold in his eyes a couple of days before he died---and that, a--
M.
Wh.
Mal.
Time:
_____
Mrs. V.   Yes, um.   I was breast
M.   What?
Wh.   Were you breast feeding him?   (TC)
Mal.   (cough)
Time: (11:30)
_____
Mrs. V. feeding him.   What? (laugh) yeah, it
M.   Oh.   'Member it uz hard for me..   to breast feed
Wh.
Mal.
Time:
_____
Mrs. V. was (laugh)   Well, I usta tell her lots of things.
M.   me. She told me so.
Wh.
Mal.   Do
Time:
_____
Mrs. V.
M.   Um, yeah, I remember the things she told me,
Wh.
Mal.   you remember that?
Time:
_____
Mrs. V.   I didn't tell you to be--I told you
M.   she didn't tell me to be good.
Wh.
Mal.   She tell you
Time:
_____
Mrs. V. to be bad, I suppose. I told you to be bad?
M.   In a way ya did.
Wh.
Mal.   to be bad?
Time:
_____
Mrs.V. h-h-h-
M.   I told myself to be bad.
Wh.
Mal.   (TC) You mean she told you to commit that mortal sin? Tell us
Time: (12:00)
_____

```
Mrs. V.
M.                                                              Take my picture.
Wh.
Mal.      what has happened since, uh---Memorial Day.
Time:
```

```
Mrs. V. She--the next thing I thought she was gettin' better, then she
M.
Wh.
Mal.
Time:
```

```
Mrs. V. starts to vomit---and she vomits every---I got nervous, I called
M.
Wh.
Mal.
Time:
```

```
Mrs.V. to my people, I says she, she vomits everything, she can't live
M.
Wh.
Mal.
Time:
```

```
Mrs. V. if she keeps vomiting---                        They, they came
M.                          All I did is wanna live.
Wh.
Mal.
Time:
```

```
Mrs. V. over and they, they ga'm porridge,        they say its da heat
M.
Wh.
Mal.                                Wa--                          Was
Time:
```

```
Mrs. V.
M.
Wh.
Mal.      this---vomiting all day long, or at night, or in the morning, when
Time:            (12:30)
```

```
Mrs. V.          Towards the afternoon it sorta started.   The n---
M.                                              I didn't go through
Wh.
Mal.      was it?
Time:
```

```
Mrs. V.          The next day I, I, I, I, during the night, I mean, and
M.       purgatory.                              Oops.
Wh.
Mal.
Time:
```

```
Mrs. V. she says, I, I, I usually sleep downstairs, she says I betcha
M.                                    (          )
Wh.
Mal.
Time:
```

Mrs. V. you're not gonna hear me she says if I want milk, I says I'll stay
M.
Wh.
Mal.
Time:

Mrs. V. down here and I'll hear you, and she asked for milk three times
M.
Wh.
Mal.
Time:

Mrs. V. and she didn't vomit. Oh, I says--   Yeah, I
M.
Wh.
Mal.   When ya gave her milk?
Time:

Mrs. V. says thank God---   No.   I says
M.
Wh.
Mal.   Did you warm the milk?   Just cold milk.
Time:

Mrs. V. thank God she s-seems to be getting better and --- the next day
M.
Wh.
Mal.
Time: (13:00)

Mrs. V. was Sunday, I usually went to the early mass, I says M-Marge I'm
M.   I want----
Wh.
Mal.
Time:

Mrs. V. going to mass, I'll be right back, don't go to mass. She says,
M.
Wh.
Mal.
Time:

Mrs. V. why? Don't you, I don't feel good. Oh, I says, you're not
M.   No, I wanted
Wh.
Mal.
Time:

Mrs. V. going to mass if she don't feel good, so, uh, I says you want me
M.   to go to mass
Wh.
Mal.
Time:

Mrs. V. make ya something?   I mean, she says, yeah,
M.
Wh.   Why didn'cha tell her?
Mal.
Time:

284

Mrs. V. make me an egg, and she ate the egg but she doesn't eat enough
M.
Wh.
Mal.
Time: (13:30)

Mrs. V. eggs. Oh, I say, thank God she's ate the egg. She starts ta
M.
Wh.
Mal.
Time:

Mrs. V. say call a doctor, call a priest, call a, oh I says, my God
M. o-o-o-h
Wh.
Mal.
Time:

Mrs. V. Marge, wha---
M. I didn't confess to the priest---when he came--I, I, I
Wh.
Mal.
Time:

Mrs. V. Before I knew it she had, she had called
M. couldn't open my mouth.
Wh.
Mal.
Time:

Mrs. V. the priest and the priest was in the house and---he gave her
M.
Wh.
Mal.
Time:

Mrs. V. (laugh) he did something to her. So---
M. No, he didn't do anything,
Wh.
Mal.
Time:

Mrs. V. He, he blessed you, I say-- No?
M. he didn't bless me...he didn't bless me, he didn't bless me
Wh.
Mal.
Time:

Mrs. V. He did so I could tell. Marge, I says, maybe you'd like to stay
M. ( ) Why didn't he bless me? I don't know.
Wh. Why not?
Mal.
Time:

Mrs. V. by Aunt Mary or somethin', cause I always thought she don't
M. I wanted him to but he didn't do it.
Wh.
Mal.
Time: (14:00)

Mrs. V. like that house---and I don't like it---my husband don't wanna
M.
Wh.
Mal.
Time:
___

Mrs. V. move, so I says maybe if you'd like to live somewheres
M.   ye-s-es
Wh.
Mal.
Time:
___

Mrs. V. else it'd be all right with me, I'd come and see you sometime.
M.
Wh.
Mal.
Time:
___

Mrs. V. Yeah, I'd go by Aunt Mary.
M.
Wh.
Mal.   You'd do almost anything for her,
Time:
___

Mrs. V.   Yeah. I'll go by Aunt Mary's. So I s-, she
M.
Wh.
Mal.   wouldn't cha?
Time:
___

Mrs. V. went over to Aunt Mary. She come home Monday--and she just
M.
Wh.
Mal.
Time:
___

Mrs. V. couldn't walk, she just couldn't walk, she was--two nurses
M.   I'm jealous of (mother)
Wh.
Mal.
Time:
___

Mrs. V. (   )
M.   In a way (   )
Wh.   You jealous of mama?   Is it 'cause we're
Mal.
Time:
___

Mrs. V.   Two nurses carried her in the hospital.
M.   I am jealous of her.
Wh.   talking to her about this?
Mal.
Time: (14:30)
___

Mrs. V. Jealous? There's nothing to be jealous of me.
M.
Wh.   Did you ever
Mal.
Time:
___

286

Mrs. V.	never, never, never, she---
M.	
Wh.	collapse like this, mother, like she has? Ya ever been sick,
Mal.	
Time:	

Mrs. V.	Yeah--ah-- No, I've never been badly sick, I guess.
M.	
Wh.	badly sick? Can you
Mal.	
Time:	

Mrs. V.	No, I, I have no---I
M.	
Wh.	tell us about the last itme you were sick? don't
Mal.	
Time:	

Mrs. Va.	don't--I, I, not badly sick, I've never been.
M.	
Wh.	remember? Mother ever been
Mal.	
Time:	

Mrs. V.	When? Oh (laugh) that time, oh yeah, the one
M.	Yes.
Wh.	sick, Marge?
Mal.	
Time:	

Mrs. V.	with the ice cream or something, I couldn't--I got a terrific
M.	o-o-o-h ( )
Wh.	
Mal.	
Time:	(15:00)

Mrs. V.	headache, one of the worse headaches ya can get and I, I was as
M.	
Wh.	
Mal.	
Time:	

Mrs. V.	though I didn't eat for two months, I had eaten breakfast, and
M.	
Wh.	
Mal.	
Time:	

Mrs. V.	dis was about three or four o'clock, and---I was terrifically
M.	
Wh.	
Mal.	
Time:	

Mrs. V.	hungry and yet there wasn't a thing I could eat, only ice cream.
M.	
Wh.	
Mal.	
Time:	

Mrs. V. I says, it was Sunday--I says to Frank if you don't go out for ice
M.
Wh.
Mal.
Time:
_____
Mrs. V. cream, as sick as I am, I'm going out---the streets lookin' for
M.
Wh.
Mal.
Time:
_____
Mrs. V. it. I took about two tea---two teaspoons of ice cream.
M.
Wh.   He went out
Mal.
Time: (15:30)
_____
Mrs. V.   He went out and got it, yeah.
M.   Did he take my picture yet?
Wh.   and got it for ya   Does he always do that
Mal.
Time:
_____
Mrs. V.   Well, he was pretty good-----I have ta, I have ta admit he
M.
Wh.   when you ask him to do something, he'll go and do it?
Mal.
Time:
_____
Mrs. V. was always pretty good.
M.
Wh.   Did he ever hit you like he--Marge says
Mal.
Time:
_____
Mrs. V. No, well, ah, well, ha-ha, that comes into something. Well
M.   yea-a-ah.
Wh.   he had?
Mal.
Time:
_____
Mrs. V. I moved twenty blocks away---the street, the street usta be---
M.   I am thinking- - - - - -too much.
Wh.
Mal.
Time:
_____
Mrs. V. they usta make ice and call it a carnival, and uh-uh, I saw the
M.
Wh.
Mal.
Time:
_____
Mrs. V. fuss it involved---and I saw that they didn't say hello to me,
M.   I think too much.
Wh.
Mal.
Time:
_____

Mrs. V. well they're making a carnival for me, and it bothered me, I
M.
Wh.
Mal.
Time: (16:00)
_____
Mrs. V. wanted to move out.   And,   Yeah, and he never
M.   The carnival, it bothered me, I thought of it,
Wh.
Mal.
Time:
_____
Mrs. V. woulda wanna move out.   So, I take her
M.   I got scared 'bout going, I thought I'd get sick, I felt sick,
Wh.
Mal.
Time:
_____
Mrs. V. twenty blocks away. There was a nice house there about three
M.   ---yeah, I felt sick.
Wh.
Mal.
Time:
_____
Mrs. V. blocks away. I'd rather stay, but I says I'm tryin' to get out
M.
Wh.
Mal.
Time:
_____
Mrs. V. of this, ain't I. I moved twenty---the same thing twenty blocks
M.
Wh.
Mal.
Time:
_____
Mrs. V. off.   Ten years ago. So I says--
M.   After this
Wh.   When was this now that you moved?
Mal.   (TC)
Time:
_____
Mrs. V. oh, twenty blocks away, w-what do I hafta get out of this city?
M.
Wh.
Mal.
Time:
_____
Mrs. V. I says I'm gonna forget, my father usta give us wine (laugh) and
M.
Wh.
Mal.
Time:
_____
Mrs. V. I drank---three---water glasses of it.
M.   Trying to kill yourself,
Wh.
Mal.
Time: (16:30)
_____

Mrs. V.　　　　　　No, I was trying to forget what the street was doin'. I
M.　　　mother?
Wh.
Mal.
Time:
_____

Mrs. V. figured by the time I come back to life---the street is finished
M.　　　　　　　　　　　　　　　　　　That's a sin, a mortal
Wh.
Mal.
Time:
_____

Mrs. V.　　　　(laugh) I'm not tryin' to kill myself---so, uh, I was acting---
M.　　　sin.　　　I know it is, I don't care.
Wh.
Mal.
Time:
_____

Mrs. V.　　　　　　　　　　　　　　　　　　　　I think I
M.
Wh.　　　Do you think she's ever tried to kill herself, Marge?
Mal.
Time:
_____

Mrs. V. was acting crazy--he, he just gave me a punch and right away I
M.
Wh.　　　　　　　　　Huh?
Mal.
Time:
_____

Mrs. V. got black, that's all. But he didn't do anything---I wouldn't,
M.　　　　　　　　　　　　　　　　　　'Member
Wh.
Mal.
Time:
_____

Mrs. V.　　　I wouldn't say he beat me up.　　　　　　　What?
M.　　　when you said---remember that time a long time ago?　　　Remember
Wh.
Mal.
Time:
_____

Mrs. V.
M.　　　that time a long time ago when, uh, you were on the bed and, uh--
Wh.
Mal.
Time:　　　　　　　　　　　　　(17:00)
_____

Mrs. V.　　　　　　　　　　　Struggle?
M.　　　some kinda struggle going on.　　　　Remember that you were on
Wh.
Mal.
Time:
_____

Mrs. V.　　　　I was on the bed and daddy was doin' something to me?
M.　　　the bed or something.　　　　　　　　　　　　Yeah
Wh.
Mal.
Time:
_____

Mrs. V. No-o, I don't remember.   Waddya mean, daddy was
M.   I do. Yes you did.
Wh.
Mal.
Time:
_____
Mrs. V. doin' something to me?   Well, I don't remember it. I
M.   Yes you did.
Wh.   Did it scare you?
Mal.
Time:
_____
Mrs. V. would say it if I remembered.
M.
Wh.   Would--
Mal.   Did you think that was a mortal
Time:
_____
Mrs. V.   Was I awake?
M.   What was a mortal sin?   Were you awa--, ha,
Wh.
Mal.   sin?   Her struggling.
Time: (17:30)
_____
Mrs. V.   Oh, well then I, something
M.   you were crazy to me, I called you crazy.
Wh.
Mal.
Time:
_____
Mrs. V. I don't remember.
M.   In my mind I thought she was crazy.
Wh.   How long have you thought
Mal.
Time:
_____
Mrs. V.
M.   How long have I thought that she was crazy? As long
Wh.   that, Marge?
Mal.
Time:
_____
Mrs. V.
M.   as I can remember   she's been---------she's been./3sec. pause/
Wh.   Have you always told her that?
Mal.   How long can you remember?
Time:
_____
Mrs. V.
M.   I, I--   How long
Wh.   Did you tell her that?
Mal.   How long can you remember?
Time:
_____
Mrs. V.
M.   can I remember? /3 sec. pause/ How long can I remember---way back,
Wh.
Mal.
Time:
_____

```
Mrs. V.
M.       way back /3sec.pause/                                    Yes.
Wh.                              Before you started school?
Mal.                                                     Before you
Time:    (18:00)
_____
Mrs. V.
M.                 No, of course not.  People can't remember that far.
Wh.                                                                    I
Mal.     walked?
Time:
_____
Mrs. V.                                    (          ) And I say--
M.                                                              Be
Wh.
Mal.     thought maybe dead people could.
Time:
_____
Mrs. V.              I, I'm being myself, I'm saying wha---
M.       yourself---be--                              be yourself,
Wh.
Mal.
Time:
_____
Mrs. V.  whether it's good or bad
M.       I can't be myself, I'm not myself, I imitate other people.
Wh.
Mal.
Time:                                                      (18:30)
_____
Mrs. V.              Wouldn't you like to get home and just live, uh,
M.       /3sec.pause/
Wh.
Mal.
Time:
_____
Mrs. V.  the way you usta live, Marge, wouldn't you---like to do that?
M.
Wh.
Mal.
Time:
_____
Mrs. V.          Maybe if you don't like the house would you like to live,
M.       Yes.
Wh.
Mal.
Time:
_____
Mrs. V.  uh---that we would move?          Well,  that's what I would like to
M.                                 Yes.
Wh.                                                          Would
Mal.
Time:
_____
Mrs. V.  see.                                          Would you
M.
Wh.      you like to move back to the old house---before the carnival?
Mal.                                      (TC)
Time:
_____

292
```

Mrs. V. like (ha) would you like to live there?
M.   Yes I would, yes I would.
Wh.   You know, I was
Mal.
Time:
_____
Mrs. V.
M.
Wh.   never quite clear as to who was upset about the carnival,
Mal.
Time:
_____
Mrs. V.   Oh, she was too young.   She was six
M.
Wh.   you or mother?   You were the one who was
Mal.
Time: (19:00)
_____
Mrs. V.   Yeah, she was six or seven--when we moved out of---
M.   Sixteen
Wh.   upset, huh?
Mal.
Time:
_____
Mrs. V. when we moved out of there it was either six or seven/5sec. pause/
M.
Wh.
Mal.
Time:
_____
Mrs. V.   Oh, but,
M.   Let me tell you something, when you had me did it hurt?
Wh.
Mal.
Time:
_____
Mrs. V. yeah, it hurts everybody, I guess.
M.   Were you awake when you had
Wh.
Mal.
Time:
_____
Mrs. V.   No no, not for her, I was--given--ether, d--
M.
Wh.   her, mother?   They
Mal.
Time:
_____
Mrs. V.   Yeah (   )
M.   Going away,
Wh.   put you asleep, huh.
Mal.   You were awake when the other (   )
Time: (19:30)
_____
Mrs. V.   Oh,
M.   going away, remember you told me that, you were going away.
Wh.
Mal.   (TC)
Time:
_____

Mrs. V. that's the (ha) operation.   I had an
M.
Wh.   What operation was that?
Mal.
Time: _____

Mrs. V. appendix operation.
M.   A bad thought. I dreamt--I ha--I had a picture about, you know,
Wh.
Mal.
Time: _____

Mrs. V.   Seein' diaper pins? What?
M.   seein' dad with you.   Bein' la--you and
Wh.
Mal.
Time: _____

Mrs. V.   Well, I just can't imagine what she--
M.   daddy.
Wh.   Struggling, you mean?
Mal.
Time: _____

Mrs. V. I, I don't remember anything, but I say yes I do remember.
M.
Wh.   Was
Mal.
Time: (20:00)
_____

Mrs. V.   I was
M.
Wh.   that the time when you thought she was killing herself--Marge?
Mal.
Time: _____

Mrs. V. killing myself?
M.   No, she never tried to--she never tried to kill
Wh.
Mal.   (TC)
Time: _____

Mrs. V.   Was daddy tryin' to kill himself?
M.   herself.   Did daddy try to
Wh.   (TC)
Mal.
Time: _____

Mrs. V.
M.   k--- yes, I thought he tried to, no, I thought those cigarettes
Wh.
Mal.
Time: _____

Mrs. V.   He did smoke a lot but he always did. He
M.   were makin' him sick.
Wh.
Mal.
Time: _____

294

Mrs. V. says he smoked a lot since he was very young.
M.
Wh.   You try to stop
Mal.
Time:
_____
Mrs. V.   No, only because I figured---he wants to smoke, it's not
M.   (   )
Wh.   him?
Mal.
Time:
_____
Mrs. V. so bad.
M.
Wh.   /5sec. pause/ Do you think daddy was tryin' to kill
Mal.
Time: (20:30)
_____
Mrs. V.   I just can't
M.
Wh.   mother when they were havin' all this trouble?
Mal.
Time:
_____
Mrs. V. imagine, unless I was sleepin' (ha)
M.   Remember that night, remember
Wh.
Mal.
Time:
_____
Mrs. V.
M.   when I called the police---no, when he called, you ca--, you called,
Wh.
Mal.
Time:
_____
Mrs. V.   Oh, I know, I know what she's tryin', (ha)
M.   he called the police.
Wh.
Mal.
Time:
_____
Mrs. V. now I know what she's tryin' to say. I, I told you, ten years
M.
Wh.
Mal.
Time:
_____
Mrs. V. in that house it ha-, it has been makin' me nervous because I
M.
Wh.
Mal.
Time: (21:00)
_____
Mrs. V. imagined---the food you can't eat it, er haven't been strugglin'
M.
Wh.
Mal.
Time:

Mrs. V. to try to eat and all (   )   I think ta-, I, I, when,
M.
Wh.
Mal.
Time:
_____
Mrs. V. communion, she was eight years old, I says Fra-, and I, I
M.
Wh.
Mal.
Time:
_____
Mrs. V. didn't live, uh, the best life in the world when I was single,
M.
Wh.
Mal.
Time:
_____
Mrs. V. I says Frank, if she hasta go through the eight years I've gone
M.
Wh.
Mal.
Time:
_____
Mrs. V. through, I hope she dies right after communion. Because I
M.
Wh.
Mal.
Time:
_____
Mrs. V. thought it was terrific, and I didn't know if it'd get worse,
M.
Wh.
Mal.
Time: (21:30)
_____
Mrs. V. that I could move on (   ) (   )   and get
M.
Wh.
Mal.
Time:
_____
Mrs. V. worse, you couldn't, I told Marge you could never eat--and
M.   o-o-o-h   w-o-o-o-w
Wh.
Mal.
Time:
_____
Mrs. V.   and, uh
M.   Yeah, Kancil street.
Wh.   Didn't you know mother had wanted to have
Mal.
Time:
_____
Mrs. V.   And uh I didn't
M.   I didn't
Wh.   you dead, you were gonna hafta suffer all that much?
Mal.
Time:
_____

Mrs. V. know wha-, I mean, I was in the kitchen, I was in the kitchen
M.   know she wanted me to, she told me to drop dead,   I got mad at
Wh.
Mal.
Time:

Mrs. V.   I was in the kitchen cookin'--whatever it was, and whatever he
M.   that.
Wh.
Mal.
Time:

Mrs. V. musta said, I hadn't had intention, whatever he musta said, I says, it
M.
Wh.
Mal.
Time:

Mrs. V. isn't--I have the kni-, the kitchen knife in my hand, I says, I certainly,
M.
Wh.
Mal.
Time: (22:00)

Mrs. V. with my mad-. I was always mad, remember? With my madness I, I, I had
M.
Wh.
Mal.
Time:

Mrs. V. the kitchen, I had no intention of hurtin' him with the knife. In two
M.
Wh.
Mal.
Time:

Mrs. V. shakes, in two shakes, he musta just, I always usta say you lift a finger
M.   (No, he tried to--)
Wh.
Mal.
Time:

Mrs. V. and its all done. Two shakes there was a cop standing right there (ha)two
M.
Wh.
Mal.
Time:

Mrs. V. cops in fact.   And they went out after that.
M.   I talked to 'em.   You
Wh.
Mal.
Time:

Mrs. V.   But I didn't go get, I wasn't in
M.   I liked em.
Wh.   called the cops?
Mal.
Time:

Mrs. V. there and I went to get a knife and, I was---cookin' in the
M.
Wh.
Mal.
Time:

Mrs. V. kitchen, and I---answered with the knife in my hand.
M.   I have dreams   'bout being
Wh.
Mal.
Time: (22:30)

Mrs. V.   That's just the way it---really was.
M.   raped.   Raped--
Wh.   About being what?
Mal.
Time:

Mrs. V.   Draped? Who's draped?   Um,
M.   I wanna be raped.   I wanna be dead.
Wh.   Uh.
Mal.
Time:

Mrs. V. you gotta believe---
M.
Wh.
Mal.   Do you feel you're being raped here, Marge?
Time:

Mrs. V. Raped? (Ha-ha)
M.   No-----what?   I feel
Wh.
Mal.   Do you feel you're being raped here?
Time:

Mrs. V.
M.   somethin' there.
Wh.   Do you feel we're sorta pushin' you around, you
Mal.
Time: (23:00)

Mrs. V.
M.   Yeah, I feel you're pushin' me around.
Wh.   and mother both?   You think
Mal.
Time:

Mrs. V.   (ha-ha)
M.   Yeah, I do. In a way I do.
Wh.   we're rapin' mother, too?   Well,
Mal.
Time:

Mrs. V.
M.   In a---   In a---   I saw a light.
Wh.   I think in a way you're right.
Mal.   I think you're very right.
Time:

Mrs. V.
M.   You see the light, yeah, I saw a light---I saw somethin' bright,
Wh.
Mal.
Time:

Mrs. V.   I think of you (   ) otherwise you're
M.   just watch there.
Wh.   Listen--ma---mother
Mal.
Time:

Mrs. V. not.   Huh.
M.   Wow
Wh.   What did you think you were coming here for?   What did ya
Mal.
Time:

Mrs. V.   To ask me a few-----to ask me a
M.   You gotta be a bum. What does that mean, a bum? What's it
Wh.   think you were coming here for?
Mal.
Time: (23:30)

Mrs. V. few questions like the other two doctor.
M.   mean to be a bum?   It means to be a whore.
Wh.   Why
Mal.
Time:

Mrs. V.
M.   Why did I think I was
Wh.   did you think you were coming here, Marge?
Mal.
Time:

Mrs. V.
M.   Cut up? Waddya mean, an
Wh.   comin' here? To get cut up, honest to God.
Mal.
Time:

Mrs. V. operation or somethin"?
M.   An operation--cut up--my whole body.
Wh.
Mal.
Time:

Mrs. V.
M.   /3sec.pause/ My whole body is, is, is, is
Wh.   Well, we'd like to tell
Mal.
Time:

Mrs. V.
M.   My whole bo-- I sin with my
Wh.   you something of what you're here for.
Mal.
Time: (24:00)

Mrs. V.
M.   whole body.
Wh.   We're doctors of people's feelings---and we want to see
Mal.
Time:
_____

Mrs. V.
M.   People's feelings
Wh.   if we can---help ya--with some of these feelings you've been
Mal.
Time:
_____

Mrs. V.
M.   Feelings, feelings,   Emotions, and other
Wh.   talking about.   Crazyness, you know---- that's right,
Mal.
Time:
_____

Mrs. V.
M.   things.   Emotions---I have emotional troubles.
Wh.   emotions.   Help you with some of your crazyness.
Mal.   And we wanted to
Time:
_____

Mrs. V. That's what I think I have for you, I mean, I don't know, uh, I,
M.
Wh.
Mal.   meet your mother.
Time:
_____

Mrs. V. I think maybe some of it is responsibility.
M.   What is it?
Wh.   Smell it.
Mal.
Time: (24:30)
_____

Mrs. V.
M.   I did.   (laughter)
Wh.   Smell it.   What does it smell like?   It's good
Mal.
Time:
_____

Mrs. V.
M.   Smells like peanut butter sandwiches, oh.
Wh.   parmesian cheese.   Peanut butter
Mal.
Time:
_____

Mrs. V.   (ha-ha)
M.   Cheese   Yeah,
Wh.   sandwiches? Smells like parmesian cheese to me.
Mal.
Time:
_____

Mrs. V.
M.   yes, I smell.   No, I'm not, honey.   No, I'm not
Wh.   We wanted to talk to you,
Mal.
Time: (female laughter)
_____

300

Mrs. V.   Oh, you
M.
Wh.   and then we're going to plan to see Marge---everyday---
Mal.
Time: (25:00)

Mrs. V. mean uh, uh, if she should come home---if she should come home.
M.
Wh.   except over the weekend, uh huh, for two weeks now. Now the
Mal.
Time:

Mrs. V.
M.
Wh.   problem that's upsetting us and that we can't do anything about,
Mal.
Time:

Mrs. V.   She's gonna be here
M.
Wh.   is that we can only do this for two weeks.
Mal.
Time:

Mrs. V. two weeks.
M.
Wh.   Yeah. After the two weeks, we hafta go--we don't
Mal.
Time:

Mrs. V.
M.
Wh.   live in Philadelphia. We're just up here for the two weeks.
Mal.
Time:

Mrs. V. I see.
M.
Wh.   We want to do what we can to help her during these two
Mal.
Time:

Mrs. V.
M.
Wh.   weeks----and we hope it'll make it easier for her to work with
Mal.
Time:

Mrs. V.   Will she go back
M.
Wh.   the other doctors that you'd be working with---and to get better.
Mal.
Time: (25: 30)

Mrs. V. to um, the other hospital, I guess.   That should be
M.
Wh.   Yeah, yeah.
Mal.
Time:

```
Mrs. V.  all right.
M.                                        what?              You gonna cut me
Wh.      But in that sense we are raping you----and --
Mal.
Time:
_____
Mrs. V.                                        No, Marge, they gonna---
M.       up?---my body, you gonna cut my body up?
Wh.
Mal.
Time:
_____
Mrs. V.                  take care of you-----Marge
M.         (          )                    Scared to death.
Wh.
Mal.                                              We're gonna take
Time:
_____
Mrs. V.
M.                                    /3sec. pause/ In that way.
Wh.                                                              I
Mal.      care of you but not in that way.
Time:                                                     (26:00)
_____
Mrs. V.
M.                                            (              )
Wh.       think one of the other things you oughtta know is--  and
Mal.
Time:
_____
Mrs. V.
M.
Wh.       I guess you already know it, but I want to tell you about it---
Mal.
Time:
_____
Mrs. V.
M.                                          this is  (          )
Wh.       that this is not just for you and just for Marge.    We're
Mal.
Time:
_____
Mrs. V.
M.        Heaven is not (          )
Wh.       doing this partly----because these doctors want to study how
Mal.
Time:
_____
Mrs. V.
M.                        I'm not.
Wh.       people get better - - - and how doctors help people---and that's
Mal.
Time:
_____
Mrs. V.
M.
Wh.       why we're takin' the movies, and that's why we're---having you in
Mal.
Time:
_____
```

Mrs. V.   Uh, will I hafta come

M.

Wh.   this special place for this two weeks---so that we can---

Mal.

Time:
___

Mrs. V. here--uh, tomorrow. she told me for two days.

M.

Wh.   That's right.

Mal.   But

Time: (26:30)
___

Mrs. V.   Yeah, that was it.

M.

Wh.   We won't be

Mal.   after tomorrow we'll be seeing--Marge alone.

Time:
___

Mrs. V.   Uh.

M.   Oh---I---

Wh.   seeing you again.   If you--if you want to do something about

Mal.

Time:
___

Mrs. V.

M.

Wh.   your nervousness you might be able to find a doctor to help you,

Mal.

Time:
___

Mrs. V.   Well, I don't know, it's just, I think it's, that's something

M.

Wh.   too.   We won't be able to help you with that, now.

Mal.

Time:
___

Mrs. V. that almost everybody---I, I'd call it moral responsibility

M.

Wh.

Mal.

Time:
___

Mrs. V. that---because I have ten brothers and sisters and I feel---I

M.   Afraid of responsibility.

Wh.

Mal.

Time:
___

Mrs. V. think of them, don't think I don't, but I feel they're not my

M.

Wh.

Mal.

Time: (27:00)
___

Mrs. V. responsibilities, my responsibility is her---and I think my

M.

Wh.

Mal.

Time:
___

Mrs. V. emotion is more responsibility---than anything else.
M.
Wh.   Your
Mal.
Time: _____

Mrs. V.
M.   (
Wh.   emotion is more responsibility than anything else. If you
Mal.
Time: _____

Mrs. V.
M.   )
Wh.   didn't have all this responsibility you think you'd be all
Mal.
Time: _____

Mrs. V.   Oh, I don't know (ha). I feel that---I feel that-
M.   Very emotional,
Wh.   right, huh?
Mal.
Time: _____

Mrs. V. see I, I miss my husband, but I saw him die, and I forgot it---
M.   very emotional, very, very, very   (   )
Wh.
Mal.
Time: _____ (27:3(

Mrs. V. and I always feel that they're trying to work something that
M.
Wh.
Mal.
Time: _____

Mrs. V. I'm, I'm never gonna see her no more or something and I don't
M.
Wh.
Mal.
Time: _____

Mrs. V. know know if she's dead or living.   That's-- Yeah.
M.   Who?   Me.   You don't
Wh.
Mal.
Time: _____

M.   Well--
M.   know if I'm dead or livin'?   Let me tell you something mothe
Wh.
Mal.
Time: _____

Mrs. V.
M.   I am alive, in hell, alive in hell, 'live in hell, wow.
Wh.   Pretty
Mal.
Time: _____

Mrs. V.
M.   They're gonna do it.   They're gonna do it.   I
Wh.   tricky, huh?   Ain't many   people can do that.
Mal.
Time:
_____
Mrs. V.
M.   know, I'm the only one---to do that.   /5sec.pause/
Wh.   Congradulations
Mal.
Time:
_____
Mrs. V.
M.   (ha) You wanna see my sin? I won't tell. I will not tell. I did
Wh.
Mal.
Time: (28:00)
_____
Mrs. V.
M.   something to my soul---there's not a soul down there.
Wh.
Mal.   I'm not interested in your sin. (TC) I'm
Time:
_____
Mrs. V.
M.   /7sec.pause/ I'm not interested
Wh.
Mal.   not interested in your sin, Marge.
Time:
_____
Mrs. V.
M.   in it either.   Because that's
Wh.
Mal.   Why are you talking about it then?
Time:
_____
Mrs. V.
M.   what sent me to hell.
Wh.
Mal.   We're not interested in what sent you to
Time:
_____
Mrs. V.
M.   Of hell.
Wh.
Mal.   hell, we're interested in what's gonna get cha out.   Yeah,
Time: (28:30)
_____
Mrs. V.   You know that you, uh, you don't have another
M.
Wh.
Mal.   back to earth.
Time:
_____
Mrs. V. home. That's your home. Wh-, when I was single grandpa's home
M.
Wh.
Mal.
Time:
_____

Mrs. V. was <u>my</u> home.   Well,
M.   I have----
Wh.   You mean hell is her home?   Kinda
Mal.   You mean hell?
Time:
_____
Mrs. V. I, I lived with my father, I couldn't go live with an aunt or an
M.
Wh.   like it was yours, huh?
Mal.
Time:
_____
Mrs. V. uncle. I'd have to live with my father. I would imagine---
M.
Wh.
Mal.
Time:
_____
Mrs. V. someplace---like this is nice.
M.
Wh.   She's kinda saying that---the devil's her
Mal.
Time:
_____
Mrs. V.
M.   The devil's my father? God is my father.
Wh.   father, isn't she, Marge?   She said she lived
Mal.
Time: (29:00)
_____
Mrs. V.
M.   Who's my father? He'd dead. What? I am not---at home.   I am
Wh.   with----hell was her home.
Mal.
Time:
_____
Mrs. V.   Would you like to---   You wouldn't like to
M.   very insecure.   Very afraid.
Wh.
Mal.
Time:
_____
Mrs. V. live with me.
M.
Wh.   Sounds like you learned it in the first grade.
Mal.
Time:
_____
Mrs. V. You wouldn't like to live with me.   You wouldn't? Oh, I
M.   Yes.
Wh.
Mal.
Time:
_____
Mrs. V. know, but I, I, I.   You
M.   Did I talk like a baby when I was a baby?
Wh.
Mal.
Time:
_____

306

Mrs. V. talked like anybody would. I know then that's it. And it
M.
Wh.
Mal.
Time:

Mrs. V. isn't as if I don't know that that's it---and I can't do nothing
M.
Wh.   Has she been talking
Mal.
Time:

Mrs. V. about it.   Huh?   No, she was--
M.
Wh.   like a baby since she collapsed?   Has she been talking like a
Mal.
Time: (29:30)

Mrs. V. I thought she was intelligent and smart.
M.   Yes, oh---oh--I'm
Wh.   baby since---
Mal.
Time:

Mrs. V.   I didn't realize
M.   intelligent. Um, I don't wanna be intelligent.
Wh.
Mal.
Time:

Mrs. V. that (   ) livin', there's nothin' I could do about it because--
M.
Wh.
Mal.
Time:

Mrs. V. I do my best towards her when---when she was home.
M.   Strange man.
Wh.
Mal.
Time:

Mrs. V.   That
M.   Strange man.
Wh.
Mal.   I had a couple of other questions. Does this make you sad?
Time:

Mrs. V. she (   ). Yes, it does, a lot. Unless I knew was --- like I
M.   (   )
Wh.
Mal.
Time: (30:00)

Mrs. V. say it would be a marriage or a career---that I knew she was
M.
Wh.
Mal.
Time:

307

Mrs. V.	contented somewhere, so that--I, I would be satisfied then. I
M.	They don't care about me.
Wh.	
Mal.	
Time:	

Mrs. V.	wouldn't hafta have her livin' with me.
M.	
Wh.	
Mal.	As long as you were sure
Time:	

Mrs. V.	Yes. Maybe like a marriage or a career--
M.	I tried to, I tried to, I tried to, feel that--
Wh.	
Mal.	where she was.
Time:	

Mrs. V.	she should make her life--
M.	
Wh.	What kind of a career had you thought
Mal.	
Time:	

Mrs. V.	Oh, I don't know. A nurse I usta say, she ( )
M.	
Wh.	for her?
Mal.	
Time:	(30:30)

Mrs. V.	/4sec. pause/ I know she shouldn't have to live with me---
M.	I never was
Wh.	
Mal.	
Time:	

Mrs. V.	Yeah, I can manage by
M.	in mortal sin.
Wh.	
Mal.	Can you get along alone?
Time:	

Mrs. V.	myself ( ) today I have the money---
M.	
Wh.	Would you live alone
Mal.	
Time:	

Mrs. V.	( ) Well, I guess I would
M.	
Wh.	if Marge---had a career or got married?
Mal.	
Time:	

Mrs. V.	I, I had a husband and a daughter.
M.	Got married Got married.
Wh.	I mean you-- Would you get
Mal.	(TC)
Time:	

Irs. V.   But

I.

Vh.   married again or go live with your brothers or sisters, er--?

Ial.

Time:
_____

Irs. V. I, I, if it's my brothers and sisters I might live with 'em, but

I.

Vh.

Ial.

Time:
_____

Irs. V. I have no--

I.   Ouch

Vh.

Ial.

                          ("end slate" bang)

Time: (31:00)
_____

309

Appendix B

THE METHOD OF CONTEXT ANALYSIS

In the 1950s the study of communication became immensely popular, but there was not yet any clarity about levels of organization and the nature of communicational phenomena. Communicational processes were being located variously in mind, brain, the reflex area, the group, and in the electronic devices of mass media, and also according to the classical methods in which a variety of disciplines were used to examine the subject. The result was a number of conflicting theories of communication.

In 1956 a multidisciplinary group established a systems methodology specifically designed to study communication.[1] They operationally defined communication in behavioral terms so that visible and audible phenomena could be studied directly. The principles of natural history method were adopted as the premises of observation, but the recordings were made on audiovisual media. Behavior was analyzed by structural methods adapted from structural linguistics but applied to all types of communicational behavior. And the unit forms of behavior were studied by newer systems approaches to synthesis and integration at the social level. This procedure was named context analysis.

Context analysis is not to be confused with content analysis — a method which evolved in the 1940s to study the content of language. The method of context analysis, then, does not fall within the traditions either of clinical-subjectivist methods or of the experimental-statistical tradition of American psychology.

The procedures of context analysis have evolved and been further explicated since 1956. Similar methodologies also developed in the 1950s. So the basic approaches of context analysis

311

are no longer unique and operations such as these I describe here are currently employed in a number of human and animal research projects.[2]

This account of context analysis overviews the full scope of operations which can be used for the detailed multidiciplinary analysis of a transaction. Many researchers do not care to use all of these operations. Some, for instance, may not be interested in cross-cultural sampling, while others may be interested only in comparing certain forms of behavior cross-culturally. Neither of these may wish to study the total structure of any given transaction. Accordingly, those readers who work within traditional disciplines may choose merely to scan this broad methodological statement, returning to those operations of specialized interest for more careful reading. Furthermore, because the criteria of context analysis may be unnecessarily stringent for many researchers' purposes even within the scope of a specialized usage, this account of the method is somewhat idealized.

On the other hand, the methodology does cross older disciplinary lines and an overview of it may encourage broader studies in human communication than the compartmentalized ones we have had in the past. Five major operations are:

OPERATION	I.	Obtaining an Audiovisual Record of a Transaction
OPERATION	II.	Mapping the Behavioral Events
OPERATION	III.	Delineating the Units of Communicative Behavior
OPERATION	IV.	Determining the Units of Transaction or Communication
OPERATION	V.	The Contextual Analysis of the Behavioral Processes

OPERATION I. OBTAINING AN AUDIOVISUAL RECORD OF A TRANSACTION

In context analysis we favor first-hand, naturalistic, and nonparticipant observation. Procedurally, we plan a sample, then make film or videotape recordings of specific examples.[3]

Step I-A. Planning an Observation

Film development is expensive and a context analysis is time consuming, so we cannot afford random and unrepresentative shooting. We select a subject transaction, choose a vantage point for observation, and try to anticipate disruptions.

1. Choosing a Type of Subject Matter

Since communication occurs among members of a group, our subject must be interactions or transactions, not individuals.

In order to examine all of the modalities of behavior in communication, we choose transactions of small or face-to-face groups. So far we have not studied electronic communication at a distance. We could not get all of the participants in our picture and they would use a contrived code derived from the natural systems of behavior we are trying to understand. We choose some communicational event which illustrates a point or is representative of a class of such transactions. In the latter case we want any example we study to be representative of the class.

For this purpose we prefer a customary, uncomplicated transaction. We try to locate a usual activity which people are used to enacting together. We seek participants who are native to the tradition of that transaction and experienced in taking part. And we make our observations under usual and favorable conditions. We prefer to study the transaction at sites where it usually occurs under customary conditions.

We have to learn something about the situation to make such decisions. We read the literature about that kind of transaction and talk to colleagues who have worked in that area. Then we interview subjects who are experienced in that kind of transaction. We visit sites where it usually occurs and make preliminary observations.

2. Choosing a Direct, Naturalistic Approach

We decide to observe the transaction directly. We have found on interviewing that participants do not know much about nonlanguage behavior. And they cannot see much of their own behavior in communication. So we decide to use interviewing as an adjunctive method of collecting data, but we will observe the events first hand.

We start with naturally occurring communicational processes before we attempt any experimental manipulation; otherwise we do not know what we are experimenting upon and what changes we have induced. So we will not bring strangers together in the laboratory and give them contrived tasks. We will go to sites where that transaction normally occurs on the occasions at which it would happen anyway. We prefer experienced, native participants

who know each other. And we will take all possible measures
to avoid being obtrusive and manipulative.

We will not participate directly in the transaction we are to
study. In part nonparticipant observation will reduce our obtru-
siveness and in part will give us a more useful perspective.

As group members we are constrained by etiquette to concentrate our attention on the speaker of the moment and we must
make the effort to take a meaningful part in this action. As observers we can watch any participant or any grouping and we are
free to concentrate on research. When we are members of the
group we cannot see ourselves, and we may be too close to the
others to see more than one or two of them at a time. So we
stand back from the subject group far enough that we can see
all of the ongoing behaviors at the same time. This will provide us the Einstellung from which to see behavioral relations
at the social level.

The reader will notice that these premises of observation
are classical for natural history methods. [4]

Step I-B. Making the Film Recording

Our techniques for film recording have been described elsewhere (VanVlack 1966). We have also written about the relative
advantages of videotape and motion pictures (Scheflen, Schaeffer,
and Kendon, 1970A), so I will merely mention a few requirements for obtaining filmed records which are desirable for a
context analysis.

1. Preparing for the Filmed Observation

We contract with our subjects in advance and prepare them
for filming. If we are to film a relatively small group in a situation that is at all private we explain our purposes and procedures to the participants in advance and seek their permission.
In this case we co-sign a written agreement with the subjects.
We usually pay them a fee and we promise that the filmed docu-
ments and other data will be confidential. We keep the promise. [5]

We set up the equipment in advance of the transaction,
choosing a camera location which is inconspicuous but at an appropriate distance from the scene. Then we clear the site of
personnel and extra equipment. There is no need for the process to be obtrusive.

The camera should be located, loaded, and turned on before
the transaction begins. There is no excuse for technicians or
staff members to be visible or audible at the scene. All equipment can be operated from an adjoining room. Nothing is

visible, then, to the participants except one or two small cameras and microphones which do not move, make noise, or give off light.[6]

We do not, on the other hand, try to conceal the cameras and microphones. It is our experience that people search endlessly for these devices if they cannot see them. It helps to allow participants to examine the equipment before a transaction. When we are recording in fixed locations such as the office or home, we try to locate the cameras there for days or weeks in advance to facilitate the adaptation of the subjects.

Contingencies can occur after our cameras have been turned on and these can cause the transaction to be unusual. To some extent we can guard against filming distorted occurrences even at the scene of observation: (1) We can postpone the filming if untoward circumstances threaten the event. In an outdoor filming for instance, we may not film if a storm is threatening or the temperature is extreme. If known deviants, aliens, or novitiates attend that day, we may wait for another occasion: (2) The research team can try to protect the scene. We stay out of the transaction and we prepare the participants so our own presence is not unduly disruptive. We station ourselves at points of entry to ward off intruders, rubberneckers, or incidental traffic, and we try to prevent undue noise.

Other interferences can be minimized. We can use fast film rather than intense lighting. We can use wide angle lens so the participants are not jammed together.

2. Recording the Complete Transaction

When feasible we film the entire transaction. First of all we record it from the beginning to the end. We turn the camera on before the transaction begins so we can record the initial encounter of the participants. In the early minutes they often negotiate their roles and establish the structure and format of the transaction. We are at a loss if we do not have this data on the record. When possible we also want to film the entire duration for it may progress in steps and we cannot generalize about later phases from the nature of the early ones.

We try to include all of the visible and audible behavior of all participants. We do not, therefore, manipulate the camera. It is placed to cover the whole scene and it is left in this position. If we want to zoom for close-ups, we use a second or mobile camera. And similarly we do not pan from one participant to the next and thus perpetuate the myth that people behave one at a time. We do not cut ourselves off from information about bodily communication by filming only the heads and upper torsos of our participants. We are not making an artistic film or studying facial expressions out of context.

3. Obtaining Information About the Context of the Scene

We make notes about events which occurred off camera during the transaction. Often we photograph the surrounding areas and neighborhood. Later we show the film to the subject participants and obtain a record of their thoughts and feelings, for these are regarded as a context of their visible and audible behavior.

Step I-C. Developing a Stratified Sample

Since one filmed example does not prove sufficient for generalization, we locate the transaction we filmed in categories of transactions and build a stratified sample.

1. Locating Our Example in a Class of Transactions

If a transaction is carried out in a number of cultural traditions, there are likely to be major variants in each of these. We must therefore either plan a cross-cultural sample or else avoid making generalizations about communication in general. At least we must identify the cultures and subcultures we sample.

Even within a single tradition there may be major institutional variants. Performances may also vary markedly among people of given gender, age groups, social position, and so on. Thus we try to identify certain categories of transactional type and collect further examples of them.

2. Determining the Representativeness of Each Example

We make every effort to pick examples that are representative of any class we are studying. To some extent we have done this by exploring the distribution of occurrences and filming usual transactions at usual sites and occasions. We also try to assess how representative the examples are after we have filmed them. We show them to experienced informants of that tradition and ask them if we have captured typical examples.

3. Obtaining a Sufficient Number of Examples

We rarely know in advance how many film recordings we need to picture a transactional type and its major variants. In some cases transactions are highly variable from one occurrence to the next. We may never obtain a rounded and comprehensive sample.

In other cases a transaction is highly ritualized. One enactment will be much like the next. If a number of experienced informants review the films and tell us that our examples are typical, we can proceed as though we had a significantly larger sample.[7] If a transaction is highly customary and standard, we do not need a large number of examples.

4. Stratifying the Sample

In practice we can rarely follow the classical principles of research design. We cannot usually know the adequate size and distribution in advance. As we study a given example we learn of other variants and we come across unexpected and atypical occurrences. In the end, we are using a stratified sample, recalibrating our original plans and adding categories as we discover their significance.

OPERATION II. MAPPING
THE BEHAVIORAL EVENTS

When we examine a communicational event we find a good many interesting dimensions for study and deduction. In fact each of these is the province of a classical discipline. Thus we might study the characteristics of the participants. We might make a variety of inferences about their feelings and motives or make deduction about neurological or cognitive processes in general. Or we might study the relationships of group members and the communicational networks in which they operate.

But we are not going to focus on these concepts. In fact we are not going to study physical systems like the group, the individual or the nervous system per se. We are going to study the behaviors of these systems. In the analysis of a group we find that individuals are the constituents, but the elements of analysis in a process like communication are behaviors.

Of the various behaviors we could study we will focus on those that are visible and audible. These are the only ones we can see on the film, and they are the ones which other participants in a transaction can actually perceive. Cognitive behaviors may mediate the processes of participation, but they are not the media or code of communication.

The subject of our analysis, then, is patterns of movement and sound — musculoskeletal and motor activities (and the sounds they produce). These are plotted on a time graph to map the events of the transaction.

Step II-A.   Recording Speech Behavior

Speech behavior is formed by ordering a number of traditional sounds. These are made by altering the column of vibrating air with various positionings of the larynx, glottis, tongue, teeth, and lips. We cannot see these motor activities directly, but we can use a coding system that has developed in structural linguistics.

In a detailed analysis of speech we record an analysis of the phonemic and morphemic structure of language (Harris 1951; Gleason 1955). We can code the nonlanguage sounds and vocal qualities by a paralinguistic coding system like that of Trager (1958). In a less-detailed analysis we may be satisfied merely to mark off the syntactic sentences and transcribe the lexical 'content,' noting as well the nonlanguage sounds and the gross speech qualifiers.

We insist upon one elaboration of the usual structural analysis of speech. We place the linguistic occurrences on an accurate time graph.

Step II-B.   Making a Topography
of the Visible Nonlanguage Behavior

We can distinguish and transcribe several types of nonlanguage behavior. In some transactions, the activity centers upon a task that involves physical objects — materials, tools, and the like. Such behavior may appear in any transaction including a conversation. M. Harris (1964) has called this type of behavior 'actonic' and he has advanced a method for its analysis which does not differ in principle from the context analysis I am describing.

If the participants speak to or otherwise service each other they also use a coded system of metacommunicative signals which Birdwhistell (1952) called 'kinesic behavior.' He has developed a coding system for this type of nonlanguage behavior. In either case the participants will employ a system of postural locations, orientations, and distances (Scheflen 1964, Hall 1963).

1. Setting Up for the Transaction

Our task now is to study the shadows of positioning and movement that are recorded on the film media, order these, and represent them on a graph. Remember that our representations will be descriptions of form — descriptions of the orientation, duration, and excursion of movement. They will not be abstracted qualities, inferences, notations about effort or style, or the like.

We have a copy of the motion picture or videotape and equipment to project the media. The motion picture has been developed by double exposure with a frame-numbered print, so that a number appears on every motion picture frame. And the videotape has been exposed with a digital clock video picture so that clock images appear in divisions of a thirtieth of a second on each video scan. Thus we can tell exactly where we are in the temporal sequences of the transaction and we can measure all intervals. We also have projectors or videotape recorders that will screen the media at normal and at slow speeds and play forward or backward at the touch of a control.

We need, in addition, a media on which to record the notations. This will have to be graphic, so we can see at a glance the location of any behavior. And it will have to be marked off in exact intervals of time.

A great many tapes of media have been tried by various workers in the field. Long sheets of graph or electroencephalograph (EEG) paper are probably the most useful. In the past I have used a metal board lined like graph paper and hung on the wall. Magnets of various shapes and colors are placed on the board to represent various bodily positions and movement patterns. We have also used representative 35mm or Polaroid still shots as mockups on a time graph.

2. Making the Transcription

The graphic media is therefore marked off in time by a series of equally spaced vertical lines. Each column then is a fixed interval of time, maybe eighth seconds for a microanalysis and one- or three- second intervals for a more gross analysis.

The graph is also divided into rows by horizontal lines. In each row we record the exact position (at that instant of time) of bodily region. We delineate a bodily region on the basis of our experience with segmental movement. If some bodily region can be moved separately it will rate a row in our topography. Thus we may have a row for the head as a whole, one for the brows, one for the eyelids, one for the eyes, and so on to the mouth, upper torso, arms, hands, pelvis, legs, and feet.

Now we screen the filmed media. We take one participant at a time and concentrate on the bodily part which we will describe on the first row. We notice that it is held for a while in a certain position and orientation, then it is moved to another place, then another. By showing the film forward and backward first at normal, then at slow speeds, we can record the exact dimensions of these patterns of movement and hold. We note exactly how long the region is held, where it is moved to, the excursion and range of the movement, and so forth.

Then we examine the next region and then the next, and record the information on the topography. Actually we place this data on the same time graph which we used for language behavior so that later we can note the co-occurrence of both language and nonlanguage behavior.

<h3 style="text-align:center">Step II-C.   Adding the Contextual Data</h3>

We add notes about certain events that are not recorded on the filmed media. Maybe a door slammed or someone called on the telephone or the temperature dropped appreciably. These events, too, we note in a special row on the time graph. And we may have interviewed our subjects by showing them the filmed record. Their comments can be placed in yet other rows in the topography.

We now have a time-segmented, simultaneous record of all of the behavior we can see and hear. The recorded material is laid out on a single graphic record. We will use this record from now on in the analysis. We can carry it home to test out certain hypotheses we have about simultaneous events. We will mark on this same record the unit segmentations as we delineate these in Operation III. We can note the location of any given behavior in the larger picture of behavior which constitutes its context.

So far, you may notice, we have proceeded in the natural history tradition. We have recorded what happened in time. We have not isolated apriori any particular kind of behavior at the expense of the others.

<h3 style="text-align:center">OPERATION III. DELINEATING
THE UNITS OF COMMUNICATIVE BEHAVIOR</h3>

We do not yet have a realistic picture of the form of behavior. The topography is laid out in rows, one for each bodily region, and we have acted so far as though there are continuous separate streams of activity in each of these regions. In fact, of course, activity is discontinuous. What seem like streams of behavior consist of discrete units which involve a number of bodily regions moved and held in concert.

These units of behavior have a customary or traditional form. The forms are species-specific for animals, and, in the case of man, they are also culturally specific.

Among nonhuman animals those of a given caste and species use the same forms of behavior in common. In man there are additional elaborations of form according to ethic group, class, and institutional tradition. Thus people of the same age group,

gender, and social position in any subcultural category will use
much the same system of behavioral forms when they are engaged in a given kind of activity or transaction. Thus we assume
that behavioral forms have evolved and are transmitted genetically and culturally from one generation to the next. Consequently, children and novitiates in a given category learn to move and
position themselves in the same general way.

The behavior of any acculturated person, then, is potentially
communicative. It is a medium for communication when it is
recognized or related to in concert.[8]

In Operation III, then, our task is to identify and describe
these customary units of behavior as they appear in our sample
of transactions. Methods for doing this have recently evolved in
the sciences of behavior. They can be called 'structural' approaches.[9] The idea of a unit form will take us beyond the dia-
chronic natural history observation we have been using to a syn-
chronic description of recurring, customary behaviors.

To make comparison of unit replications we will begin as we
would in a statistical analysis, but we will go beyond isolation of
variables techniques. We will develop descriptions of forms in
context.

In this section we will still operate at the organismic level,
defining the separate communicative contributions of one participant at a time. We do not reach the social level and communicational structure until Operation IV.

Step III-A. Delineation
of a Sample Unit

In practice there are two general ways to make use of filmed
data and the topography of a transaction. We can study all of the
unit forms as a first step to analyzing the structure of the transaction (Operations III and IV). Or, more simply, we can focus
on but one type of behavior in order to enlarge a sample of its occurrences. Eventually (Appendix B) I describe the more extensive procedure, but in this section I proceed as though we were
studying but one unit type. This makes it simpler to convey an
idea of the methodology. Then in Step III-B I will explain how all
units are studied.

Here, in summary, are the steps employed to study one unit
form: We sketch out its apparent boundaries on the topography,
noting when the movement began and ended and how many bodily
parts seemed to be associated in its enactment. Then we search
the record for similar forms which may be recurrences or replications. We compare each of these by a series of criteria to
determine if they are indeed regular replicates. Then we determine

whether or not they are customary in some traditional distribution and whether or not they are communicative in a transaction.

A-1. The Preliminary Identification

If we are already interested in some given act we search the
record for each of its appearances and we circle each of these,
including all doubtful cases. If we have no preconceived idea we
can select any movement at all for study.

Marking Off the Segment of Movement. In either case we
scan the topography and notice precisely when the movement first
appeared and when it ended. The movement started from some
given position of that bodily part and ended at the same or at some
other position. This is the segment we mark off — the movement or change from the initial to the terminal position. Ordinarily we have no difficulty in identifying this segment of movement. A body part is moved and then brought to rest at its baseline position or at some other comfortable or useful place. Many
actions, once initiated, almost have to be completed in a reasonable interval of time. We must put out the match after we have
struck it and it is embarrassing to hold our arms out for long periods, frozen midway in the completion of a gesture.

A sequence of movements is not the irreducible segment of
action; several subelements are necessary to complete an act.
To smoke a pipe we must take it out, fill it, light it, put out the
match, and puff. To make a gesture we have to raise the arm,
carry out a sequence of hand and finger movements, and eventually lower the arm. In doubtful cases we can leave the record
of that particular occurrence incomplete at this point. We can
identify exactly the usual segmentation when we compare many
enactments of that unit type.

In practice we often find that our topography is inadequate
for this task. We discover that we forgot to note when a shift
occurred from one position to another or that we did not code
exactly some dimension of the movement. In the end, we go
back to the original film again and again to correct and amplify
our record.

Identifying the Associated Segments: Now we look over each
row of the topography to discover movements of other bodily regions which accompany this segment. We may find several kinds
of relations here. The adjoining bodily regions may be involved
as a pattern of activity 'spreads' over the face or successively
involves one, and then the other hand. Or the associated movement may occur at a widely removed area. Some speakers, for
instance, shake a foot when they speak. Or regional movements

may occur 'within' each other. Thus the arm is moved, then the hand, then the fingers, and the fingers are stopped, the hand is held, and then the arm is positioned at rest. Later I will introduce a model for integrating such occurrences.

The identification of associated movements does not have to be highly precise at this point in the analysis. We can mark the doubtful cases and leave questions of coincidence open, for we are now making only a preliminary assessment. We will not know exactly what elements are combined in a given unit type until we have compared a number of recurrences.

Since the complex of movements we have identified is a tentative one, we will not waste time measuring it or describing it carefully. We only note its characteristics sufficiently so that we can recognize other examples when we scan the record. In order that we can find this instance again, we do mark it on the topography putting a dotted line around the probable configuration and numbering it.

A-2. Determining the Regularity of This Complex

Collecting a Sample of Possible Recurrences. We now scan our total record and look for other, similar complexes of movement which may be replications of the same unit form.

There are technical aids we can use in this comparison. Ekman (1969) cuts segments of videotape on which comparable forms appear and splices these together for easier comparison. I often make a short description and a series of representative still photographs of each type of segment and mount these on a chart so the forms will be fresh in my memory as I search for apparent replications.

If we do not find repetitions in our film there is no way we can go on with the analysis. We have to take other films and search these for examples. To determine the regularities of a unit form we must compare a number of examples.

Ordinarily we do not have any difficulty collecting tens or even hundreds of apparent recurrences. In a half-hour transaction the average participant uses possibly a dozen different hand gestures, a similar number of facial sets, and even fewer kinds of head-eye orientations, head movements, or brow placements; he uses the same forms over and over.

How many replications we need to examine depends, of course, on the variability. In some cases each recurrence is so alike in form that we have little doubt about the identity of the set, but in other cases the forms are highly variable and may have to be compared with hundreds of examples and carefully tested by the criteria described later in this Appendix.

We now align and compare all examples of our apparent replicates using any additional techniques we wish: any measurements of means and standard durations, rows of photographs, judges, and so forth. We put probable members of the set to the following comparative tests.

Test 1. The Interdependency of Elements. We compare the complexes we have marked off to see if each one is made up of the same constituent segments. For example: In courtship women simultaneously cock their heads, widen their palpebral fissures, smile, and finger their hair with their palm exhibited toward their partner.

If these segmental acts invariably appear together, if no one appears without the others, then the elements of the complex are interdependent and the complex is a regular unit of behavior. The composition of this entity is not in such a case, incidental, but an irreducible unit at the lowest level of integration.[10]

But this is not the case in the example I gave above. Women sometimes preen their hair and present the palm without smiling and head cocking. In this case the hair preening is the lowest unit of interdependent behavioral elements. The whole constellation is a more complex unit at a higher level of integration.

Test 2. The Identity of Form. The same set of bodily regions could be interdependent but still be assembled differently in various cases. In order to claim an identity of replicates we require that the same elements of behavior be combined in each instance to form the same general morphology or Gestalt. The replicates of a form must fall within a range of excursion, rate, rhythm, and duration, for instance. We can measure each of these dimensions accurately, since each frame of the film is numbered, and we can also make spacial measurements from film.

Test 3. Regularities in the Context of Each Occurrence. Because behavioral units are ordered in a transaction by physical and by traditional constraints which correspond to the rules of syntax in a language, the replicates of a unit type occur in the same context or contexts. Each occurs after particular antecedents and before certain successors in a sequence of events. Each occurs in given situations (see Operation V).

Test 4. Contrastibility to Other Forms. The possible replicates of a unit form will contrast obviously or noticeably from the replicates of some other unit forms, even though the two types may be similar to superficial inspection, and even though overlap occurs between extreme variants.

Replicates of any unit type, then, must have (1) the same form, (2) the same conditions of occurrence, and (3) distinguishably different form than some other class of behavioral events. If behavior were not regular in this way it could not be the basis of communication. The forms of behavior in a code must be recognizable and identifiable at a glance. And each must be easily distinguishable from others or there would be too much ambiguity to allow recognition.

A-3. Determining Whether the Unit is Traditional and Communicative

If the same unit form is used by a number of participants in some cultural or subcultural group it is traditional.

If an informant of that culture recognizes the unit we have depicted, we can assume that it is communicative. If he does not, then either we have wasted time defining an artificial configuration or else the unit is one not consciously recognized in that culture. In this case we check its relation to the performances of other people in the actual transaction (see Operation IV).

If we now have assurance that we have depicted a unit with cultural and communicative reality, we invest the time for a careful description. Now we can make careful measurements and do a statistical analysis. We describe and measure the component subunits and depict these with photographs or drawings. We systematically describe the major variations and identify the range of recognizable variants. And we describe the contexts of usual occurrence.

Step III-B. Delineating All of the Units in a Transaction

If we are to study the over-all structure of the transaction and visualize communicational units, we must now repeat the procedures for unit delineation for all of the behaviors we have recorded on film. If we plan in advance to do this, we carry out Step III-A more efficiently using alternative steps I review here.

B-1. Marking Off the Known Units

Many of the unit forms of the behavioral streams on our topography are already well known in common culture or they have been carefully described in previous context analyses. The structural linguists have already identified the forms of English speech and researchers in behavior have described actonic, kinesic, and postural forms in certain cultures. And in many cases we or our informants can immediately recognize some customary forms and describe them in detail.

There is no point repeating the analysis of these units unless we are uncertain about their form. After all, the biochemist does not repeat the history of chemistry by resynthesizing each component molecule each time he works with a macromolecule.

So we draw a clearly visible line around the rows and columns on the topography in which we have recorded a known and clear unit. Then we turn our attention to the undefined area of activity between these blocks.

B-2. Preparing a Complementary Distribution

When we are to analyze all of the units in each participant's contribution, we save time by going through the whole topography and tentatively marking off each of the elemental complexes of movement. Then we line up all those which seem alike and compare this set to other sets of similar complexes.

Each complex type may be represented by a symbol. I have used a small magnet of a certain shape and color for each type and plotted these on a large steel board hung on the wall. Then we can sit back and spot patterns of repetition at a glance. If the variants are numerous and complicated we take representative still photographs of each one and annotate these with descriptions and measurements. These become mock ups on a large chart. The apparent replicates of Type A are placed in one column, the apparent replicates of B in the next, and so forth.

Such a comparative representation of types and variants is called a complementary distribution (Z. Harris 1951).

B-3. Cataloguing Unit Types

If a type of unit does not occur often enough in a given transaction to do a structural analysis, we collect occurrences from a number of transactions. In this case we may scan all of the videotapes and motion pictures in our library, and sometimes we borrow the films of other investigators. We photograph and describe each replicate we find and file this data to build a sample. We call such data collection cataloguing.

OPERATION IV. DETERMINING THE UNITS OF TRANSACTION OR COMMUNICATION

So far we have developed a picture of the customary or communicative units that each person has contributed to the transaction, and we have plotted these on a time graph. Hence we know when and where each unit occurred in relation to the others. But we do not yet know how these units were ordered in the part that each participant took; nor have we shown how parts were related in communication. We are ready to take these steps now.

In visualizing communication we can no longer work only with the behavior of each individual separately, but we can exercise an option of priority in our steps toward such a view.

1. We can show the integration of all communicative units in one person's total part in the transaction and then study how the parts were related in the over-all transactions.

2. We can take each unit we have now delineated and examine its relation to the units of other participants at that moment.

Actually we elect to move back and forth between these options of procedures, refusing to adhere rigidly to either one, and we will do this because of the way behavior is usually integrated in a transaction. At any given moment in a transaction some bodily region of a participant may be more closely related to someone else's activity than it is to the activities of the rest of his own body. So the unit performance of a participant does not necessarily follow the anatomical integrity of the body and we lose perspective if we insist upon seeing the total contributions of each person as a whole. Similarly the part of a participant may change character as the transaction proceeds, so we do not want to conceptualize it as an entity without respect to the transactional or communicational relations of the transaction.

We, therefore, proceed as follows: We delineate units of movement in a communicative modality. A modality is defined as all of the regional movements which a participant uses interdependently at some moment of time.

Then we study the relations between units of behavior in the various modalities of each participant, thus defining the smallest unit of communicational relation. As a final step, we study the relation between these units until we can visualize the structure of the entire transaction.

Step IV-A. Delineating a Modality

We observe all of the communicative units in the performance of each participant at any moment of time and we draw a line about those which occur together. Sometimes the entire body is moved as a unit: when a participant rises to leave, for instance, sometimes the entire upper body is moved in concert. The participant turns from speaking to A and addresses B, for instance, but he turns from the waist and does not change the positioning and orientation of his pelvis and legs. And sometimes a participant moves only his eyes, looking, for example, from A or B without otherwise moving.

This pattern of movement has a duration. The bodily regions are moved to a new location, held there a while, and then moved back again or moved to another spot. We mark these off collectively as a complex segment of activity through time. Since all component bodily regions sometimes are not moved at exactly the same time, we overview the complex and include shifts that seem to be associated. As in the case of smaller units, there are cases in which we are not sure that we are delineating an entity, but we make an educated guess that we will test later.

Now we repeat the procedures I outlined in Operation III. We scan the entire record (and maybe additional films) to find like complexes which involve the co-occurring change and positioning of multiple bodily regions. We test each example for isomorphism of structure, regularity of context, contrast to similar forms, and customary usage. Then we describe, photograph, and mark off each regularly occurring unit type on the topography.[11]

Hierarchical structure of this unit. As we examine these units a feature of behavior structure becomes increasingly apparent. Units of this complexity are made up of customary subunits, which are units in their own right when we focus on them one at a time. For example, a movement of the entire upper body occurs as a unit. This unit is composed of subunits of head-eye shift, turning of the upper torso, and positioning of the hand. In other circumstances one of these subunits — for instance, a shift in head-eye orientation from one speaker to another — may be an independent unit in its own right. It could have occurred without any shift in the torso or hands. And in still other instances the eye shift alone is a unit of behavior, occurring without any perceptible movement of the head or the body.

In the act of behavior, we conclude, complex patterned movements are composed by integrating some number of patterned and customary subunits in an orderly way. The process of integration is crudely analogous to the way a builder puts together customary units of material to make standard rooms, apartments, modules, and housing projects. In systems theory such integrations are said to be hierarchical and we would hold that both material and behavioral systems are so constituted.[12] In such terminology each stage or degree of complexity is called a level.

We have visualized a behavioral integration by managing our conception of time and space in a systematic way. That duration of time which is required to complete a segment of behavior is visualized as an operational 'now' and we conceptualize all sequential events within this 'now' as a unit of structure, which we name or represent with a symbol or a picture. We similarly manipulated our conception of space. We declared all bodily regions that are interdependently related in an activity as members of the same 'here'. Having described their relations as an entity we no longer enumerate them separately. To visualize a hierarchy

of units we enlarge our definition of 'here' and 'now' progressively
level by level. [13]

We can now explicate the principle of data reduction in a
structural method like context analysis. We do not reduce the
complexity of a behavioral experience by disregarding most of
the variables or abstracting some feature of the whole. Instead,
we discover the form and composition of a customary pattern of
behavior; then we can visualize a hundred or a thousand elements
of behavior as a single entity or unit. A unit seen as a whole is
less complex than its subunits. Thus we recognize, code, and
convey with a single word an image of integrations as complex
as football, marriage, or a culture.

We might at this point wish to construct the total part which
some participant took in the transaction. Spacially a part would
consist of some configuration of modalities which corresponded
to the multiple simultaneous activities which one participant
carried out. Temporarily the part would embrace a sequence
of modal constellations. How the part could be analyzed is obvious and needs no further documentation here. Relationships,
too, are to be studied by principles which are now familiar.
Furthermore, we are now dealing with a relative, small finite
number of units, because by now we have already unitized thou-
sands of microbehaviors. Accordingly we can now move rapidly in the analysis of the transaction.

Step IV-B. Studying the Relations Between Modalities

Imagine now that we have marked off on the topograph each
unit of modality behavior for each participant. We inspect the
topography to determine how each unit of this type is related to
each of the other such units.

Some units at this level of integration are immediately familiar. There are relations of tactile contacting, synchronous
movements, conversational interchange, tête-à-tête orientations,
and so on. We can mark these off with a dotted line and then
check all recurrences as we did on Operation III.

We see at first glance two kinds of relations:

1. Enactments in a modality often co-occur

At approximately the same time two or more participants
may do something together. They may enact an isomorphic unit,
addressing each other in the same head-eye orientation, for
instance, or they may perform coterminous units which are
very different in form. One may speak, for instance, while the
other lowers his head and taps his foot.

2. Enactments in a modality may occur alternately in a sequence

One participant may speak, then the other speaks, and so forth, or the participants may take turns in enacting some subunit of a task or making moves in a game. This alternation is usually called interaction and sometimes a participant 'goes around the room' addressing each of the other persons or lighting each of the other's cigarette.

Procedurally, we do not care whether the subunits of a relation co-occur or alternate. In either case they constitute a communicational unit if they occur regularly in customary integration. [14]

In fact, units of communicational relation are at once alternative and co-occurring. For example, participants may take turns speaking while they assume the same posture, and nod their heads rhythmically, and any customary sequence of joint participation appears as a co-occurring relation once it is unitized at the next level of integration.

In a large group we usually discover that multiple simultaneous relations occur among various modalities in various subgroupings. For example, there may be a conversation involving three people but one or two others are dissociated. These two may be engaged in a unit of holding hands and gazing. Two of the conversants may be exchanging glances related to the comments the third is making, and exactly the same postures may relate these two.

Thus at this level multiple simultaneous communicational units occur. Some number of communicative performances may appear that are not visibly related to any other enactments. And we may also find activities which we cannot even demonstrate to be customary or communicative.

Step IV-C. Studying the Structure of the Transaction

Ordinarily a configuration of multiple communicational relations like this will prevail for a few minutes, and there will then be a shift in the type of activity. These constellations of conjoint participation disappear and a very different arrangement is assembled. When we have delineated the units of relation for the entire film recording, we are likely to note that two, three, or a half dozen such constellations succeed each other in the course of the transaction.

When the configuration of modality relations differ at each stage of a transaction we must regard each stage as a unit of communicational behavior. This unit occurs at an intermediate level between the relation of modalities and the transaction as a whole. I have called this unit a relation of positions in other writings. Now our task is to delineate these units which appear as stages of the transaction.

C-1. Enlarging our Sample

We cannot tackle this job with the data of one transaction. Our methodology depends upon the ability to compare a number of unit occurrences. Because a unit as large as a stage occurs but once or twice in a given transaction, we must enlarge our sample and film other transactions.

We must collect this additional data systematically to be certain that we have other examples of the same kind of transaction. Knowing that transactions are culturally and situationally specific, we can expect people of the same background to enact the same kind of transactions, provided they come together at the same kind of site and occasion. So we will return to the same sites to film again.

The easiest approach is to film the same subjects again. In our present project we place video cameras in the home and leave them there for six or eight weeks, filming a number of repetitions of the same transactional types to begin with. And we leave the cameras in site while we study transactions. Then we can go back and enlarge our sample by simply pressing a recording switch.

We also record transactions in an analogous site where people of the same type congregate. To do this we relocate our cameras in another household where a family of the same social, institutional, and ethnic background lives.

By sampling in this way we hold cultural tradition, social position, and the physical ecology relatively constant. We can then allow personality type, mood, and other organismic factors to vary and we can vary the occasion and situational contingencies by selecting when to record.

We carry out a structural analysis of these additional recordings using the methods I have already outlined. Then we compare our data on each of the transactions studied.

Certain common features in each transaction are immediately apparent. Certain kinds of people take the specialized parts. They form given kinds of relations, terminate these, and assume others in a customary progression. Given tasks or subjects of conversation appear in each phase.

If we do not find such regularities we have failed to record a like series of transactions. Maybe our subjects are unusual,

or we have not found an analogous site. In any event we will have
to go back and make further recordings until we do have a comparable sample.

C-2. Identifying the Stages in the Transaction

When we compare like transactions we ordinarily find clear
steps toward a point of completion, or at least a specific constellation of subtasks will appear at the end of which the transaction is terminated. In the case of transactions which feature
a product or a physical task performance, the stages to completion are usually apparent. In conversational activities there is
usually a sequence of topics and a number of speaker opportunities. In courtship, for example, progression by customary
stages is evident. In planned social engagement there may be
stages of initial contacting, some number of separate conversate
conversations, a group conversation, the serving of food.

There may be no progression of stages in some given enactment of a transaction, but we can often identify a clear reason
for this. Someone from the outside may interrupt, for example,
or some participant does not take this expected part and the
others leave off their performances to deal with his behavior.

C-3. Studying Regularities and Variations

We can now examine the regular and variable features of a
type of transaction.

Specifying the invariable unit performances of a transaction.
If a task is to be completed there are certain stages or subtasks
which must be performed in order to satisfy the physical requirements for completion and to maintain the traditional expectancies
of the others. There are, then, certain minimal, necessary unit
performances in a transaction. We can identify these when we
know the progression of stages, for the activity does not move on
toward its goal until these fundamental steps are enacted. We
next abstract these units of behavior that occur in every example
in which the transaction progressed to completion.

Discovering the allowable alternatives. Except in the case of
highly ritualized transactions, however, there is leeway in the
composition of necessary steps. Some range of allowable alternatives occurs. The progression is forwarded by any one of some
set of substitutable unit enactments or allomorphs. For example,
in a usual supper it may not matter what edible food is served or
it may be that it has to be cooked food. Otherwise the eating will
not continue. But on Christmas the participants may not be willing to eat meat other than turkey.

In a given kind of conversation certain topics may be forbidden but there will be some number of allowable topics. All of those which do occur without disrupting the progression constitute a set of allowable alternatives. We sometimes say that these are allomorphic or equivalent at this level.

Our task, then, is to discover the allowable or at least the usual range of alternatives. We do this at each of the larger levels for the transaction we are studying; i.e., we find the usual, alternative stages in the progression; the usual, alternative relations within a stage, the usual alternative modalities within a relation, and so on. After we have described the necessary units and alternatives, we can abstract the customary program of that type of transaction (Scheflen 1968).

Defining the normal variants in performance style. Members of a culture know the usual units and allomorphs of familiar transactions. Although they may not be very conscious of this knowledge, they can quickly spot an incongruent or deviant performance, and they signal such occurrences by comment, kinesic act, or a refusal to continue. So we can also discover the variations in form which are acceptable or allowable in a given population.

I will call those variations in unit form which pass in a transaction stylistic variants. They are often associated with participant traits, such as age, health, status or skill, mood, personality type, region of origin, or previous cultural membership.

Identifying various types of intercalated behavior. There also appear in most transactional performances supplementary or intercalated behaviors; behaviors that are not ordinarily or necessarily unit elements in the program of that transaction. I have so far studied three kinds of these in my research on transaction.

1. Unit performances appear in a transaction which belongs to the programs of other types of transactions. Such behaviors can often be explained as attempts by a participant to change the definition of the situation (Goffman 1957), or the consequences of some misunderstanding about what transaction is called for. We might infer 'motives' in the case of these supplementary performances.

2. Certain actonic sequences may be intercalated to maintain or alter the ecology of the situation. Someone may rearrange the furniture, for example, or turn up the heat.

3. Certain intercalated kinesic acts or lexical comments refer to the ongoing performances and relations and serve to correct, regulate, control, or reduce the ambiguity of these communicational processes. Following Bateson (1955) I will call such behavioral intercalations, metacommunicative behaviors and metabehavior. These behaviors will further concern us in Operation V.

C-4. Identifying Instances of Communicated Variation

Now that we have identified the regular or traditional forms
of a transaction and the recurring variations, we carry out a
final task in the definition of transactional structure — we study
relations between commonly occurring variations. We examine
the common allomorphs, stylistic variations, and intercalated
behaviors to see which of these are repeatedly associated. We
use the now-familiar procedures of context analysis to examine
the social context of each variation. In some cases we will find
that a variation occurs in the performance of one participant
alone. There is no evidence at the time of a spread or interaction of variation among the participants.

In other cases the occurrence of variation in the performance
of one participant is associated with the occurrence of variation
in the activities of others. In fact, a flurry of variant performances may appear at times in the transaction and sometimes
these seem to disturb the progression of the transaction or even
break up the group.

When variations in multiple performances are associated we
can assume that an interaction or a communication of variant or
deviant performances has occurred. We note such instances
prominantly on our record, but we must be careful how we explain them. It may be that Smith and Jones are not reacting to
each other, but rather performing variantly in the face of events
in other contexts.

OPERATION V. THE CONTEXTUAL ANALYSIS
OF THE BEHAVIORAL PROCESSES

Bear in mind that we now have acquired a structural view of
one kind of customary transaction type. We know the fundamental units of communicative behavior and the necessary relations
among these which replicate the program. And we know the recurring variations that occur red in our sample.

There is a good deal more we would like to know about the
communicational behavior we have described. In presystems
terms we would like to know the determinants of the events. Or
conversely we would like to know what consequences, effects,
function, or meaning these events have. In systems terms we
would like to know the dynamics or systematics of communicational processes in context analysis. We explain communicational events by relating them to larger systems of events or contexts. [15]

We are not satisfied to explain with simple determinisms and linear causation. As we do not settle for a motivational or a social or a cultural explanation, we must deal with all the contexts from which these classical constructs are derived. We will not rest with finding first causes of behaviors, but will repeat the examination of unit-context relations — this time relating unit occurrences within our filmed record to events in other systems of behavior.

Elsewhere I have described a model of interrelation (Scheflen 1970) so here I will merely describe methodological steps in the study of contexts. Starting with a look at yet other aspects of the immediate transaction (Step V-A), we then move to ways in which less immediate contexts can be scanned and sampled (Step V-B).

Step V-A. Studying the Immediate Contexts of the Transaction

By the time we have visited a number of sites and made a number of filmed records of a given type of transaction we will have abstracted the main features of the context of occurrence. As I already pointed out a given transaction occurs at usual sites on usual occasions and ordinarily involves particular kinds of people. With more careful observation we can also identify the stable features of the immediate context — those that remain unchanged throughout its enactment. In contrast, then, contextual changes which take place during the performance can often be associated with variations in relations and in the communicative behavior of the transaction.

Visible Elements of the Immediate Context

Two aspects of the immediate context may be represented on the films we have made.

1. **Visible elements of the immediate ecology.** Our films will show walls, furniture, props, and tools if these are used in the transaction. In addition the actonic behaviors of the transaction will show direct relations to these objects, and the territorial behaviors of the participants will be interdependent with the physical boundaries and obstacles at the site. In many cases we will also have data about climate at the site and here again the participants' behaviors may reflect these ecological states and changes.

2. **Perceivable indicators of suborganismic states and changes.** Participants will provide indicators of their suborganismic states by autonomic signs, utterances about these matters, and by the qualities of behavior and demeanor.

Subjectivist Data about the Immediate Context

We can also interview subjects about their sensations, affects, thoughts, and perceptions during the transaction. We can also ask them about immediate contextual situations. At present we show participants the video or filmed records of the transaction asking them in detail about their usual and variant performances.

Step V-B. The Study of Broader Contexts

We also obtain what information we can about the larger contexts of the transaction and try to relate the features of or changes in these larger contexts to the events of the performance. To some extent we can gather such information by further study of the transaction itself, but we also have to enlarge our sample, thereby studying still other occurrences.

The Representation of Broader Contexts in the Transaction Itself

Many of the behaviors of the transaction itself make reference to broader contexts. Elements of decor and dress, statements made in the transaction, indications of approval and disapproval, and subjectivist comments on interviewing may provide information about the traditional practices, rules, and values of the culture in which that transaction ordinarily occurs. These behaviors may tell us about the social organizations under whose auspices the transaction is held.

Often one or more participants belong to somewhat different traditions or to different social networks. They thus have different commitments in the transaction which may relate to variations or deviations in their behavior. In these cases we may have to seek data about discrepancies between the memberships and identifications of the participants. I have elsewhere claimed that performance styles and predilections for certain allomorphs and parts discernible in a transaction provide information about the background of each participant and thus allow us to predict the qualities of his performance. I also suggested that these features of behavior be called paracommunicative (Scheflen 1971).

But because these kinds of information depend upon inference, we next will make direct observations of the broader context.

Strategic Sampling as a Quasi-Experimental Approach

We can expand our sampling in four directions to account for most of the variants we have been studying: (1) The same transaction type can be examined in other ecosystems. (2) The same transaction can be studied with people of other social positions and relationships. (3) The same participants can be studied in other kinds of transactions. (4) Analogous transactions can be examined in other cultures.[16]

These directions provide a view of contextual factors that are known to influence the form of behavior:

1. Ecological conditions of the transaction. The sites, occasions, and ecological conditions at the time of meeting will determine the type of transaction. In some instances transaction type is ritualized and the same communicational events occur again and again at prescribed sites and occasions. In other cases given transactions are held whenever certain contingencies 'call for' their enactment.

2. Social relationships and social organization. The durable and pre-existing relationships among people will determine their relations and parts of the transaction.

3. Traits of the participants. In addition to cultural origins and social position, participants vary in physical and affective state, age, gender, skill, etc.

4. Culture. We know that the form of behavior and relations are shaped by the cultural and subcultural memberships of participants, including ethnic background, social class, region, and institutional tradition.

By planning to make observations under such conditions we can in effect hold three kinds of contexts relatively constant while we observe variations in the fourth. For example, if we can find analogous transactions among participants of roughly equivalent position which occur under comparable physical conditions, we can observe a number of cultures and subcultural origins, and gain a rough idea about the variations which are incident to tradition.

We can observe the same subjects engaged in other transactions at the same site to identify the influence of the program of transaction, and so forth.

If we select a sufficient number of carefully selected examples, we can achieve a quasi-experimental result without creating the artificial relationships and tasks of a laboratory experiment.[17] Such methods have been called naturalistic experiments.

The Scanning of Existing Film Records

There are already a great many films and videotapes of human behavior we can use to scan broader contexts. In some instances one can use commercial films or videotapes, but often these are fragmented into overly short sequences and are replete with close-up shots which preclude the study of communication. But the network of researchers in the audiovisual field has now become large enough that it is possible to borrow hundreds of research films or tapes made in a large variety of cultures and situations.

We scan these rapidly. When we spot a familiar unit or relation we check the context quickly to make sure we are not dealing with a morphologically similar form which actually occurs in different cultural contexts and therefore has a different significance.

To record these observations we can make still photographs from the movie or videotape and describe the contexts with other photographs or written descriptions. If we are to study a form more carefully we can request the film owner's permission to copy a segment of the medium.

By this time, however, we are much less dependent on film recordings to make our observations. We are more experienced observers and we have baselines in our mind with which we can make a rapid comparison. We can now make some of our observations in everyday life without film recording.

The Final Product of a Context Analysis

The outcome of a context analysis is a set of systematic descriptions implemented as much as possible with segments of representative movies, videotape, or still photographs. The following types of descriptions accrue:

The structure of a type of transaction and the usual, programmatic alternatives are depicted hierarchically.

Common, repetitive variants are also described and related to ecological contexts and social structures.

Certain variants related to traits of the performers and certain cross cultural variants are described.

Particular unit types of communicative behavior and relations may be singled out for more careful description. Common variants of these in various types of context are also described. From the analysis of their relations to context we may also derive the functions and meanings of these forms.

In general we can claim that customary units are enacted to maintain transactions, institutions, and cultures, and that variants restore dynamic equilibrium and adapt organismic, social, and ecological systems. In this framework we can try to formulate the functions of unit performances.

Many units also have meaning in the traditional linguistic and cognitive systems of a culture. Variants in style and the choice of allomorphs related to individual and cultural differences are also meaningful in deriving information about the participants, and such assessments on the part of participants may influence the transactional performance itself. The research may formulate the meaning of units by the study of subjectivist contexts in both of these dimensions.

BIBLIOGRAPHY

Abraham, K. 1949. Selected papers on psychoanalysis. London: Hogarth Press.

Abrahams, J., and Varon, E. 1953. Maternal dependency and schizophrenia. New York: International University Press.

Ackerman, N. W. 1966. Treating the troubled family. New York: Basic Books.

Alexander, F., and French, T. 1946. Psychoanalytic therapy. New York: Ronald Press.

Altman, I., and Haythorn, W. 1967. The ecology of isolated groups. Behavioral science 12 (May): 169-182.

Altman, S. A. 1966. Social communication among primates. Chicago: University of Chicago Press.

Ardrey, R. 1966. The territorial imperative: A personal inquiry into the animal origins of property and nations. New York: Atheneum.

Ashby, W. R. 1952. Design for a brain. New York: Wiley.

Ashby, W. R. 1956. An introduction to cybernetics. New York: Wiley.

Austin, W. M. 1962. Research seminars.

Bacon, C. 1960. Personal Communication.

Bales, R. F., Borgatta, E. F., and Hare, A. P., eds. 1955. Small groups: studies in social interaction. New York: Knopf.

Barker, R. G. and Wright, H. F. 1954. The midwest and its children: The psychological ecology of an American town. Evanston, Ill.: Row, Peterson.

Barker, R. G. 1963. The stream of behavior. New York: Appelton Century Crofts.

Bartlett, F. C. 1932. Remembering. Cambridge, Mass.: Cambridge University Press.

Bateson, G., and Mead, M. 1942. Balinese character. New York: New York Academy of Science.

Bateson, G. 1954. Films of family interviews made in the home. Unpublished.

Bateson, G. 1955. The message, 'This is play.' In Group processes, II, ed. B. Schaffner. Madison, N. J.: Madison Printing Co.

Bateson, G., Jackson, D. D., Haley, J., and Weakland, Jr. 1956. Toward a theory of schizophrenia. Behavioral Science, 1 (Oct) : 251.

Bateson, G. 1958. Naven. 2nd ed. Stanford: Stanford University Press.

Bateson, G. 1962. Personal communication.

Bateson, G. 1962. Research seminar. Eastern Pennsylvania Psychiatric Institute.

Bateson, G. 1969. Chapter 1. In The natural history of an interview, ed. N. McQuown. New York: Grune and Stratton. Forthcoming.

Bender, L. 1945. Organic brain conditions producing behavior disturbances. In Modern trends in child psychiatry, ed. N. D. C. Lewis and B. L. Pacella. New York: International University Press.

Benedict, R. 1946. Patterns of culture. Boston: Houghton Mifflin.

Berelson, B. 1952. Content analysis in communication research. New York: Free Press.

Berger, M. M. 1958. Nonverbal communications in group psychotherapy. International journal of group psychotherapy. 8 (Apr): 161-78.

Berne, E. 1964. Games people play. New York: Grove Press.

Bertalanffy, L. V. 1950. An outline of general systems theory. Brit. J. Phil. Sci. 1:134.

Bertalanffy, L. B. 1960. Problems of Life. New York: Harper.

Bibring, E. 1954. Psychoanalysis and the dynamic psychotherapies. American Journal of Psychoanalysis. 2:745.

Birdwhistell, R. L. 1952. Introduction to kinesics. Louisville,
Kentucky: University of Louisville Press.

Birdwhistell, R. L. 1959. Contribution of linguistic-kinesic
studies to the understanding of schizophrenia. In Schizophrenia, ed. A. Auerback. New York: Ronald Press.

Birdwhistell, R. L. 1960. Kinesics and communication. In
Exploration in communication, ed. E. Carpenter and M.
McIuhan. Boston: Beacon Press.

Birdwhistell, R. L. 1961. Paralanguage: 25 years after Sapir.
In Lectures on experimental psychiatry, ed. H. Brosin.
Pittsburgh: University of Pittsburgh Press.

Birdwhistell, R. L. 1962. Unpublished.

Birdwhistell, R. L. 1963. Personal communication.

Birdwhistell, R. L. 1964. Communicational anthropology in the
residency setting. In The teaching of psychotherapy. International Psychology Clinics, I, 2 (Apr), ed. F. H. Hoffman.

Birdwhistell, R. L. 1965. A continuous multi-channel process.
In Conceptual bases and applications of the communicational
sciences. University of California Press.

Birdwhistell, R. L. 1966. Some relations between American
kinesics and spoken American English. In Communication
and culture, ed. A. G. Smith. New York: Holt, Rinehart
& Winston.

Birdwhistell, R. L. 1967. Personal communication.

Birdwhistell, R. L. 1969. Chapter 3. In The natural history of
an interview, ed. N. McQuown. New York: Grune and
Stratton.

Bleuler, E. 1950. Dementia praecox or the group of schizophre-
nias. Zinkin, Jr., tr. New York: International University
Press.

Bloomfield, L. 1933. Language. New York: Holt.

Bock, Phillip B. 1962. The social structure of a Canadian
Indian reserve. Doctoral thesis, Harvard University.

Bowen, M. 1966. The use of family therapy in clinical practice.
Comprehensive psychiatry. 7 (Oct) : 345.

Broadbent, D. E. 1965. Information processing in the Nervous System. Science 150 (Oct 22): 457-62.

Brody, M. 1959. Observations on 'direct analysis.' New York: Vantage Press.

Brosin, H. 1968. Chapter 4. In The natural history of an interview, ed. N. McQuown. New York: Grune & Stratton.

Bullowa, M., Jones, L. G., and Duckert, A. R. 1964. The acquisition of a word. Language and speech 7 (Apr) : 107-11.

Bychowski, G. 1952. Psychotherapy of psychosis. New York: Gruen & Stratton.

Carmichael, H., and Haggard, E. 1955. Films made of psychoanalytic sessions. Unpublished.

Carnap, R. 1942. Introduction to semantics. Cambridge: Harvard University Press.

Carnap, R. 1947. Meaning and necessity. Chicago: University of Chicago Press.

Chance, M. R. A. 1962. The nature and special features of the instinctive social bond of primates. In The social life of early man, ed. S. L. Washburn. London: Methuen.

Chappel, D. 1949. The interaction chronograph: Its evolution and present application. Personnel 25:294.

Charny, E. J. 1966. Postural configurations in psychotherapy. Psychosomatic Medicine 28 (Jul):305-15.

Cherry, C. 1961. On human communication. New York: Science Editions.

Chomsky, N. 1957. Syntactic structures. The Hague: Mouton.

Chomsky, N. 1966. Three models for the description of language. In Communication and culture, ed. A. G. Smith. New York: Holt, Rinehart & Winston.

Colby, M. D. 1960. An introduction to psychoanalytic research. New York: Basic Books.

Condon, W. S., and Ogston, W. D. 1966. Sound film analyses of normal and pathological behavior pattern. Journal of nervous and mental disorders 143 (Oct) :338-47.

Condon, W. S., and Ogston, W. D. 1967. A segmentation of behavior. Journal of psychiatric research 5 (Nov) :221-35.

Condon, W. S. 1968. Interactional syncrony.

Darwin, C. 1955. The expression of emotions in man and animals. New York: Philosophical Library. Paralanguage (see 196-212), subject file.

Davis, M. 1968. Bronx state hospital. Unpublished manuscript.

Davitz, J. R., and Davitz, L. J. 1958. The communication of feeling by content-free speech, Journal of communication 9:6-13.

Deutsch, F. 1951. Thus speaks the body. Part III, analytic posturology. Psychoanalysis quarterly 20:338.

Deutsch, F. 1952. Analytic posturology. Psychoanalysis quarterly 21:196-214.

Devereux, G. 1956. Therapeutic education. New York: Harper.

Diamond, S. G., and Schein, M. D. 1966. The waste collectors. New York: Columbia University. Department of Anthropology Paper.

Dittman, A. T. 1962. The relationship between body movement and moods in interviews. Journal of consultant psychology 26:480.

Duncan, S. 1966. 'Paralinguistic analysis of psychotherapy interviews.' Paper read at American Psychological Association meeting.

Duncan, S. 1964. Nonverbal communication. Psychological bulletin 72(2):118-37.

Efron, D. 1941. Gesture and environment. New York: King's Crown.

Einstein, A. 1933. On the methods of theoretic physics. In The world as I see it, ed. A. Einstein. New York: Covice, Friede.

Ekman, P. 1964. Body position, facial expression and verbal behavior during interviews. Journal of abnormal and social psychology 68(Mar) :295.

Ekman, P. 1965. Differential communication by head and body cues. Journal of personality and social psychology 2:725-35.

Ekman, P. 1967. Nonverbal behavior in psychotherapy research. In Research on psychotherapy, III. ed. J. Shlien. American Psychiatry Association.

Ekman, P. 1969. Communication through nonverbal behavior.

Ekman, P. 1969. Personal communication.

Eldred, S. H., and Price, D. B. 1958. A linguistic evaluation of feeling states in psychotherapy. Psychiatry 21:115-21.

English, O. S., Bacon, C. L., Hampe, W. W., and Settlage, C. F. 1961. Direct analysis and schizophrenia. New York: Grune & Stratton.

English, O. S., Scheflen, A. E., Hampe, W. W., and Auerbach, A. H. 1966. Strategy and structure in psychotherapy. Behavioral studies monograph, 2. Philadelphia: Eastern Pennsylvania Psychiatric Institute.

Erikson, K. 1966. The wayward puritans: A study in the sociology of seviance. New York: Wiley. 550.

Exline, R. V. 1963. Explorations in the process of person perception. Journal of personality 31(Mar) :1-20.

Fearing, F. 1953. Toward a psychological theory of human communication. Journal of personality 22:71-88.

Fisher, S. 1961. Body image and upper in relation to lower body sector reactivity. Psychosomatic medicine 23:400.

Ford, D. H., and Urban, H. B. 1963. Systems of psychotherapy. New York: Wiley and Sons.

Frank, I. K. 1960. Tactile communication. In Exploration and communication, ed. E. Carpenter, and McIuhan. Boston: Beacon Press.

Frazee, H. E. 1953. Children who later became schizophrenic. Smith College Studies of Social Work. 23:125-49.

Freud, A. 1946. The ego and the mechanisms of defense. New York: International Universities Press.

Freud, S. 1949. On psychotherapy. Collected papers 1 (1904), London: Hogarth, p. 249.

Freud, S. 1949. The dynamics of the transference. Collected papers 2 (1912). London: Hogarth Press, p. 312.

Freud, S. 1913. The Interpretation of dreams. New York: MacMillan.

Freud, S. 1949. The unconscious. Collected papers 4 (1915), London: Hogarth Press.

Freud, S. 1933. New Introductory lectures in psychoanalysis. New York: W. W. Norton.

Freud, S. 1949. Mourning and melancholia. Collected papers 4 London: Hogarth Press.

Freud, S. 1959. Psychopathology of everyday life. New York:
The New American Library.

Fromm-Reichmann, F. 1950. Principles of intensive psychotherapy. Chicago: University of Chicago Press.

Galvin, J. 1956. Mothers of schizophrenics. Journal of nervous
and mental disorders 123:568-70.

G.A.P. Report. 1970. The dual tradition: clinical and research.
New York: Group for the Advancement of Psychiatry.

Gleason, H. A. 1955. An introduction to descriptive linguistics.
New York: Holt, Rinehart and Winston.

Goffman, E. 1955. On face-work: an analysis of ritual elements
in social interaction. Psychiatry 18:213-31.

Goffman, E. 1956. The presentation of the self in everyday life.
Edinburgh: University of Edinburgh Press (Social Science
Research Center Monographs 2).

Goffman, E. 1961. Encounters. Indianapolis: Bobbs-Merrill.

Goffman, E. 1963. Behavior in public places. Glencoe, Illinois:
The Free Press.

Goffman, E. 1961. Asylums. New York: Doubleday.

Gottschalk, L. A., ed. 1961. Comparative psycholinguistic
analysis of two psychotherapeutic interviews. New York:
International Universities Press.

Grinker, R. R., ed. 1956. Toward a unified theory of human
behavior. New York: Basic Books.

Haggard, E. A., and Isaacs, K. S. 1966. Micromomentary
social expression as indicators of ego mechanisms in psychotherapy. In Methods of research in psychotherapy, ed.
L. A. Gottschalk and A. H. Auerbach. New York: Appleton
Century Crofts.

Haley, J. 1959. The family of the schizophrenic: a model
system. Journal of nervous and mental disorders 129:357-74.

Hall, E. T. 1959. The silent language. New York: Doubleday.

Hall, E. T. 1963. A system for the rotation of proxemic behavior. American anthropology 65:1003-1026.

Hall, E. T. 1966. The hidden dimension. New York: Doubleday.

Hampe, W. W. 1967. Territory defense and fear of the therapist.
Voices 3(Fall):47-52.

Hare, P. A. 1962. Handbook of small group research. New York: Free Press.

Harris, M. The nature of cultural things. New York: Random House.

Harris, Z. 1951. Methods in structural linguistics. Chicago: University of Chicago Press.

Harris, Z. S. 1952. Discourse analysis. Language. 28:1.

Hayakawa, S. I. 1941. Language in action. New York: Harcourt, Brace.

Horowitz, M. J. 1966. Body image. Archives of general psychiatry 14(May):456-60.

Hewes, G. W. 1955. World distribution of certain postural habits. American anthropology 57, 2(Apr) :231.

Hewes, G. W. 1957. The Anthropology of posture. Scientific american 196(Feb) :123-32.

Hill, L. B. 1955. Psychotherapeutic intervention in schizophrenia. Chicago: University of Chicago Press.

Hockett, C. F. 1958. A course in modern linguistics. New York: MacMillan.

Jackson, D. D. 1962. Family therapy in the family of the schizophrenic. In Contemporary psychotherapies, ed. M. I. Stein. Glencoe, Illinois: Free Press.

Jaffe, J. 1958. Language of the dyad. Psychiatry 21:249.

Jaffe, J., Feldstein, S., and Cassotta, L. 1956. A stochastic model of speaker switching in natural dialogue. Paper read at Conference on Verbal Communication.

Jakobson, R., and Halle, M. 1956. Fundamentals of language, The Hague: Mouton.

Johnson, A. M. 1953. Factors in the etiology of fixations and symptom choice. Psychoanalysis quarterly 22:475.

Joos, M. 1950. Description of language design. Journal of acoustic society of America 22(Nov) :701-08.

Kaufman, I. C., and Rosenblum, L. A. 1966. A behavioral taxonomy for macaca nemestrina and macaca radiata. Primates 7:205-58.

Kendon, A. 1965. Some functions of gaze direction in social interaction. Acta-Psychologica 26:22-63.

Kendon, A. 1970. Movement coordination in social interaction. Acta Psychologica 32:100-25.

Kendon, A. 1971. Some relationships between body motion and speech. In Studies in dyodic communication, ed. A. Siegman and B. Pope. New York: Pergammon Press.

Klopfer, P. H. 1962. Behavioral aspects of ecology. Englewood Cliffs, N.J.: Prentice-Hall.

Köhler, W. 1947. Gestalt psychology. New York: Liveright.

Korzybski, A. 1948. Science and sanity. Lakeville, Conn.: International Non-Aristolelian Library.

Krasner, L., and Ullman, L. P., eds. 1965. Research in behavioral modification. New York: Holt, Rinehart and Winston.

Kubie, L. S. 1964. The teleological fallacy in dynamic psychology. Journal of nervous and mental disorders 138(Feb) 103-04.

Langer, S. K. 1953. Introduction to symbolic logic. Second ed. New York: Dover.

Lawson, C. A. 1963. Language — communication and biological organization. In General systems, ed. L. Bertalanffy, and A. E. Rappoport.

Levi-Strauss, C. 1951. Language and the analysis of social laws. American anthropology 53:155-63.

Levi-Strauss, C. 1963. Structural anthropology. C. Jacobson, tr. New York: Basic Books.

Levy, D. 1943. Maternal overprotection. New York: Columbia University Press.

Lewin, K. 1951. Field theory in social science. New York: Harper.

Lidz, T., Cornelison, A. R., Fleck, S., and Terry, D. 1957. The intrafamilial environment of the schizophrenic patient. Part I: the father. Psychiatry 22(Nov) :329.

Limentani, D. 1956. Symbiotic identification in schizophrenia. Psychiatry 19:231.

Loeb, F. F. 1968. The microscopic film analysis of the function of a recurrent behavioral pattern in a psychotherapy session. Journal of nervous and mental disorders. 147:605-17.

Lomax, A. 1960. The folk songs of North America. New York: Doubleday.

Lorenz, K. 1935. Der Kumpan in der Umvelt des Vogels. Journal of ornithology 83:137-213.

Mahl, G., Danet, B., and Norton, N. 1956. Reflection of major personality characteristics in gestures and body movements. American psychology 14:357.

Mahler, M. S. 1958. Austism and symbiosis. International of psychoanalysis 39:77-85.

Mahler, M. S. 1963. Certain aspects of the separation-individualion phase. Psychoanalysis quarterly 29:317-27.

Maruyama, M. 1959. Morphogenesis and morphostasis. Mimeographed (Nov).

Maruyama, M. 1963. The second cybernatic: Deviation-amplifying mutual causal processes. American scientist 51 (Jun):164-80.

McBride, G. 1964. A general theory of social organization and behaviour. St. Lucia: University of Queensland Press.

McBride, G. 1966. Seminars at the Center for Advanced Studies in the Behavioral Sciences. Stanford, California.

McBride, G. 1968. On the evolution of human language. Social science information. 7(5):81-85

McBride, G. 1970. Social adaptation to crowding in animals and man. In The impact of civilization on the ecology of man, S. U. Boyden (ed.). Canberra: A. N. U. Press, 142-54.

McQuown, N. E. 1964. Seminar at Eastern Pennsylvania Psychiatric Institute.

McQuown, N. E., Bateson, G., Birdwhistell, R. L., Brosen, H. W., and Hockett, G. F. 1971. The natural history of an interview. Microfilm Collection of Manuscripts in Cultural Anthropology. Chicago: University of Chicago Library.

Mead, M. 1964. Continuities in cultural evaluation. New Haven: Yale University Press.

Mendel, D., and Fischer, S. 1956. An approach to neurotic behavior in terms of a three generation model. Journal of nervous and mental disorders 123(Feb):171.

Menninger, K. 1958. Theory of psychoanalytic technique. New York: Basic Books.

Miller, J. G. 1960. Information input overload and psychopathology. American journal of psychiatry 116(Feb):695-704.

Miller, J. G. 1965. Living systems — basic concepts. Behavioral science 10(Jul):193-411.

Miller, G. A., Galanter, E., and Pribram, K. H. 1960. Plans and the structure of behavior. New York: Holt.

Mills, T. M. 1953. Power relations in three-person groups. In Group dynamics, research and theory. Evanston, Illinois: Row, Peterson.

Mowrer, O. H. 1954. The psychologist looks at language. American psychology 9:660-94.

Mowrer, O. H. 1950. Learning theory and personality dynamics. New York: Ronald Press.

Nadel, S. F. 1957. The theory of social structure. London: Glenn & West.

Newell, A., and Simon, H. A. 1956. The logical theory machine: a complex information processing system. I. R. E. transactions on information theory. 2:61-79.

Newell, A., Shaw, J. C., and Simon, H. A. 1958. Elements of a theory of human problem solving. Psychology review 65:151-66.

Ogden, C. K., and Richards, J. A. 1949. The meaning of meaning. London: Routledge, Kegan, and Paul.

Osgood, C. E., ed. 1954. Psycholinguistics: a survey of theory and research problems. Baltimore: Waverly Press.

Osgood, C. E. 1963. On understanding and creating sentences. American psychology 18(Dec):735-52.

Osgood, E., and Sebeok, T. A., eds. 1964. Psycholinguistics: a survey of theory and research problems. International journal of American linguistics, Memoir 10.

Parsons, T. 1951. The social system. Glencoe, Illinois: Free Press.

Parsons, T. 1961. Introduction. In Theories of society, 1, ed. T. Parsons et al. Glencoe, Illinois: Free Press.

Percy, W. 1961. The symbolic structure of interpersonal process. Psychiatry 24:39.

Pike, K. L. 1954. Language. Part I. Glendale, California: Summer Institute of Linguistics.

Pike, K. L. 1957. Toward a theory of structure of human behavior. General systems 2:135-41.

Pittenger, R. E., and Smith, H. L. Jr. A basis for some contributions of linguistics to psychiatry. Psychiatry 20(Feb):1, 1957. Paralanguage, Subject. 61-78.

Pittenger, R. E., Hockett, C. F., and Danehy, J. J. 1960. The first five minutes. Ithaca, N. Y.: Paul Martineau.

Pribram, K. H. 1954. Toward a science of neuropsychology. In Current trends in psychology and the behavioral sciences, ed. R. A. Patton. Pittsburgh: University of Pittsburgh Press.

Pribram, K. H. 1963. Reinforcement revisited: a structural view. Nebraska Symposium on Motivation.

Pribram, K. H. 1965. Proposal for a structural pragmatism. In Scientific psychology, ed. B. B. Wolman. New York: Basic Books.

Pribram, K. H. 1966. Some dimensions of remembering: Steps toward a neuropsychological model of memory. In Marcomolecules and behavior, ed. G. Gaito. New York: Academic Press.

Pribram, K. H. 1967. Personal communication.

Pribram, K. H., and Melges, F. T. 1969. Emotion: The search for control. In Handbook of neurology, North Holland Publishing Company.

Quine, W. 1960. Word and object. New York: Wiley.

Radcliffe-Brown, A. R. 1956. Structure and function in primitive society. Glencoe, Illinois: Free Press.

Redfield, R., ed. 1942. Levels of integration in biological and social systems. Biological symposium, 8. Lancaster: J. Cottell Press, 1-240.

Rogers, C. 1958. A process conception of psychotherapy. American psychology. 13:142.

Rosen, J. N. 1953. Direct analysis. New York: Grune & Stratton.

Rotter, J. B. 1954. Social learning and clinical psychology. Englewood Cliffs, N. J.: Prentiss-Hall.

Sapir, E. 1921. Language. New York: Harcourt, Brace.

Sapir, E. 1956. In Culture, language and personality, ed. D. G. Mandelbaum. Berkeley: University of California Press.

Sarles, H. B. 1967. Relational linguistics. Unpublished mimeo.

Saporta, S., ed. 1961. Psycholinguistics. New York: Holt, Rinehart and Winston.

Schaeffer, J. H. 1969. Video tapes in anthropology: The collection and analysis of data. Unpublished doctoral thesis, Columbia University.

Scheflen, A. E. 1958. Research methodology in psychiatry. Pennsylvania medical journal 61(Jul):867.

Scheflen, A. E. 1960. A psychotherapy of schizophrenia: A study of direct analysis. Springfield, Illinois: Charles Thomas.

Scheflen, A. E. 1963. Communication and regulation in psychotherapy. Psychiatry 26(May):126.

Scheflen, A. E. 1964. The significance of posture in communication systems. Psychiatry 27(Nov):316-31.

Scheflen, A. E. 1965. Quasi-courting behavior in psychotherapy. Psychiatry 28(Aug):245-57.

Scheflen, A. E. 1965. The institutionalized, the institution-prone and the institution. Psychiatry quarterly 39(Apr): 203-19.

Scheflen, A. E. 1966. Natural history method in psychotherapy: communicational research. In Methods of research in psychotherapy, ed. L. A. Gottschalk and A. H. Auerbach. New York: Appleton Century Crofts.

Scheflen, A. E. 1967. On the structuring of human communication. American behavioral scientist. 10(Apr):8-12.

Scheflen, A. E. 1968. Human communication: behavioral programs and their integration in interaction. Behavioral science 13(Jan):44-55.

Scheflen, A. E. 1969. Templates, blueprints and programs of human behavior.

Scheflen, A. E.; Kendon, A.; and Schaeffer, J. 1971. Audiovisual media in research.

Scheflen, A. E. 1972. The Stream and Structure of Communicational Behavior. Bloomington: Indiana University Press.

Schoggen, P., and Schoggen, M. F. 1968. Behavioral units in observational research. Paper read at American Psychological Association Meeting in San Francisco.

Schneirla, T. C. 1951. The levels concept in the study of social
organization in animals. In Psychology at the crossroads,
ed. J. H. Rohner and M. Sherif. New York: Harper.

Searles, H. G. 1955. Dependency processes in the psychotherapy of schizophrenia. Journal of American psychoanalysis
association 3:19.

Sebeok, T. A. 1965. Animal communication. Science 147(Feb
26):1006-1014.

Sebeok, T. A. 1963. Coding in animals and man. The informa-
tional model of language. In Natural language and the computer, ed. P. L. Garvin. New York: McGraw-Hill.

Sebeok, T. A., Hayes, A. S., and Bateson, M. C. 1964.
Approaches in semiotics. The Hague: Mouton and Company.

Sechehaye, M. 1956. A new psychotherapy in schizophrenia.
New York: Grune & Stratton.

Sechehaye, M. 1951. Symbolic realization. New York: International University Press.

Shands, H. 1960. Thinking and psychotherapy. Cambridge:
Harvard University Press.

Shannon, C. E., and Weaver, W. 1949. The mathematical
theory of communication. Urbana, Illinois: University of
Illinois Press.

Sherman, M. H., Sherman, S. N., Mitchell, C., Stauch, I.,
and Ackerman, N. W. 1968. Nonverbal cues and the re-
enactment of conflict in family therapy.

Simmel, G. 1902. The number of members as determining
the sociological form of the group. American journal of
sociology 8:1.

Simpson, G. G. 1962. The status of the study of organisms.
American scientist 50 (Mar):36-45.

Singer, M. T., and Wynne, L. C. 1965. Thought disorder and
family relations of schizophrenics. Archives of general
psychiatry 12:187-200.

Skinner, B. F. 1957. Verbal behavior. New York: Appleton
Century Crofts.

Sokolov, E. N. 1960. Neuronal models and the orienting reflex.
In The central nervous system and behavior, ed. M. A. B.
Brazier. New York: Third Conference, Josiah Macy Jr.
Foundation, 187-276.

Sommer, R. 1965. Further studies of small group ecology. Sociometry 28(Dec): 337-48.

Sommer, R. 1966. Man's proximate environment. Journal of social issues 22(Oct): 59-70.

Southhall, A. 1959. An operational theory of roles. Human relations, 12: 17.

Speck, R. 1967. Conference on schizophrenia at Hahnemann Medical College (Oct).

Spiegel, J. P. 1954. The social roles of doctor and patient in psychoanalysis and psychotherapy. Psychiatry 17(Nov): 369-76.

Spiegel, J. P., and Bell, N. W. 1959. The family of the psychiatric patient. In American handbook of psychiatry, S. Ariete, ed. New York: Basic Books.

Stevens, S. S. 1950. Introduction: a definition of communication. Journal of accoustical society in America 22(Nov): 689-90.

Talmon-Garber, Y. 1959. Social structure and family size. Human relations 12: 121.

Thorpe, W. H. 1961. Bird song. Cambridge: Cambridge University Press.

Tolman, E. C. 1948. Cognitive maps in rats and men. Psychological review 55: 217-89.

Tolman, E. C. 1951. A psychological model. In Toward a general theory of action, ed. T. Parsons and E. A. Shils. Cambridge, Massachusetts: Harvard University Press.

Tolman, E. C. 1932. Purposive behavior in animals and men. New York: Century.

Trager, G. L. 1958. Paralanguage: A first approximation, In Studies in linguistics, 13: 1-2, ed. W. M. Austin.

Trager, G. L., and Smith, H. L. Jr. 1956. An outline of english structure. In Studies in Linguistics, ed. W. M. Austin. Occasional papers, No. 3.

Ulmann, S. 1962. Semantics — introduction to the science of meaning. New York: Barnes and Noble.

vanVlack, J. D. 1966. The research cinematographer. In Methods of research in psychotherapy, ed. A. Auerbach and L. A. Gottschalk. New York: Appleton Century Crofts.

Watson, J. S., and Crick, F. H. C. 1953. Nature 171:737.

Watson, R. 1962. Personal communication.

Watzlawick, P., Beavin, J. H., and Jackson, D. D. 1967. Pragmatics of human communication. New York: Norton.

Wertheimer, M. 1925. Drei Abhandlungen Zur Gestalt Theorie.

Whitaker, C. A. 1958. Psychotherapy with couples. American journal of psychotherapy 12:18-23.

Whitaker, C. A., and Malone, T. P. 1959. Research seminars.

Whitaker, C. A., and Malone, T. P. 1953. The roots of psychotherapy. New York: Blahiston.

Whitaker, C. A., and Malone, T. P., and Warkentin, J. 1956. Multiple therapy and psychotherapy. In Progress in psychotherapy, ed. F. Fromm-Reichmann and J. L. Moreno. New York: Grune & Stratton.

Whorf, B. L. 1956. Language, thought and reality. In Selected writings of Benjamin Lee Whorf. New York: Wiley.

Wiener, N. 1961. Cybernetics. Second edition. New York: Wiley.

Wolpe, J. 1958. Psychotherapy by reciprocal inhibition. Stanford University Press.

Wynne, L. C., Ryckoff, I. M., Day, J., and Hirsh, S. I. 1958. Pseudomutuality in the family relations of schizophrenia. Psychiatry 22:205.

Wynne-Edwards, J. C. 1962. Animal dispersion in relation to social behavior. New York: Hafner.

NOTES

Introduction

1. See vanVlack, 1966, for principles of research cinema-tography.

2. There were psychological or psycholinguistic theories (Fearing 1953; Mowrer 1954; Skinner 1957; Davitz and Davitz 1959; Saporta 1961; Gottschalk 1961; Osgood 1963; Osgood and Sebeok 1964); neurophysiological theories of information process-ing (Ashby 1952; Newell and Simon 1956; Broadbent 1958; Wiener 1961); interactional concepts and information theory variants of these (Shannon and Weaver 1949; Chappel 1949; Bales, Borgatta, and Hare 1955; Miller 1960; Colby 1960; Cherry 1961; Percy 1961; and Hare 1962); constructs about language structure (Z. Harris 1951; Pike 1954; Gleason 1955; Jakobson and Halle 1956; Hockett 1958); methods for studying speech content (Barelson 1952); and more philosophical ideas about communication and meaning (Korzybski 1948; Hayakawa 1941; Ogden and Richards 1949; Ullman 1962; Whorf 1956; Carnap 1942, 1947; Quine 1960).

3. Parsons (1951, 1961) made formulations such as this in sociology (Goffman 1956, and others 1961; Southall 1959; Nadel 1957). They were also made by Redfield (1942), Bateson and Mead (1942), Benedict (1946), Baleson (1958), Birdwhistell (1952, 1960, 1961, 1966, 1969), and Levi-Strauss (1951, 1956) in anthropology; by Pike (1954, 1957) in linguistics; by Wynne-Edwards (1962), Schneirla (1951), and Simpson (1962) in biology;

by Barker and Wright (1954) , Barker (1963) , and Schoggens
(1968) in social psychology; by Grinker (1956) , Brosin (1968) ,
and Speigel and Grinker (1956) in psychiatry. At present, such
views are sometimes used in ecology or environmental psychology
(Altman and Haythorn 1967) .

4. The term, context analysis, emerged in 1955 at the
Center for Advanced Studies in the Behavioral Sciences. That
year Gregory Bateson, Ray Birdwhistell, Henry Brosin, Frieda
Fromm-Reichmann, Charles Hockett, and Normal McQuown
carried out a detailed analysis of a filmed transaction which,
unfortunately, is still not published (McQuown et al. 1971) . This
method evolved in the analysis, though it has antecedents and has
been developed further since 1955.

Early methods evolved in structural linguistics (Sapir 1921,
1956; Bloomfield 1933; Harris 1951) , and general principles
emerged in anthropology (Radcliffe-Brown 1956; Benedict 1946) .
In the behavioral science era these approaches have been applied
to all types of behavior and made specific for nonlanguage behavior (Pike 1954, 1957; Birdwhistell 1952, 1959, 1965, 1966, 1970;
Bateson 1971; McQuown et al. 1971; Lawson 1963; Charny 1966;
Loeb 1968; Condon and Ogston 1966; Bullowa et al. 1964; Bock
1962; Harris 1964; Diamond and Schein 1966; Ekman 1964;
Kendon 1965, 1968; and others.

5. We are currently placing video cameras in the homes of
urban families and making records of family behavior. The cameras are kept in the home for weeks until camera adaptation
seems to have occurred; then several days of video recording
are taken. These video tapes are then analyzed through methods
such as context analysis. The family members are shown the
tapes and systematically interviewed about their behavior.

6. Dr. O. Spurgeon English, the project director, Dr.
Warren Hampe, and Mrs. Jeanne Speiser, the administrator,
attended every session and discussion. Dr. Catherine Bacon
attended all but one session. Dr. Morris W. Brody was present
at several sessions. To minimize the number of persons present, Doctors Scheflen and Birdwhistell stayed away from most
sessions except to arrange for the motion picture recording.
On filming days a camera crew of three was also present. Assistants and visitors were excluded. Figure 1 shows the seating arrangement and the setting of the sessions.

Chapter 2

1. Certain colleagues have been surprised at the regularity of many behaviors in Session I. Some have said that the behaviors of these participants must be more stereotyped than is
usual in transaction. I do not believe this is the case. As I will
describe later, such regularity in nonlexical behavior is characteristic of psychotherapy. Mrs. V's performance seems
more stereotyped than one usually sees and the tendency for cy-
cling is more pronounced than it usually is in a transaction.
Marge's behavior and Whitaker's, however, seem to me to be
more varied than usual.

I think the surprise at regularity arises from the operations
of the method. Ordinarily we do not pay attention to regularity
when we are engaged in a transaction. Only change elicits an
orienting reflex (Sokolov 1960) and calls an action to our conscious attention. Language behavior is the modality which usually shows high variability and we habitually pay attention to
content in a conversation. We can take for granted much of the
nonlanguage behavior which regulates, and maintains relationships, and paces the performances. We can thus gain the illu-
sion that behavior is highly variable. In fact it is typical in the
psychological sciences and in common culture to emphasize the
individuality and pleomorphism of human behavior. The operations of reviewing film again and again and searching for patterns leave us with a somewhat different viewpoint.

2. Physically (M. Harris 1964), the body has to be positioned before some part of it can be moved and oriented. The
face is directed toward someone before he is addressed, and the
hands must be held to a task before the work can be done. If the
act is a gesture, the hands must be held where others can see
them.

In systems terms, a shift in position can indicate that a
parameter has been introduced. Often a position is held until
some task best accomplished in that position has been completed
or abandoned. In conversation, for example, the face-to-face
address facilitates seeing and hearing. In some cases the unit
markers do not serve any obvious function and may be a consequence of custom.

Such logical-physical considerations also determine in some
degree the sequencing of behaviors. It is not possible to perform
certain acts until others have been completed (M. Harris 1964).
The carpenter does not nail up the board until he has cut it and
the cook does not fry the eggs until she has taken them from the

refrigerator. And, analogously, one positions the total body on a base, then positions the upper body, then the arms and head.

3. The contexts of a unit can also be seen as its necessary conditions of appearance. When we notice a familiar context, we can predict some of the units that will occur and can know what is expected of us. A given context elicits the enactment of a particular unit. A context is a stimulus, a highly integrated one, to be visualized as a Gestalt.

In context analysis we determine the function of a given type of unit by observing its occurrence in a context. We collect a corpus or recurrences of a given behavioral unit and determine by observation the circumstances under which it regularly appears and its regular consequences in the communicational process (see Appendix B). The meaning or significance of a given unit of behavior, then, is defined by the effects or consequences of its occurrence in some larger context.

We recognize a position not only on the basis of its configuration but also by its location in a particular context. This is the way we recognize a casual acquaintance. We vaguely remember his appearance and count on seeing him in context.

4. 'A' behavior can also be defined as some change in the state of a system. The change will be patterned or else the system will move to a state of entropy. A cell secretes, the heart rate increases, an organism turns and utters a sound. At some levels change seems to be continuous, like the cycles of cardiac contraction and dilation, but at the organismic level most changes are intermittent. They consist of a stop-go-stop sequencing, an action followed by a pause.

5. The hierarchical structuring is analogous to the organization of behavior in living systems in general (Bertalanffly 1950, 1960; Ashby 1952, 1956; Miller 1965). Integrations of cellular behavior form the outputs of organs and these are organized into organic systems. Collectively these integrations constitute the organization of life at the organismic level. And the integrated behavior of individuals constitutes communication and focal organization at multiple social levels.

Note that these are multiple levels of behavioral integration within the level of organismic observation.

6. Motion pictures are taken at twenty-four frames per second, and in our research films every frame is numbered so that durations can be accurately measured. We can also impose grids and exactly measure the range and excursion of a movement.

But it does not seem necessary to report mathematically what is so obvious in experience. The fact is that we can recognize instantly a proper recurrence of a customary morph, and in doing the research we rarely have trouble deciding to which class of morphs any particular replication belongs. So it is the configuration of the behavioral morph that will concern us here, rather than its statistical measurements.

Since the possible range of usual occurrences is limited, codification systems have been developed for American microbehavior: for language (Z. Harris 1951; Gleason 1955; Hockett 1958), for paralanguage (Trager 1958), and for body language (Birdwhistell 1952, 1966, 1969).

Chapter 3

1. Some participants also split their bodily activities along a vertical axis, moving the right side in relation to someone on that side and the left side in another relationship (Scheflen 1960). It has been shown experimentally that differences in galvanic skin reflexes between the upper and lower halves of the body and those between its two sides, correspond to differences in body-image concepts (Fisher 1961).

2. I do not have a conjecture about it: Early in Session I Marge had said 'cheese' or 'jeez' when her mother was talking about her father's death (2:23 minutes; page three of the multi-modality transcript.) In interview later Whitaker said the object in his hand was a bit of cheese and he told Marge it was Parmesan cheese when he held it for her to smell. My hunch is that Whitaker was making reference to Mrs. V, that Mrs. V was the Italian or Parmesan cheese. This idea would be far-fetched except that such behavior is one kind of tradition in psychotherapy and Whitaker and Malone have used and advocated this tradition. In the work of Sechehaye a symbolic act is deliberately used to convey an idea to a patient which cannot be explicated in language or which, it is felt, the patient cannot understand in the conscious media of language (Sechehaye 1951, 1956; Whitaker and Malone 1953, 1959; Bacon 1960). Whitaker did not know why he did this but considered the above speculation justifiable.

3. These kinds of representational acts often occur as prestages or preparatory phases of the bond-servicing activities they represent. But these representations do not necessarily escalate into fully developed conjoint activities. Their development may be inhibited by the presence of other people and the explicit

definition of the ongoing transaction. This is the case in psychotherapy. Furthermore these sequences of representational activities are customary programs of action in their own right. Thus we have flirtation patterns and dominance contests in common culture that are not merely preludes to sex and fighting. If we can regard these as sublimated activities we have to note that the sublimation was made centuries ago in cultural evolution. Maybe each child has to learn the ability to sublimate as he grows up, as Freud (1933) suggested, but the patterns are already provided in the cultural heritage — they are not novel inventions of each individual.

4. In relationships of men and women, the lowered eyelids are characterized as 'feminine' and 'demure,' sometimes 'coquettish.' McBride (1966) says that all cows in a herd keep their lids lowered except the dominant female.

As a matter of fact some of the dominance and submissive behaviors I have described here may be characteristic for all homo sapiens and for other primates (McBride 1966, 1969). I have studied this behavior in a Bushman conversation and have seen it in many films of primate troops. It has been catalogued for rhesus macaques by Kaufman and Rosenblum (1966).

The holding of some bodily part in an erect and higher position seems to be characteristic of the dominance group member in many species of mammals (McBride 1966). The psychoanalyst might be interested in the symbolism of this generalization.

Chapter 4

1. In nonconversational transactions the occurrence of multiple simultaneous activities is much more pronounced. We are now studying family behavior in the home by using video cameras which are left in position for weeks. Family members in the sample so far rarely sit and talk, even when friends drop in. They watch television, cook or sew, pace, arrange furniture, make tactile contact, and talk, all at the same time.

2. It seems safe to assume that a rhythmical, oscillatory movement is equivalent to a stationary transfix. This principle seems to hold true at all levels of behavioral integration. Thus a speaker may hold his head still to maintain an orientation or he may sweep it back and forth rhythmically in addressing a row of vis-à-vis participants. And he may nod his head rhythmically up and down when he is listening. In either case he defines and holds a given positioning and a given orientation. (At the level

of the position, a participant may pace the floor so his postural transfix is oscillatory.)

In a systems concept either statis or oscillation will maintain a dynamic equilibrium. The oscillation, however, may have an additional function. The rhythmical moving of a body part sometimes sets a beat that is adopted by the group as a whole. Thus the oscillation may be regulatory, marking time as well as space.

3. I am assuming that the participant seeks to act communicatively. One can think of many situations where this is not the case. It is often said that the schizophrenic patient characteristically 'does not want to' act communicatively, preferring to be noncommunicative and avoid relationships. The other patient with whom Whitaker and Malone worked in Philadelphia adamantly refused to speak to them, look at them, or even stay in the room. Marge, however, did appear to work hard at conveying her ideas to the men.

Chapter 5

1. Birdwhistell (1962) has described three types of address which he calls modes of communicating:

In 'intrapersonal modes,' the performer holds his head and eyes down, underprojects his voice, and converges short of his listeners — usually a few feet before himself and in the direction of the floor. He is likely in this mode to slouch, cross his legs, and clutch his own hands or arms. He may also feel or stroke himself or play with an object.

In the interpersonal mode, or the mode of direct address, the participant holds his head up and he looks at his vis-à-vis. He projects his voice and converges his eyes appropriately for the interpersonal distance.

In the extrapersonal mode the speaker may hold his head up looking above or beyond his vis-à-vis and he projects his voice beyond them. Normally this mode can be used to enlist the attention of someone outside the immediate circle of interaction, but some speakers use it to direct general remarks and some people use it habitually.

2. Any type of phenomenon could be coded substances or behavioral events. What counts is not the media, but the form and arrangement. The DNA molecule is coded, not because it contains particular atoms, but because the atoms are arranged and

integrated in particular ways, (Watson and Crick 1953). We could speak of bricks, glass, and wood as being coded if they were put together according to some blueprint hence replicated in a familiar, particular structure. Seeing a hospital, post office, or domicile conveys information among Americans, who recognize these at a glance in any small town or city. So when we speak of coding, we refer not to intent or meaning, nor to the neuronal pathways that mediate behavior, but to the shape and order of the actions.

3. This ordering of elements to context can be abstracted in various terms, depending on the activity in question. Lawfulness is abstracted in language as syntax (Chomsky 1957; Gleason 1955) and in various other actions, such as building codes, law, techniques, ethics, etiquette, mores, rules of the game, and, broadly, culture.

4. Suppose a young animal observes time and time again that the herd takes flight whenever a particular predator approaches. When one day it begins to take flight at sight of the predator without the prompting from others of the herd, we can say he has learned a context-pattern association.

5. Psychotherapy is intermediate in this regard. There is a body of literature on techniques, ethics, and the like. But systematic descriptions of sessions from first-hand observation have rarely been made and it is not a popular idea that specific behavioral units and steps are generally used. Therapists tend to stress the innovative, individualistic aspects of their work.

6. It is important to include emotion or affect in this generalization. To be sure there must be affective states, expressed in visible behavior, which predate language in the development of the child and these may be indicated in a format performance without concealment. But even these states have been named, described, and theorized about for centuries and the conceptions, part observation and part myth, are learned and learned and believed in common culture.

In fact we are not only taught how to behave, but also how to look, think, and feel at a transaction; certain roles are to be performed with solemnity, others with levity, and so forth; we may even learn to deny that we feel any other way. In fact we probably can learn to modify affect to suit a particular occasion. We learn to 'come up for a party, get into a mood, sadness for a funeral, or develop quiet for a confession.

Pribram and Melges (1969) have pointed out that affect is
meditated cortically, contrary to the older idea that it was sub-
cortical. If we forget these observations we can get trapped in
the traditional myth that affective metabehavior is, then, somehow more real, more true, or more genetic than other forms of
behavior and cognition. Maybe this is so where a subject is con-
cealing or lying, but ordinarily, I suspect, an 'emotional' response is merely cognitive experience for which the idea is not
conscious.

Chapter 6

1. For the most part I have studied psychotherapy sessions
in America and a few in England and France. The participants
of these sessions have been mainly Americans of British and
Irish extraction, Eastern European Jewish-Americans and Southern Italian-Americans. Most have been middle class. We have
also studied informal conversations, games, parties, and other
transactions. On occasion I have examined conversational activities in nonwestern cultures; those recorded on films taken in
eastern Nigeria, New Guinea, Bali, Samoa, and so forth.
The over-all bodily orientations which I am about to describe
appear to occur generally, but there are marked differences in
posture, spacing, rhythm, and other features of the relations.
We are now studying relations among lower-class members
in the home. In this situation there are some striking differences. Family members rarely stand or sit purely for the purpose of holding discourse. What they do is carry on running
commentaries while they engage in tasks, games, hobbies, and
watching TV.

2. As far as I know the term, complementarity, was first
used to describe relations by Bateson (1938) (Watslawick, Bevin,
and Jackson 1967).

3. For several years I had been working on the relationship
of people who sit in identical postures and had discovered that
they have a complementary relationship in interaction. I was
planning to illustrate this concept by suggesting as an analogue
to these postures the structure of the helices in the DNA molecule. Coincidentally, I happened to hear a lecture by the biochemist Dr. David Drabkin, who called this molecular relationship a complementarity, and to illustrate this complementarity
he showed a slide of a Greek statue. A man and a woman were
depicted standing in exactly the parallelism of postures that I had
been studying.

4. We do not, of course, speak of postural isomorphism any time two or more people sit in the same posture. This could occur from coincidence. We use this designation when members of a group repeatedly assume a striking degree of congruence, move in and out of this congruence at the same time, and so maintain a kind of rhythmical coordination of postures.

5. Sommer (1965) came to similar conclusions studying college students. Of those interviewed, eighty-eight per cent chose a face-to-face relation for an informal chat. Only eleven per cent said they would use a side-by-side position and in experimental trials only eight per cent actually did so.

In mammals the vis-à-vis position appears to be used in 'bond servicing.' Such activities include grooming, dominance displays, courtship routines, and call signals (Thorpe 1961; Sebeok 1965; McBride 1964; Kaufman and Rosenblum 1966). From examining films of primates and conversational behavior in nonwestern societies I have gained the idea that the face-to-face relation is an automatic releaser of social engagement, fighting, grooming, sexual intercourse, play, etc. In a resting period, animals stand or sit so that they do not come eye to eye, and people have rules for gaze avoidance (Kendon 1965). For example, when strangers pass in public places they do not hold eye-to-eye contact beyond a fleeting moment. Goffman (1963) calls this 'civil inattention.'

6. If we watch multiple performances of a role we can abstract the traditional format just as a musicologist can listen to many performances of a folk song and reconstruct the score which each singer must have learned (Lomax 1960). I have tried to abstract formats which appeared to govern the performances in Session I with the hope that these are analogous to come cognitive representation which the performer holds (see Chapter 8).

7. This is the way machine transmission had been depicted by the information theorists (Shannon and Weaver 1949). Since the interactional model was common to the two views, the concepts and terms of information theory were extrapolated to human communication. It became customary, then, to speak of 'A' transmitting a message to 'B' who decoded it and encoded a message for transmission back to 'A,' who then decoded that, and so on. This approach became known as 'communication theory' (Miller 1960; Cherry 1961; Colby 1960).

Chapter 7

1. Sommer (1966), observing at the organismic level, has described 'personal space' as an invisible area into which others do not penetrate except in intimate activities. Hall (1966) has shown zones of distance in face-to-face relations. Thus, people have territoriality, as other animals do (Ardrey 1966; Wynne-Edwards 1962).

Chapter 8

1. I would guess that the maintenance of characteristic styles and symbols of membership are necessary for categorical recognition in a complex society. In total institutions the members wear uniforms and also display insignia of status or rank and specialty. Though the indications of category are less overt in a nontotal institution, the idea is retained. The colored pencils of the engineer, the types of white coats and instruments in medicine, and other features of social category are well known. It is, of course, efficient in a society to be able to recognize one of the same category and to know instantly his status and competence. It may also have been self-preservative in past eras to distinguish friend and foe, relative and nonrelative. In any event, I would guess that people are trained to retain distinguishing features of categorical membership as they are trained to maintain group loyalties. Maybe this is one reason that style and manner tend to be stable traits.

2. As is also the case with paralanguage, kinesic signals have been seen in psychology and psychiatry as expression of idiosyncratic states or personality expression (Mahl 1966; Berger 1958; Exline 1963; Ekman 1967; Gottschalk 1961). There is no reason to doubt that the styles of performing these signals and perhaps the number deemed necessary reflect personality qualities. But one must also recognize their cultural regularity and see their significance for identifying regions. They are only idiosyncratic if they are not usual in some cultural category.

3. The structural linguist can make a list of all speech forms in some universe, e. g., in all of the languages of the world or all of the Indo-European languages. Such a list would be termed an etic distribution. Only certain of such forms will actually occur, however, in a given language tradition, that is,

in the language of a particular people. A list of the actually occurring forms in a real language would be called an emic set.
Pike (1954, 1957) has pointed out that such a set of forms is
actually a system of forms. Each has particular meaning and
significance; it occurs in lawful integration with the other forms
of the set. Pike also extended the idea of emic and etic distribu-
tions to behavioral forms of all types.

The distinction between etic and emic behavioral relations
must be made on operational grounds. If we observe the behavioral forms used by a given people we will develop an emic catalogue; if we observe a kind of behavior cross-culturally we will
catalogue the etic forms for an activity. Thus language, kinesic,
actonic, and cognitive forms occur in all cultural categories.
Those which occur among a given people will be emic elements
in an emic system of forms.

It is possible to define these operations somewhat differently
ly as M. Harris (1964) has done. The forms can be observed
cross-culturally and an etic listing obtained. Then the participants can be interviewed to determine the meaning they attribute
to the behaviors observed. The informants will describe the
meaning of their behavior in emic terms, i.e., within their own
specific cultural systems. Thus the meaning is emic. Hence,
Harris terms the direct behavioral observations etic and the
subjectivist ideas about these forms, emic.

In context analysis we determine the meaning or significance
of a behavior by observing its consequences or functions in a
transaction, so we think of both the form and its relations in a
given culture as emic. To identify the subjectivist's ideas about
a behavior's significance, I label them metacommunicative.

4. Among families who migrate from Europe to America
certain forms of behavior seem to be more resistant to acculturation than others. Lexication and dress, for instance, tend
to acculturate rapidly, but not postural and kinesic form, spacing patterns, pitch, stress and juncture behavior, and some
kinds of paralanguage. These elements may remain 'diagnostic'
of the European culture of origin for two or three generations.
It is possible that they do not become 'Americanized' as rapidly
because they are not conscious in common culture and therefore
are not taught.

5. Theoretically, if we had sufficient direct observations
of the behavior of Mrs. V and Marge we could describe the larger
integration of their behavior and thus carry our view of contexts
level by level to their total life experience. As it is we can only
deduce these and we do not know how many levels are involved.

Langer (1953) suggested that contexts could be categorized by their immediacy to ongoing events. Accordingly I will designate roughly three 'zones' or contexts, each having an unknown number of levels: (1) The immediate contexts of an individual's performance consist of his and others' definitions of the transaction in progress: (2) The mediate contexts consist of his active repertoire and the systems of events which maintain it: and (3) The remote contexts consist of his total repertoire and the cultural and genetic systems of transmission in which his experience occurred.

6. The term, life situation, refers to one aspect of a participant's mediate contexts. It implies simplistic environment or social determinism. From a behavioral viewpoint a context includes, as well, the learned systems of values and beliefs, the plans and motivations, and the organismic states of the individual. The mediate contexts of a person's life are seen, then, as complex systems of behavior. Lewin's concept of the life space depicts such interrelations more accurately than a concept of life situation (Lewin 1951). Strictly speaking, we visualize a context in behavioral terms — there are no people or objects in it, only behaviors. Thus we convert all dimensions of a context into the same logical type, and visualize its elements as the all inclusive behaviors of people and ecological systems.

7. I do not want to attempt any hard and fast distinction between paracommunicative inference and paracommunicative behavior. I do not know enough about the behaviors in question and the matter seems to be relative. We would hardly say that a recent Italian immigrant was speaking Italian in order to communicate that he was Italian. But there are situations which might raise such a question. If an Italian-American politican who spoke English well were to speak Italian, for instance, we might well say that he was doing so to indicate his Italian sympathies.

Chapter 9

1. How the various modalities are distributed depends upon the task at hand. In the normal instrumental chores of society, such as running machinery and building houses, the body parts necessary for the modality are busy at the task, so speech is used for whatever social coordination is necessary. In vocal tasks, such as conversing and teaching, the specialization of the two modalities may be reversed. Here speech is used in the

task itself, while postural-kinesic behaviors are used for social coordination.

2. Both the plan and the program, as I have used the term in this volume, are abstractions of traditional behavioral structures. The program describes sequences of behavioral forms which an observer has repeatedly seen in a given context. The plan is a cognitive representation which the participant has seen on a number of occasions and presumably has abstracted as a cognitive map which he can imitate and modify. The structure of the two should therefore correspond. We store our map of the program on paper; we do not know how the plan is stored. Pribram thinks it is 'held' peripherally in a molecular hologram for a few minutes, then transferred centrally and maintained in a circuit which depends upon the proliferation of olegodendroglia (Pribram 1966).

3. We could maintain the view that performances are continuous at some level of organization and in some logical type of behavioral mode. The concept of the reverberating circuit suggests that neuronal impulses at suborganismic levels maintain the pattern continuously. At a point when a context is perceived or an image of it is activated, a plan becomes preconscious or conscious and hence organismic. It may then be activated in the neuromuscular system and thus become communicative. Organismic control, then, is exercised at the points of entry to consciousness and then to actualization. Some relationship between images and contexts is critical, then, in a process of 'clutching' or gateing. Thus the thought does not cause the activation of behavior; nor does the plan.

Chapter 10

1. Birdwhistell (1962) has claimed that there are counterdependent roles for people who need to take care of dependent people. Such counterdependent people, having taken charge during childhood of overdependent people, grow up to assume public roles of parental type, such as doctor, nurse, pastor, and so on. Psychotherapists generally describe such factors in their own histories.

Counterdependent partnerships have been described in deviations other than schizophrenia. Johnson (1953) pointed out a counterdelinquent character in the parents of delinquents. And many authors have described a typical spouse of the alcoholic as one who nags him into escape from the home, provides funds

for his alcohol, and nurses him back after a bender. Berne
(1964) suggests that in alcoholism three or more people are engaged in maintaining it.

2. Erikson (1966) reports that the number of deviants was
fixed in New England towns for a hundred years. He thinks deviants are necessary to demonstrate and contrast socially acceptable and unacceptable behavior. Erikson also gives evidence
that army squads in training support a deviant and hide him from
the authorities. Erikson believes these deviants serve as a
cause celebre and function to bring about social cohesion. In
general, the deviant is pointed out as a bad example and public
discussion of his behavior, including courtroom dramas, may
serve the purpose of reinforcing and evaluating the morals and
laws of a society.

Chapter 11

1. A relationship may persist for years, of course, but it
appears in its closed and reciprocal form only for short intervals in order to feed, court, teach, and so forth. It then must
open to attend to others or permit the partners to leave each other physically, at least for a time. Bateson (1962) and Birdwhistell
(1963) have claimed that a persistent dyad which markedly curtail-
es access to others is a pathological social structure (see Chapter
10).

2. In the study of Session IX we found out what happened
when a therapist moves in without invitation. Malone tried this
when Marge was dissociated. She immediately crossed her legs,
moved back on the sofa, covered her face, and fell silent.

3. There are well-known instances in which an entire and
complex pattern of behavior is qualified by a metasignal in such
a way that the qualified pattern has emerged as a quite different
activity in the culture. Fights, for example, may be qualified
by a series of metasignals and thus become games or mock fights,
somewhat similar in gross appearance to real fights but very different in outcome, significance, and context of occurrence.
Males of longstanding friendship can slap each other and call
each other names that would in another situation elicit rage and
battle. In seduction and flirtation the two patterns appear as
similar. The first results in courting and often in sexual intercourse, while the second may be carried out publicly and is not
expected to lead to intimate physical contact (Scheflen 1965).

4. The issue, 'who started it,' is usually academic and un-determinable; it may also be trivial. If a given behavior is called for in a conventional format, it occurs. It is not only misleading to claim that a specific person caused the activity, but it is prob-ably a misconception even to say that the parties caused it jointly. We would not say that the orchestra leader caused Beethoven's Fifth Symphony or that the leading actor in Hamlet caused the death of Polonius. I am always suspicious of a favorite line of research in human transactions — one that tries to determine who initiated, who caused, who decided, and who led in behavior-al sequence.

5. Maneuvers like this have been used by many other ther-apists of schizophrenia since the late 1950s. Bacon (1960) calls them symbolic interpretations. Thus words and acts are con-nected by replicating them together without lexical explanation. These techniques presumably derive from the work of Sechehaye (1951, 1956); she presented symbolic gifts to a schizophrenic patient, gifts selected on the basis that symbolized permissions and instructions which the patient could not comprehend or use in the form of language. Sechehaye called her approach 'sym-bolic representation.' Thus again is applied the conception that a child has prelanguage symbolism in which objects and repre-sentational acts have experiential referents just as words later have. This idea probably stems from Freud's concept (1913) of primary process.

6. At some point in a transaction a shift in activity occurs because some previous activity has been brought to completion or sufficiency.
In Session I we can guess that Whitaker and Malone had learned enough from Mrs. V and that Marge had come into a re-lationship considered adequate for conducting future sessions. I will elaborate the basis for such an inference later.
A converse statement of the pacing of a transaction could also be postulated. A given time was allotted for Session I — a usual arrangement for a psychotherapy session and for many other kinds of transactions. If a second phase is supposed to occur in a time-limited transaction, there comes a point when the phase must be attempted — whether or not the initial bus-iness has been completed and even if the participants are not ready for the shift.

Chapter 12

1. Pipe signaling included the following behaviors: ostentatiously blowing puffs of smoke, tamping the pipe, lighting it, making the shape of the bowl with the hands.

2. The progression of steps reminded me of the psychoanalytic theory of a girl's psychosexual maturation. In this theory the daughter moves from an infantile dependency upon the mother to a relationship with the father. Possibly the infant-mother relationship is at first primarily reciprocal and closed, progressively becoming more complementary and open to the influence of the father. The father-daughter relationship presumably develops reciprocality with sexual aspects, but ideally it, too, becomes more complementary and open as the daughter learns about courtship and prepares to move into the next order of relationship with her potential mate. Such courtship relationships, at first closed and reciprocal, must also become complementary and open to other people and other experiences.

Appendix B

1. Context analysis was developed in 1956 at the Center For Advanced Studies in the Behavioral Sciences in Stanford, California. The inventors were Gregory Bateson, Ray Birdwhistell, Henry Brosin, Frieda Fromm-Reichmann, Charles Hockett, and Norman McQuown et al. 1970). Since 1956 the method has been further developed by Birdwhistell (1961, 1966), this author (1966), and younger workers such as Condon and Ogston (1966), Kendon (1969), Charny (1966), and others.

2. A number of methods like context analysis also developed. Pike (1954) applied the analytic methods of structural linguistics to behaviors of many types and Birdwhistell (1952) published a coding system for non-lexical behavior in communication. Goffman (1957) published 'The Presentation of the Self in Everyday Life,' that advanced a similar framework for behavioral observation in sociology. Ethology developed rapidly in the 1950s and behavioral descriptions were provided by Wynne-Edwards (1962), Chance (1962), and others. Schneirla (1951) explicated the principle of behavioral synthesis. In American psychology holistic behavioral description was developed by Barker and Wright (1954) and Schoggen and Schoggen (1968). In British psychology

behavioral description was recommended by Bartlett (1932) and carried out from film recordings by Crossman and by Kendon (1965).

3. The addition of audiovisual recording to natural history method began with the audiotape recording of speech samples in linguistics. In anthropology the use of motion picture recording was developed by Bateson and Mead (Bateson and Mead 1942; Bateson 1954). The first context analysis was carried out from a motion picture film of an interview which Bateson made in the home (McQuown et al. 1971).

4. In the physical sciences such observation has characterized astronomy and is the basis of field theory. In zoology natural history observation has been characteristic for Darwin, Wallace, Agassis, the classical ornithologists and the modern ethologists. In psychology James, Kafka, Lewin, Bartlett, and others have used this approach, as have descriptive psychiatrists like Kraeplin, Bleuler, and Meyer. Freud also used the principles of context. Naturalistic and nonparticipant observation has also been traditional in anthropology and linguistics. Sociologists such as Weber have also used natural history approaches.

5. We keep the films locked up and show them only to the professional staff, qualified visitors, and students. On occasions we loan films or videotapes to other research projects, but we require the head of that project to assume our responsibility for confidentiality. We do not publish films or photographs unless we go back to the participants for additional permission in writing.
There are, I believe, additional, more subtle responsibilities to subjects. We cannot extract elements of film out of context in such a way that acts seem ridiculous, humorous, or discrediting. We should not use confidential data in ethnocentric, political, or entertaining contexts. On rare occasions we have captured illegal actions on our film. In practice we provide the participants the right to destroy any film which they consider damaging (no subject has ever exercised this option).

6. When I travel around to movie and video studios in hospitals and academic institutions I usually see set-ups that are so grotesque and unnatural that I wonder if someone did not plan them unwittingly to disrupt a transaction and avoid finding its patterns. Monstrous mechanical gadgets stick out from wall brackets and grind endlessly as some artistic photographer imagines he is catching the real action. Microphones are hung

from the ceiling as if normal participants were professional actors booming their voices to a large theatre. In order to get everybody in, the participants are forced into a tiny circle of straight chairs that would produce aggression or panic in any territorial organism. Flood lights cover the scene. Wires and technicians run everywhere and someone periodically holds up a clacker, bangs it, and sends shudders through the participants. It is no wonder that skeptics quote Heisenberg to us and thus compare the impingement of audiovisual gadetry to the bombardment of the electron.

7. This view of the necessary sample size can be attributed to Franz Boas. He once described the funeral ceremony of a native tribe on the basis of viewing one example. He was challanged about the adequacy of his sample. Boas allegedly replied, 'There were 300 members of that tribe present, no one of which gave the slightest indication that anything unusual was occurring. The n is therefore 300.'

8. All members of the species use certain general behavior in common. All talk and eat, for example, and accordingly we say such behavior is coded genetically. But in any given cultural tradition specific forms of behaving are used. For instance, members of a given culture use and share a specific language just as they use customary foods, ways of preparing foods, and arrangements for eating. So we say that a system of specific forms is coded culturally within a cultural tradition. There are subcultural traditions related to region, class, religion, occupation, and so forth and each one has a specific system of behavioral forms that are variants of the general cultural patterns, and individual members of these traditions and subtraditions may have unique experiences which are reflected in their styles of enactment and their total repertoires of communicative behavior. Behavioral form, then, is genetically, culturally, subculturally, and idiosyncratically patterned. Said otherwise, there are general human systems of communicative behavior, culturally specific sybsystems of form, and so on. Dichotomies such as genetic vs cultural factors are artifacts of traditional e..planation among the various sciences of man. All behavior therefore is relatively communicative. The recognizability of one person's behavior is relative to the experience of the observer. Thus any observer can recognize talking and eating anywhere in the world, but he cannot share the conversation or eating ceremonies in an alien culture unless he gains experience with its formats. Even in his own culture he may have difficulty with people of different classes or regions, and he misses nuances

even among his closest relatives. I use the term communicative here when speaking of the behavior of one person out of the context of the transaction. Thus behavior which follows the basic pattern of some given culture is called communicative. When someone with experience in that culture has, in fact, recognized the behavior and/or behaved in concert with it, I say that communication has occurred, and I use terms like communicational or transactional.

9. The methods of structural analysis derive from the operations of the structural linguists (Sapir 1921, Bloomfield 1933, A. Harris 1951, Gleason 1955, Trager and Smith 1956, Chomsky 1957). Birdwhistell (1952) first applied these operations to the study of nonlanguage communicational behavior. Pike (1954) applied structural approaches to behavior of all types; M. Harris (1964) to task behavior and I applied them to posture (1964). Structural methods are also used widely in ethology.

10. The relations are determined by what in mathematics is called the Method of Agreement and Difference (also formulated as Mill's canons). Simple stated, if A appears every time B appears and vice versa if A does not appear when B is absent, then A and B have relations of interdependence and represent an entity. The relations are examined by direct observation of multiple instances of occurrence and nonoccurrence.

11. Schaeffer (1970) has developed an ingenious technique for doing this. He plots the behavioral topography on graph paper. Each unit delineation is then recorded in color on a transparent sheet of plastic which is superimposed on the original graph. As each level of integration is specified these are drawn on another sheet of plastic in a different color and sheets are progressively laminated. Sheets can be taken off or added one at a time to demonstrate the analysis or synthesis of the hierarchy.

12. Behavioral changes in a physical system are ordered in a way which is analogous to the structuring of physical systems themselves. We generalize that within any level of organization (of physical systems) there are successive levels of integration (of behavior or change in state). Thus we describe physical states of living systems analytically by successively viewing smaller and smaller groups, then individuals, then organ systems, cells, molecules, and atoms. Or in synthesis we say that certain molecules are organized to form a cell, certain cells are organized to form an organ, organs to organisms, and so forth. Presumably these levels of organization correspond to stages in evolution.

One could argue that the difference between these two kinds of systems is purely relative to the way we conceive them. Ordinarily durations of state, which are short relative to our observational period, are described by the use of verbs and conceived as behaviors. More durable states of negentropy are named with nouns and considered things. So we speak of a smile or an utterance as a behavior, but we speak of the collective behaviors of college education as a noun and we think of the total organismic behaviors of one person as a physical system. But we can well switch this conventional way of conceptualizing. A behavioral form may last a hundred generations being successively utilized in the adaptation of hundreds of different organisms, each of which are successive recreations of the behavioral structure of genetic and cultural systems.

13. At our present stage of knowledge, at least, levels in this hierarchy are not absolute, but are relative to each other. We can consider the smallest or least complex level as that at which totally interdependent relations of behavior occur. From this lowest level of intergration we can identify and specify successively complicated compositions of these fundamental units.

14. In other places I have called this unit a relation of point units — a point unit being defined as a unit of behavior in one modality of one participant. I have different names here because we have approached the delineation of these units from the social level (Scheflen 1971).

15. Notice that I am not using the model of an organism in his environment. Instead the model is that of a behavior in its contexts. The switch in models is useful in that it enables us to view both suborganismic and extraorganismic events as contexts of a communicative behavior. Furthermore the interface between systems and therefore the relations between systems is mediate by behavior. A focus on behavior then obviates the necessity of concentrating on the physical structure of brain, organism, group, and ecosystem.

16. We are currently selecting 'representative' families from four urban subcultures: Italian-American, southern Black-American, Puerto Rican-American, and Eastern European Jewish-American. All subjects of young married people and households with several small children, are all upper lower class. We place videocameras in three or four sites in the homes of subject families and leave them there for weeks, thus collecting many recurrences of customary household activities under a variety of circumstances.

17. Differences between the naturalistic and experimental approaches to communication and differences in the selection of contextual parameters have led to two major schools of thought about communicative behavior. In the psychological sciences contextual factors are manipulated and culture is ignored, so the language and nonlanguage behaviors are seen as expressions of personality differences or differences in organismic reaction. In anthropological and structural research naturalistic operation is used. The emphasis is on isomorphism in a culture and individual differences are often neglected.

Duncan (1969) has made a detailed comparison of these two points of view. Though adherents of these viewpoints tend to confront each other, they in fact hold complementary data, each having examined different kinds of communicational contexts.